To my father, Dan Harris, who showed me the joys of hiking
and inspires me as a writer

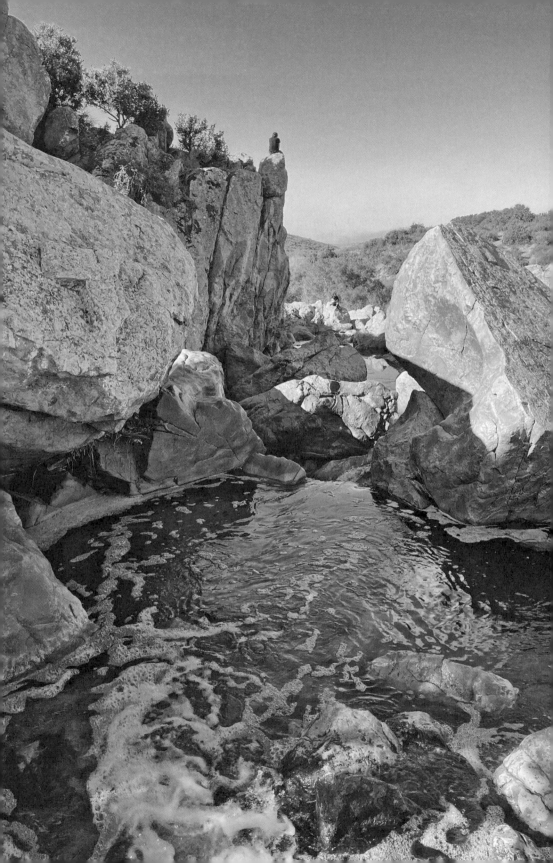

101 HIKES in Southern California

4th Edition

Exploring Mountains, Seashore, and Desert

David Harris
prior editions by **Jerry Schad**

WILDERNESS PRESS ... *on the trail since 1967*

101 Hikes in Southern California

1st EDITION 1996
2nd EDITION 2005
3rd EDITION 2013
4th EDITION 2022

Editor: Kate Johnson
Interior and cover photos: David Harris except where noted on page
Maps: Scott McGrew and David Harris
Cover design: Scott McGrew
Book design: Larry B. Van Dyke
Proofreader: Emily Beaumont

Library of Congress Cataloging-in-Publication Data

Names: Schad, Jerry, author. | Harris, David, 1973- author.
Title: 101 hikes in Southern California : exploring mountains, seashore, and desert / Jerry Schad and
    David Harris.
Other titles: One hundred one hikes in Southern California
Description: Fourth edition. | Birmingham, AL : Wilderness Press, [2022] | Includes index. |
Identifiers: LCCN 2021034566 (pbk.) | LCCN 2021034567 (ebook) | ISBN 9781643590318 (pbk.) |
    ISBN 9781643590325 (ebook)
Subjects: LCSH: Hiking—California, Southern—Guidebooks. | Trails—California, Southern—
    Guidebooks. | California, Southern—Guidebooks.
Classification: LCC GV199.42.C22 S687 2021 (pbk.) | LCC GV199.42.C22 (ebook) |
    DDC 796.5109794/9—dc23
LC record available at lccn.loc.gov/2021034566
LC ebook record available at lccn.loc.gov/2021034567

Published by 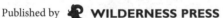 **WILDERNESS PRESS**
          An imprint of AdventureKEEN
          2204 First Ave. S., Ste. 102
          Birmingham, AL 35233
          800-678-7006; FAX 877-374-9016

Visit wildernesspress.com for a complete listing of our books and for ordering information. Contact us at our website, at facebook.com/wildernesspress1967, or at twitter.com/wilderness1967. To find out more about who we are and what we're doing, visit blog.wildernesspress.com.

Manufactured in the United States of America
Distributed by Publishers Group West

Cover photos: (front) Springtime in Malibu Creek State Park (see Hike 8, page 34); (back) The Diving Board on Cucamonga Peak (see Hike 36, page 101)
Frontispiece: Los Peñasquitos Narrows (see Hike 79, page 197)

SAFETY NOTICE: Although Wilderness Press and the author have made every attempt to ensure that the information in this book is accurate at press time, they are not responsible for any loss, damage, injury, or inconvenience that may occur to anyone while using this book. You are responsible for your own safety and health. The fact that a trail is described in this book does not mean that it will be safe for you. Be aware that trail conditions can change from day to day. Always check local conditions and know your own limitations.

Preface

Just beyond the limits of Southern California's ever-spreading urban sprawl lies a world apart. In snippets of open space here and in sprawling wilderness areas there, California's primeval landscape survives more or less untarnished. In hundreds of hidden places just over the urban horizon (and sometimes within the cities themselves), you can still find nature's radiant beauty unfettered—or at least not too seriously compromised—by human intervention.

Our purpose in writing this book is to entice you to explore some of these hidden places. In its pages you will find updated versions of trips previously published in the authors' *Afoot & Afield* series of guidebooks on Los Angeles, Orange, and San Diego Counties and the Inland Empire—a total of 101 hikes described in detail. The overview map on pages x–xi reveals how the majority of hikes chosen for this book cluster around the region's major urban areas. As a result, no matter where you live within Southern California, you can likely access 50 or more of these hikes in less than a 2-hour drive.

Users of the *Afoot & Afield* titles will already be familiar with the format and layout of this book. Each hike description includes a capsulized summary, and each trip is plotted on an easy-to-read map. Photos of scenery and interesting features on or near the trails are sprinkled throughout.

The book was originally written by Jerry Schad, the grand master of Southern California hiking guidebooks. Unequaled in his knowledge of the region's wild places and in enviable physical condition, Jerry was abruptly diagnosed with kidney cancer in 2011 and passed away in the same year. At his request, I have revised this book to keep it up-to-date with changing conditions while endeavoring to retain Jerry's lively writing and insightful descriptions. This edition introduces color maps and photographs to make the book easier to use and to do justice to our beautiful places in Southern California.

I revisited all of the trailheads in this book, rehiked many trails, and reviewed the content with rangers when possible to ensure that the information contained herein is current. Based on this fieldwork, I have replaced 15 of the hikes covered in the third edition with outstanding substitutes. The hikes removed were:

2: Happy Camp Canyon *Mostly of local interest*

6: Charmlee Wilderness Park *Recovering after the 2018 Woolsey Fire*

28: Lewis Falls *Enjoyable but short and not a destination hike*

31: Fish Canyon Falls *Chronic access issues; currently closed after the 2016 Fish Fire*

39: Aspen Grove *Trail to the second and third groves wiped out by 2015 Lake Fire*

56: Antsell Rock *Zen Center Trail badly damaged by 2013 Mountain Fire*

59: Hills for Everyone *Long-term closure after trail damage*

61: El Moro Canyon *Replaced with Laurel Canyon for more varied views*

64: Trabuco Canyon Loop *Burned in the 2018 Holy Fire and currently inaccessible*

77: Blue Sky Ecological Reserve *Mostly of local interest*

82: Agua Caliente Creek *Lightly visited*

89: Corte Madera Mountain *Sensitive area with limited parking*

90: Noble Canyon Trail *Heavily used by fast-moving mountain bikers*

93: Culp Valley *Lightly visited*

98: Ghost Mountain *Lightly visited*

In their place, I have added the following great hikes:

 8: Malibu Creek State Park *A bit of everything: pools, rock formations, oaks, wildflowers, M*A*S*H set*

 9: Topanga Overlook *Unsurpassed views of the Santa Monica Bay*

16: Mount Hollywood Loop *A popular route in one of America's largest urban parks*

18: Mount Lukens *Great views; restored after being cut from previous editions due to the Station Fire, from which it has now recovered*

25: Strawberry Peak *A classic and fun peak climb*

31: Silver Moccasin Trail *An epic 50-mile backpacking trip across the San Gabriel Mountains*

35: Baldy via Bear Ridge *A strenuous and spectacular climb via the original trail on the mountain*

39: Heart Rock *Striking waterfall and the best hike near Lake Arrowhead*

41: Grand View Point *A popular trail above Big Bear with forest, lake, and mountain views*

55: Murray Canyon *Waterfalls, palm oases, and cacti in this classic desert hike*

63: Trans-Catalina Trail *A major destination backpacking trip*

64: Lower Aliso Canyon *Popular introduction to Chino Hills State Park*

66: Crystal Cove Beach Walk *Unsurpassed beach walk, with tidepools and whale-watching*

67: Laurel Canyon Loop *Most popular trail in Laguna Coast Wilderness Park*

88: Three Sisters Falls *Popular waterfall in San Diego County*

I also made major changes to the following hikes:

15: Mount Lee (now HOLLYWOOD sign via Cahuenga Peak) *Rerouted hike via the Wisdom Tree because of trailhead closure*

34: Old Baldy Loop *Replaced the out-and-back from the ski lift with the classic loop*

82: Woodson Mountain *Switched to the more scenic western approach*

87: Cedar Creek Falls *Added new approach from the west avoiding long dirt roads*

93: Garnet Peak Loop *Extended to make one of the best loop hikes in San Diego County*

I would like to thank the team at Wilderness Press for making this book possible. My editor, Molly Merkle, envisioned the new edition. Kate Johnson copyedited it and guided it through the production process. Scott McGrew drew the new color maps. Any remaining errors are my own. During the fieldwork, I enjoyed the company of Werner Zorman, Elizabeth Thomas, Craig Clarence, and my family.

Roads, trailheads, and trails continue to change every year. You can keep me apprised of recent developments or changes by writing to me in care of Wilderness Press at info@wildernesspress .com. Your comments will be appreciated.

—David Harris
Upland, California
February 2022

Contents

101 Hikes Southern California

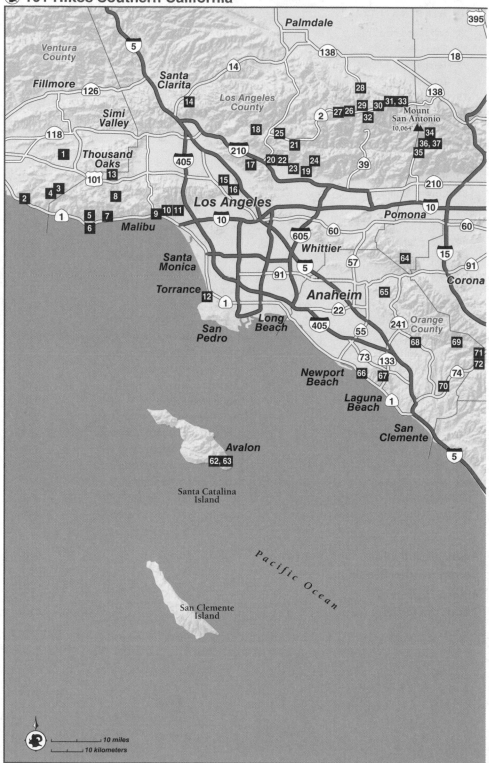

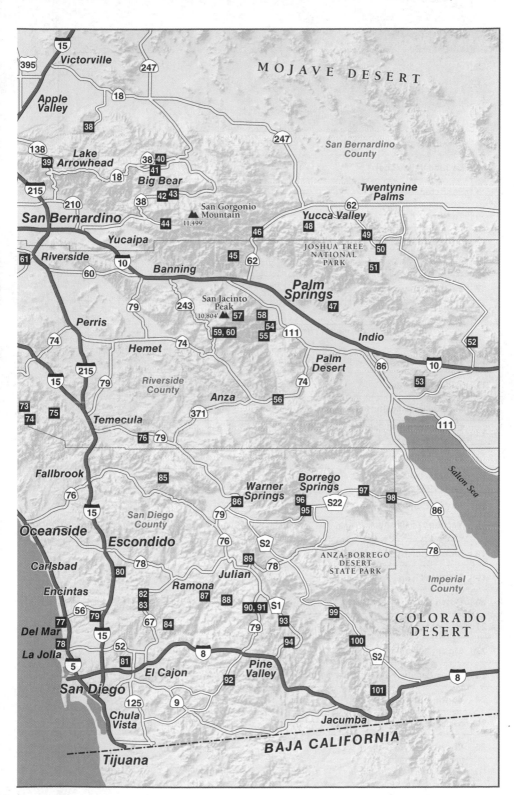

OVERVIEW OF HIKES

NO.	HIKE	DISTANCE (in miles)	ELEVATION GAIN (in feet)	TRAIL TYPE	DOGS ALLOWED	GOOD FOR KIDS	MTN. BIKING	BACKPACKING
1	Paradise Falls	2.7	400	↻	🐕	🧒		
2	La Jolla Valley Loop*	11	1,950	↻				🥾
3	Sandstone Peak	6	1,400	↻	🐕			
4	The Grotto	2.8	650	↗	🐕	🧒		
5	Zuma Canyon	9	1,700	↻				
6	Point Dume to Paradise Cove	2.1	200	↗		🧒		
7	Solstice Canyon Park	2.4	350	↗	🐕	🧒		
8	Malibu Creek State Park	5	300	↗				
9	Topanga Overlook	7	1,700	↗				
10	Temescal Canyon	2.8	850	↻		🧒		
11	Will Rogers Park	2.0	350	↻	🐕	🧒	⊙	
12	Malaga Cove to Bluff Cove	2.0	200	↻		🧒		
13	Cheeseboro and Palo Comado Canyons	10	1,200	↻	🐕		⊙	
14	Placerita Canyon*	5	700	↗	🐕	🧒		
15	HOLLYWOOD Sign via Cahuenga Peak	2.8	1,000	↗	🐕	🧒		
16	Mount Hollywood Loop	5	1,000	↻	🐕	🧒		
17	Verdugo Mountains: South End Loop	6	1,500	↻	🐕		⊙	
18	Mount Lukens: Grizzly Flat Loop	13	3,400	↻	🐕			
19	Mount Wilson	15	4,800	↗	🐕			
20	Down the Arroyo Seco	10	-2,600	↗				🥾
21	Mount Lowe	3.2	500	↗	🐕	🧒		
22	Mount Lowe Railway	11	2,800	↻	🐕			🥾
23	Eaton Canyon Falls	3.4	400	↗	🐕	🧒		
24	Santa Anita Canyon Loop	9	2,300	↻	🐕			🥾
25	Strawberry Peak	7	2,700	↗				
26	Cooper Canyon Falls	3.2	800	↗	🐕	🧒		

All or part of trail was closed at press time. See hike profile for details.

OVERVIEW OF HIKES

NO.	HIKE	DISTANCE (in miles)	ELEVATION GAIN (in feet)	TRAIL TYPE	DOGS ALLOWED	GOOD FOR KIDS	MTN. BIKING	BACKPACKING
27	Mount Waterman Trail	8	1,400/-2,250	✓	✓			✓
28	Devil's Punchbowl*	1.4	300	✓	✓	✓		
29	Mount Williamson	4.4	1,600	✓	✓			✓
30	Mount Baden-Powell Traverse	8	2,400	✓	✓			✓
31	Silver Moccasin Trail	52	14,600	✓	✓		✓	✓
32	Mount Islip	8	2,400	✓	✓			✓
33	Down the East Fork	16	-4,800	✓	✓			✓
34	Old Baldy Loop	10.5	3,900	✓	✓			✓
35	Baldy via Bear Ridge	13	5,800	✓	✓			✓
36	Cucamonga Peak	12	4,300	✓	✓			✓
37	The Three T's	13	5,000	✓	✓			✓
38	Deep Creek Hot Springs	3.8	950	✓	✓			
39	Heart Rock	1.8	200	✓	✓	✓		
40	Cougar Crest Trail	5	800	✓	✓	✓		
41	Grand View Point	7	1,100	✓	✓	✓	✓	
42	Forsee Creek Trail*	13	3,700	✓	✓			✓
43	Dollar Lake	12	2,700	✓	✓			
44	San Gorgonio Mountain	18	5,700	✓	✓			✓
45	Whitewater Canyon	4	400	✓	✓	✓		✓
46	Big Morongo Canyon	1–3	50–300	✓		✓		
47	Pushwalla Palms	6.5	1,000	✓				
48	Black Rock Panorama Loop	6.5	1,200	✓				
49	Wonderland of Rocks Traverse	6	200/-1,200	✓				
50	Ryan Mountain	2.8	1,000	✓		✓		
51	Lost Horse Mine	4.2	500	✓		✓		
52	Lost Palms Oasis	7.5	700	✓				

All or part of trail was closed at press time. See hike profile for details.

OVERVIEW OF HIKES

NO.	HIKE	DISTANCE (in miles)	ELEVATION GAIN (in feet)	TRAIL TYPE	DOGS ALLOWED	GOOD FOR KIDS	MTN. BIKING	BACKPACKING
53	Ladder Canyon	4.3	750	↺		🧍		
54	Murray Hill	7	1,900	↗			⚙	
55	Murray Canyon	4	500	↗		🧍		
56	Pines to Palms	15	-3,500	↗				🥾
57	San Jacinto Peak (easy)	11	2,600	↗				🥾
58	San Jacinto Peak (hard)	21	10,600	↗				🥾
59	San Jacinto Peak (middle)	15	4,400	↗				🥾
60	Tahquitz Peak	9	2,400	↗	🐕			🥾
61	Mount Rubidoux	3.3	500	↺	🐕	🧍	⚙	
62	Lone Tree Point on Catalina	6	1,800	↗		🧍		
63	Trans-Catalina Trail	38.5	8,000	↗				🥾
64	Lower Aliso Canyon	6	800	↺			⚙	
65	Santiago Oaks Regional Park	1–3	100–400	↺	🐕	🧍	⚙	
66	Crystal Cove Beach Walk	5	100	↺		🧍		
67	Laurel Canyon Loop	3.5	700	↺		🧍		
68	Whiting Ranch	4.4	500	↗		🧍	⚙	
69	Santiago Peak*	16	4,000	↗	🐕			
70	Bell Canyon Loop	3.3	400	↺		🧍		
71	San Juan Loop Trail	2.1	350	↺	🐕	🧍	⚙	
72	Sitton Peak	9.5	2,150	↗	🐕			🥾
73	Tenaja Falls	1.4	300	↗	🐕	🧍		🥾
74	Tenaja Canyon	7	1,100	↗	🐕			🥾
75	Santa Rosa Plateau Ecological Reserve*	6	650	↺		🧍		
76	Agua Tibia Mountain	15	3,200	↗	🐕			🥾
77	La Jolla Shores to Torrey Pines Beach	5	Flat	↗				

All or part of trail was closed at press time. See hike profile for details.

OVERVIEW OF HIKES

NO.	HIKE	DISTANCE (in miles)	ELEVATION GAIN (in feet)	TRAIL TYPE	DOGS ALLOWED	GOOD FOR KIDS	MTN. BIKING	BACKPACKING
78	Torrey Pines State Natural Reserve	up to 4	up to 600	loop		✓		
79	Los Penasquitos Canyon	6	200	loop	✓	✓	✓	
80	Bernardo Mountain	7	1,000	out-and-back	✓		✓	
81	Cowles Mountain	2.8	950	out-and-back	✓	✓		
82	Woodson Mountain	7	2,000	out-and-back	✓		✓	
83	Iron Mountain	6	1,200	out-and-back	✓	✓	✓	
84	El Capitan Open Space Preserve	12	4,000	out-and-back	✓		✓	
85	Doane Valley	3.3	300	loop		✓		
86	Eagle Rock	6	700	out-and-back	✓	✓		
87	Cedar Creek Falls	6	1,100	out-and-back	✓	✓		
88	Three Sisters Falls	4	1,000	out-and-back	✓	✓		
89	Volcan Mountain	3.2–5	900–1,300	out-and-back	✓	✓	✓	
90	Cuyamaca Peak	5.5	1,650	out-and-back	✓		✓	
91	Stonewall Peak	4.5	850	out-and-back		✓		
92	Horsethief Canyon	3.2	500	out-and-back	✓	✓		✓
93	Garnet Peak Loop	12	1,700	loop	✓			
94	Sunset Trail	7	700	loop	✓	✓		
95	Hellhole Canyon	5.5	900	out-and-back		✓		✓
96	Borrego Palm Canyon	2.9	450	out-and-back		✓		
97	Villager Peak	14	5,000	out-and-back				✓
98	Calcite Mine	4.2	800	loop		✓	✓	
99	Moonlight Canyon Loop	1.5	350	loop		✓		
100	Mountain Palm Springs	2.1	350	loop		✓		
101	Mortero Palms to Goat Canyon	6	2,400	out-and-back				✓

All or part of trail was closed at press time. See hike profile for details.

Southern California Mountain Ranges

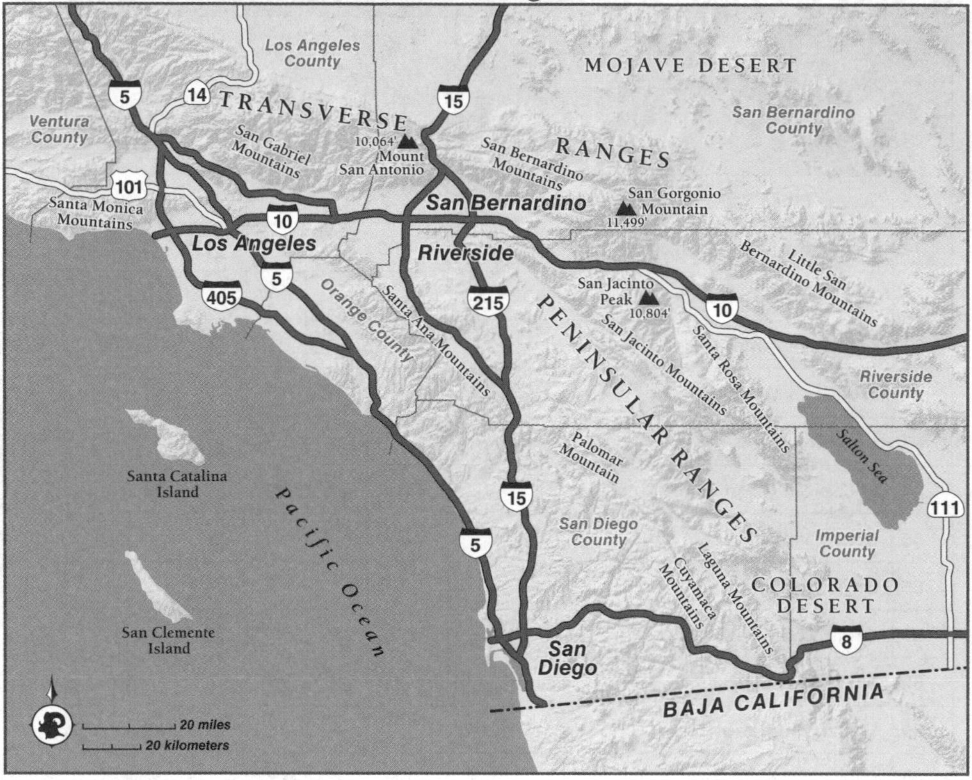

Southern California's Wilderness Rim

Southern California sits astride one of the earth's most significant structural features—the San Andreas Fault. For more than 10 million years, earth movements along the San Andreas and neighboring faults have shaped the dramatic topography evident throughout the region today. The very complexity of the shape of the land has spawned a variety of localized climates. In turn, the varied climates, along with the diverse topography and geology, have resulted in a remarkably plentiful and diverse array of plant and animal life.

Living on the active edge of a continent has advantages and disadvantages that cannot be untangled. Like the proverbial silver lining of a dark cloud, the rumpled beauty of our youthful, ever-changing coastline, mountains, and desert redresses the ever-present threat of earthquakes, fires, and floods. Because much of Southern California is physically rugged, not all of it has succumbed to the plow or the bulldozer. When you've had the pleasure of hiking beside a crystal-clear mountain stream minutes from downtown LA or cooling off in the spray of a cottonwood-fringed waterfall just beyond suburban San Diego, you'll realize that not many regions in the world offer so great a variety of natural pleasures to a population of many millions.

Let us, in the next couple of pages, briefly explore the principal wild and semiwild natural

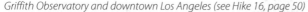

Griffith Observatory and downtown Los Angeles (see Hike 16, page 50)

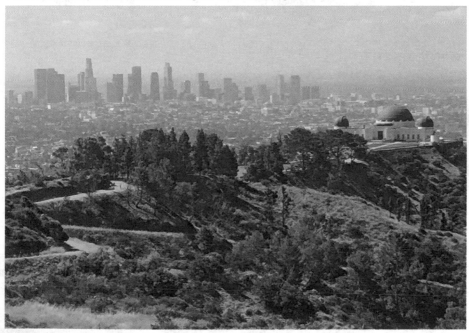

areas bordering Southern California's coastal plain. When linked together, these natural areas form a broad, curving crescent around Southern California's urban population—now more than 20 million strong. About 90% of the hikes found in this book fall into this unpopulated or sparsely populated crescent.

The Santa Monica Mountains

WE START WITH the Santa Monica Mountains, which rise abruptly from the Pacific shoreline west of (or up the coast from) Los Angeles. They, along with the San Gabriel and San Bernardino Mountains, are part of the Transverse Ranges, so named because they trend east–west and stand crosswise to the usual northwest–southeast grain of nearly every other major mountain range in California. This anomaly, it is thought, is largely due to compression along the San Andreas Fault. There is a kink in the San Andreas Fault north of Los Angeles where the fault, running southeast from the San Francisco Bay Area, jogs east for a while before resuming its course toward the southeast. Compression against this kink has caused the land south of it to crumple and wrinkle upward. The devastating January 1994 Northridge earthquake was just one small episode in the slow but fitful uplift of the Transverse Ranges.

Compared to other Southern California ranges, the Santa Monicas are modest in size—barely more than 3,000 feet high—but their rise from the sea is dramatic. They are a shaggy-looking range, clothed in tough, drought-resistant vegetation that falls into two principal categories: coastal sage scrub and chaparral. The *coastal sage scrub* plant community lies mostly below 2,000 feet in elevation, on primarily south-facing slopes in the Santa Monica Mountains and elsewhere in the coastal ranges of Southern California. Characterized by various aromatic sages (California sagebrush, black sage, and white sage) along with buckwheat, laurel sumac, lemonade berry shrubs, and prickly pear cactus, sage scrub is fast disappearing in the Santa Monicas and elsewhere as urbanization encroaches on it. Much of the sage-scrub vegetation is dormant and dead-looking during the warmer half of the year but green and aromatic during the cool, wet half.

The *chaparral* plant community is commonly found between 1,000 and 5,000 feet in elevation—almost anywhere there's a slope that hasn't burned recently. Chaparral needs

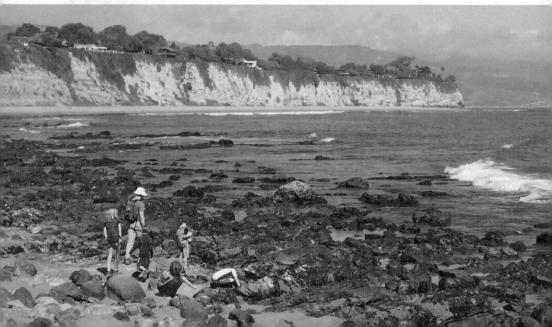

A strip of rocky coastline near Point Dume harbors tidepools and an array of plant and animal life (see Hike 6, page 30).

more moisture than sage scrub, so in the Santa Monicas it's often found on the shadier, north-facing slopes and other spots protected from the full glare of the sun. The dominant chaparral plants include chamise, scrub oak, manzanita, toyon, mountain mahogany, and various forms of ceanothus (wild lilac). Yuccas, known for their spectacular candle-shaped blooms, often frequent the chaparral zones. The chaparral plants are tough and intricately branched evergreen shrubs with deep root systems that help the plants survive during the long, hot summers. Chaparral is sometimes called elfin forest—a good description of a mature stand. Without benefit of a trail, travel through mature chaparral, which is often 15 feet high and incredibly dense from the ground up, is almost impossible.

A touch of the *southern oak woodland* and *riparian woodland* communities is present in the Santa Monicas and sparsely distributed nearly everywhere else in coastal Southern California. The Santa Monica Mountains include the southernmost stands of the valley oak, a massive, spreading tree that is as much a symbol of the Golden State as the redwoods farther north. The southern oak woodland is very parklike in appearance, especially in the spring when attended by new growth of grass and wildflowers. Riparian (streamside) vegetation includes trees such as willows, sycamores, and alders that thrive wherever water flows year-round—typically along the bottom of the larger canyons. Strolling through the riot of growth in riparian zones is the nearest thing to a jungle experience you can have in arid Southern California. Both types of habitat have declined all over California as a result of urbanization and agricultural development, and the attendant exploitation of water resources.

Wildfire plays a dominant role in the ecology of the Santa Monica Mountains, and indeed almost everywhere else in coastal Southern California. Sage scrub and chaparral vegetation readily renews itself after fire. Before modern times, wildfires would incinerate most hillsides every 5–15 years, and thick stands of chaparral seldom developed. Over the past century, however, the active prevention and suppression of fires has led to longer growth

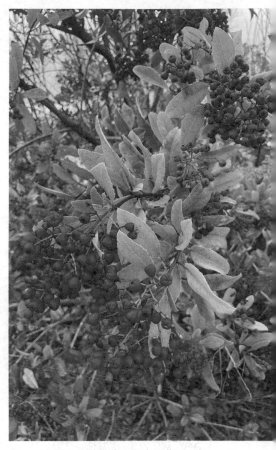

Toyon (California holly, for which Hollywood is named) is a common chaparral plant.

cycles and abnormally large accumulations of deadwood. Once started, today's wildfires in chaparral zones are often difficult or impossible to control.

From Malibu east into LA's west side, the Santa Monicas are steadily filling up with custom houses and subdivisions, all of which are in jeopardy from firestorms during the dry summer and fall seasons. Large and small wildfires will forever torment those who seek to establish permanent residence here.

Today the Santa Monicas are a patchwork quilt of private lands (many already built upon or slated for future development) and public lands, protected from urban development by inclusion within Santa Monica Mountains

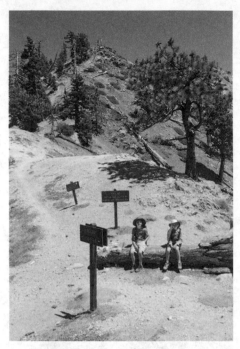

Windy Gap (see Hike 32, page 92)

National Recreation Area, a unit of the national park system.

The San Gabriel Mountains

TURNING OUR ATTENTION farther north and east, we find the San Gabriel Mountains, another segment of the east–west–trending Transverse Ranges. Behind the south ramparts of the San Gabriels, whose chaparral slopes rise sheer from the Los Angeles Basin and the San Gabriel Valley, stands a series of high peaks, the tallest of which—Old Baldy, also known as Mount San Antonio—exceeds 10,000 feet in elevation. Yawning gorges slash into the range, in one place offering more than a mile of vertical relief between the canyon bottom and the adjacent ridge.

Geologists figure that the San Gabriels are being squeezed horizontally about a tenth of an inch each year, and being thrust upward much more rapidly than that. Caught in this tectonic frenzy, the San Gabriel Mountains are surging upward as fast as any mountain range

on the planet. They are also disintegrating at a spectacular rate. Although the San Gabriels consist mainly of durable granitic rocks, much like those in the sturdy Sierra Nevada, the San Gabriel rocks have been through a tectonic meat grinder. The tops of the San Gabriels are fairly rounded, but their slopes are often appallingly steep and unstable. An average of 7 tons of material disappears from each acre of the front face each year, most of it coming to rest behind debris barriers and dams in the L.A. Basin below.

The San Gabriel Mountains themselves are relatively young as upthrust units—only a few million years old. This is not true of the ages of most of the rocks that compose them. Some rocks exposed here are representative of the oldest found on the Pacific Coast—more than 600 million years old.

Botanically, parts of the San Gabriel Mountains are extremely attractive, especially in zones above 4,000 feet that receive enough precipitation. There the *coniferous forest,* which has two phases in Southern California, thrives. The yellow pine phase forms tall, open conifer forest of bigcone Douglas-fir, ponderosa pine, Jeffrey pine, sugar pine, incense-cedar, and white fir. These species are often intermixed with live oaks, California bay (bay laurel), and scattered chaparral shrubs such as manzanita and mountain mahogany. Higher than about 8,000 feet, in the lodgepole pine phase, lodgepole pine, white fir, and limber pine are the prevailing trees. These trees, somewhat shorter and more weather-beaten than those below, exist in small, sometimes dense stands interspersed with such shrubs as chinquapin, snowbrush, and manzanita.

Excluding relatively small parcels of private land, the bulk of the higher San Gabriel Mountains lies within Angeles National Forest. Hundreds of square miles of wilderness or near wilderness in the San Gabriels are available within easy reach of millions of LA residents. In 2014, President Obama designated 346,177 acres of the national forest as the San Gabriel Mountains National Monument. This designation has not yet come with much in the way of new resources. Within Angeles National Forest are five wilderness areas closed

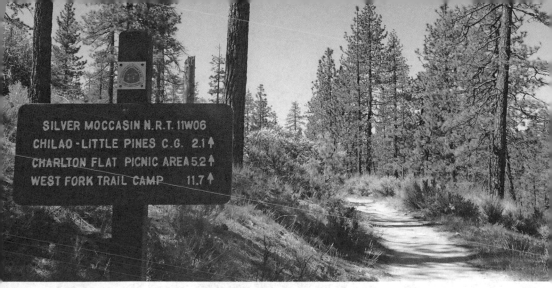

The Silver Moccasin Trail runs the length of the San Gabriel Mountains (see Hike 31, page 87).

to mechanized travel: Cucamonga Wilderness, San Gabriel Wilderness, Sheep Mountain Wilderness, Pleasant View Wilderness, and Magic Mountain Wilderness.

The 2009 Station Fire devastated the western portion of the San Gabriel Mountains, charring more than 160,000 acres. Some trails took nearly a decade to reopen, and others have been abandoned. Some forested areas may have permanently been succeeded by chaparral due

to the fire and climate change. The 2020 Bobcat Fire burned 115,000 acres in the central portion of the range, impacting many trails.

The San Bernardino Mountains

FARTHER EAST, ACROSS the low gap of Cajon Pass, the Transverse Ranges soar again as the San Bernardino Mountains. With Lake Arrowhead, Big Bear Lake, and winter ski areas, the

Wading up the East Fork Narrows (see Hike 33, page 94)

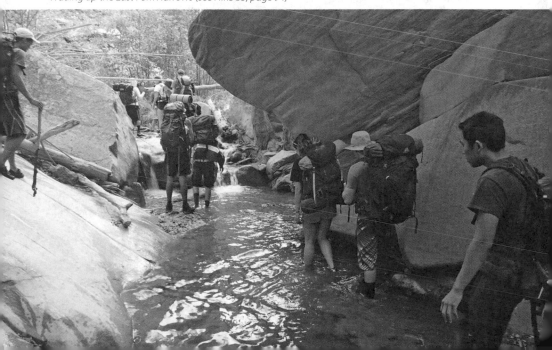

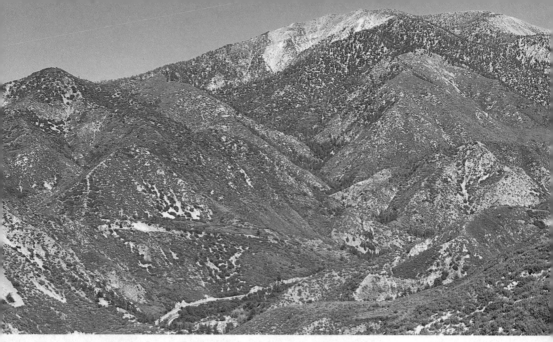

Old Baldy's Bear Ridge rises from San Antonio Canyon (see Hike 34, page 97).

mid-elevations (5,000–8,000 feet) draw millions of day-trippers and vacationers annually. Hikers and backpackers can explore the 10,000-foot-plus peaks of the San Gorgonio Wilderness, including 11,500-foot San Gorgonio Mountain itself—Southern California's high point. There it's possible to ascend through the yellow pine and lodgepole belts to treeline and above.

As in the San Gabriel Mountains, islands of private land in the San Bernardinos are surrounded by large sections of national forest.

San Bernardino National Forest encompasses much of the San Bernardino Mountains, as well as the San Jacinto and Santa Rosa Mountains to the south.

The most dramatic change taking place in the high mountains of Southern California—especially the San Bernardinos—is a massive die-off of coniferous trees. The high-elevation areas in Southern California have been receiving less precipitation in recent decades. A string of very dry years beginning in 1998–99

The Great San Bernardino Ridge towers behind Big Bear Lake (see Hike 40, page 109).

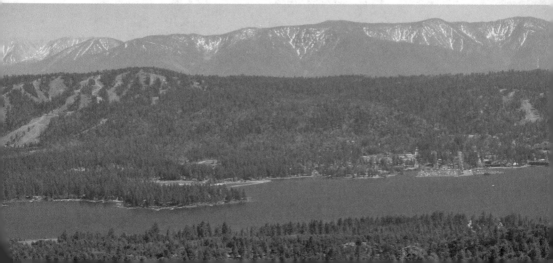

triggered an acute infestation of bark beetles, which eventually resulted in sudden death for millions of drought-stressed pine, fir, and cedar trees. Wildfires in October 2003 and 2007 destroyed millions of these dead and dying trees, and many others are being removed by logging operations in an overall effort to thin the forest to attain a more healthy level of tree density.

San Bernardino National Forest encompasses 823,816 acres, including the San Jacinto Mountains and the eastern end of the San Gabriel Mountains in San Bernardino County. In 2016, President Obama designated the 154,000-acre Sand to Snow National Monument, spanning from the edge of Joshua Tree National Park west to the high peaks of the San Gorgonio Wilderness.

The Mojave Desert

NORTH AND EAST of the San Gabriel and San Bernardino Mountains lies the vast, arid sweep of the Mojave Desert, a zone only partly included in this book. The Mojave, sometimes known as the high desert for its generally high average elevation, becomes far less populated and more diverse in its natural features as we move toward eastern California. A few of the hikes in this book explore the transitional region between high mountain and high desert.

There, at elevations of 3,000–5,000 feet, thrives the *pinyon/juniper woodland*, largely characterized by the rather stunted-looking one-leaf pinyon pine and the California juniper.

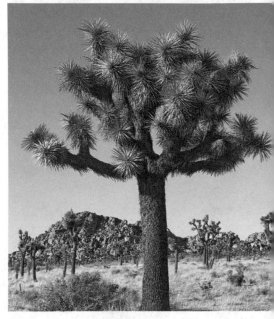

Joshua tree

Large sections of the Mojave, again in the elevation range of about 3,000–5,000 feet, are dominated by *Joshua tree woodland*. An outsize member of the yucca family, the Joshua tree is the indicator plant of the Mojave. Joshua Tree National Park preserves some, but hardly all, of the finest stands of these odd, tree-size plants.

The San Jacinto Mountains

MOVING SOUTH FROM the San Bernardino Mountains and Joshua Tree National Park, we find the northwest–southeast–trending San Jacinto Mountains and their southerly extension, the Santa Rosa Mountains. These lofty ranges comprise the northern ramparts of what geologists call the Peninsular Ranges—so named because they extend more or less continuously south across the Mexican border and comprise the spine of the long, thin peninsula of Baja California.

As the highest peak in the entire Peninsular Ranges province, 10,800-foot San Jacinto Peak would outrank all other Southern California peaks were it not for the slightly higher San

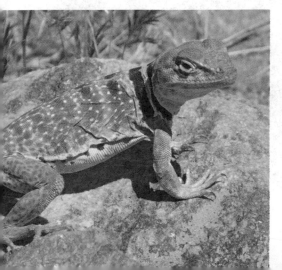

Collared lizard

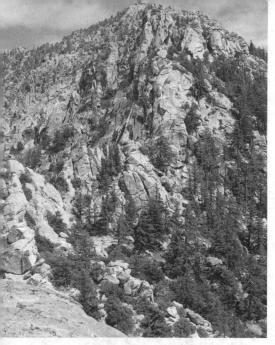

Tahquitz Peak's granite ramparts resemble the Sierra Nevada Mountains (see Hike 60, see page 153).

Gorgonio massif looming just 20 miles north. For sheer dramatic impact, however, San Jacinto wins hands down. Viewed from I-10 outside Palm Springs, the north and east escarpments of San Jacinto appear to rise nearly straight up from the desert floor—10,000 feet in 10 miles or less.

Every plant community we have mentioned so far, except Joshua tree woodland, thrives at one level or another on the mountain.

San Jacinto's pine-clad western slopes shelter several resort communities (such as Idyllwild); otherwise, nearly all of the mountain's upper elevations lie within national-forest wilderness or state wilderness areas.

Congress designated the 280,071-acre Santa Rosa and San Jacinto Mountains National Monument in 2000, spanning both this range and the fascinating desert peaks and canyons to the east.

The Colorado Desert

EAST OF THE northernmost Peninsular Ranges lie Palm Springs, the Coachella Valley, and the Salton Trough (Salton Sea). They are within the domain known as the Colorado Desert—California's low desert—so called because it stretches west from the lower Colorado River, which divides California from Arizona. A 1,000-square-mile chunk of the Colorado Desert lies within Anza-Borrego Desert State Park, by far the largest state park in California. Especially close and convenient for San Diegans, Anza-Borrego's vast acreage ranges from intricately dissected, desiccated terrain known

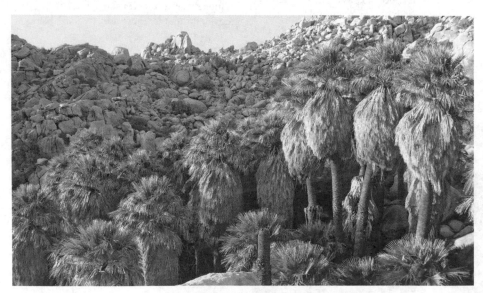

Mortero Palms Oasis in Anza-Borrego Desert State Park (see Hike 101, page 244)

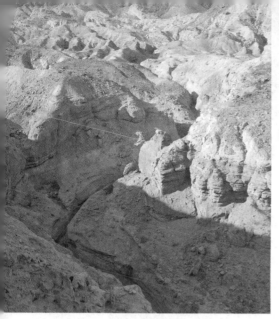

Explore a slot canyon in Anza-Borrego Desert State Park (Hike 98).

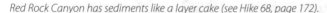

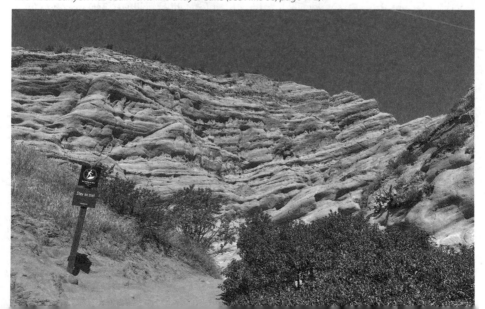

Palomar Ranges—each attaining heights of a little more than 6,000 feet. Chaparral blankets the slopes of these mountains, while the typical yellow pine assemblage of oak, pine, cedar, and fir dominates the higher elevations. Farther north and west, bordering the rapidly expanding urban zones of southwestern Riverside and southern Orange County, lie the Santa Ana Mountains. They are the northernmost coastal expressions of the Peninsular Ranges.

Suburban sprawl has crept into the foothills of these far-southern ranges and in some cases threatens to degrade the higher elevations as well. Fortunately, large parts of this mountainous region lie within the jurisdiction of Cleveland National Forest and various state parks.

All the mountain ranges rimming San Diego have recently been hard-hit by both drought and wildfire. The 300,000-acre Cedar Fire, which blazed an elongated path across central San Diego County in October 2003, burned through primarily chaparral and oak woodland, and through prime oak and coniferous forest, mostly in the Cuyamaca Mountains. The chaparral and oak woodlands of lower elevation, adapted to periodic fires, have largely recovered. The formerly lush Cuyamaca Mountains may never look quite the same.

as badlands to the pinyon-juniper and yellow pine forests of the Peninsular Ranges.

The Laguna, Cuyamaca, Palomar, and Santa Ana Mountains

EAST AND NORTH of San Diego, the Peninsular Ranges consist of a number of parallel ranges—primarily the Laguna, Cuyamaca, and

Red Rock Canyon has sediments like a layer cake (see Hike 68, page 172).

Health, Safety, and Courtesy

Good preparation is always important for any kind of recreational pursuit. Hiking the Southern California backcountry is no exception. Although most of the Southland's natural environments are seldom hostile or dangerous to life and limb, there are some pitfalls to be aware of.

Preparation and Equipment

AN OBVIOUS SAFETY requirement is being in good health. Some degree of physical conditioning is always desirable, even for the trips in this book designated as easy or moderate. The more challenging trips require increasing amounts of stamina and technical expertise. Running, bicycling, swimming, aerobics, or any similar exercise that develops both your leg muscles and the aerobic capacity of your whole body are recommended as preparatory exercise.

For the longest hikes in this book, there is no really adequate way to prepare other than hiking itself. Start with easy- or moderate-length trips, and then work gradually toward extending both distance and time.

Several of the hiking trips in this book reach elevations of 7,000 feet or more—altitudes at which sea-level folks may notice a big difference in their stamina and rate of breathing. A few hours or a day spent at altitude before exercising will help almost anyone acclimate, but that's often impractical for day trips. Still, you might consider spending a night or two at a campground with some altitude before tackling the likes of 11,500-foot San Gorgonio Mountain. Altitude sickness strikes some victims at elevations as low as 8,000 feet. If you become dizzy or nauseated, or suffer from congested lungs or a severe headache, the antidote may be as simple as descending 1,000–2,000 feet.

Your choice of equipment and supplies on the longer hikes in this book can be critically important. The essentials you should carry with you at all times in the remote backcountry are the things that would allow you to survive, in a reasonably comfortable manner, for one or two unscheduled nights out. It's important to note that no one ever plans these nights! No one plans to get lost, injured, stuck, or pinned down by the weather. Always do a "what if" analysis for a worst-case scenario, and plan accordingly. These essential items are your safety net; keep them with you on day hikes, and take them with you in a small day pack if you leave your backpack and camping equipment behind at a campsite.

Chief among the essential items is *warm clothing*. Inland Southern California is characterized by wide swings in day and night temperatures. In mountain valleys susceptible to cold-air drainage, for example, a midday temperature in the 70s or 80s is often followed by a subfreezing night. Carry light, inner layers of clothing consisting of polypropylene or wool (best for cool or cold weather) or cotton (adequate for warm or hot weather but very poor for cold and damp weather). Include a thicker insulating layer of synthetic fill, wool, or down to put on whenever you need it, especially when you are not moving around and generating heat. Add to these items a cap, gloves, and a waterproof or water-resistant shell (a large trash bag will do in a pinch)—and you'll be quite prepared for all but the most severe weather. In hot, sunny weather, sun-shielding clothing, including a sun hat and a light-colored, long-sleeve top, may also be essential.

Water and *food* are next in importance. Most streams and even some springs in the mountains have been shown to contain high levels of bacteria or other contaminants. Even though most of the remote watersheds are probably pristine, it's wise to treat by filtering or chemical methods any water obtained outside of developed camp or picnic sites. Unless the day is very warm or your trip is a long one, it's usually easiest to carry (preferably in a CamelBak or sturdy plastic bottles) all the water you'll need. Don't underestimate your water needs: During a full day's hike in 80°F temperatures you may require as much as a gallon of water. Know, too, that many springs and watercourses—even some shown as being permanent on topographic maps—may run dry at some point during the summer. Food is necessary to stave off the feeling of hunger and keep your energy stores up, but it is not nearly as critical as water in emergency situations where you are in danger of dehydration.

Farther down the list but still essential are a *map and compass* or *GPS*, a *flashlight*, a *fire-starting device* (waterproof matches or a lighter), and a *first aid kit*.

Items not always essential but potentially useful and convenient are sunglasses, a pocket-knife, a whistle or other signaling device, toilet paper, and sunscreen. Sunglasses are an essential item for travel over snow.

Every member of a hiking party should carry all these essential items because individuals or splinter groups may end up separating from the party for one reason or another. If you plan to hike solo in the backcountry, being well equipped is very important. If you hike alone, be sure to check in with a park ranger or leave your itinerary with a responsible person. That way, if you do get stuck, help will probably come to the right place—eventually.

Most hikers carry cell phones, which allow you to make emergency calls, as well as take photos and serve as a backup flashlight. Remember you may not always have coverage while hiking, and the cell phone becomes useless when you run out of charge. Consider carrying a small USB battery pack and cable in case of emergency, but remember to periodically recharge the battery pack. Satellite communicators such as the Garmin inReach or Spot

can give you two-way communication outside of cell coverage but have monthly subscription fees. Personal Locator Beacons (PLBs) can send an emergency SOS via satellite, are cheaper, and have no monthly fees. These can be a prudent investment, especially if you hike frequently, with children, or in bad weather.

Special Hazards

OTHER THAN THE possibility of your getting lost or pinned down by a rare sudden storm, the most common hazards found in the Southland are steep, unstable terrain; icy terrain; spiny plants; rattlesnakes; mountain lions; ticks; and poison oak.

Falls

Exploring some trails—especially those of the San Gabriels—may involve traveling over structurally weak rock on steep slopes. The erosive effects of flowing water, of wedging by roots and by ice, and of brush fires tend to further pulverize the rock. Slips on such terrain usually lead to sliding down a hillside some distance. If you explore cross-country, always be on the lookout for dangerous runouts, such as cliffs, below you. The sidewalls of many canyons in the San Gabriels may look like fun places to practice rock-climbing moves, but this misconception has caused many deaths over the years.

Snow and Ice

Statistically, mishaps associated with snow and ice have caused the greatest number of fatalities in the San Gabriel and San Bernardino

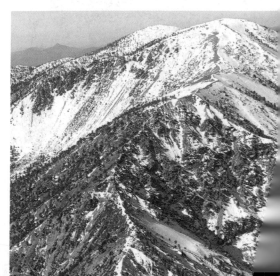

Old Baldy's Devil's Backbone is treacherous in winter (see Hike 35, page 99).

Mountains. This is not because our local mountains are inherently more dangerous than the Sierra Nevada, the Cascades, or other ranges; rather, it is because the novelty of snow and easy access by way of snowplowed highways attract inexperienced lowlanders, who never picture their backyard mountains as true wilderness areas. Icy chutes and slopes capable of avalanching can easily trap such visitors unawares. Visitors can explore the gentler areas of the high country on snowshoes or skis, but the steeper slopes require technical skills and equipment such as an ice ax and crampons, just as other snow-covered mountain ranges do.

Puncturing Plants

Most desert hikers will sooner or later suffer punctures by thorns or spines. This is most likely to happen during close encounters with the cholla, or jumping, cactus, whose spine clusters readily break off and attach firmly to your skin, clothes, or boots. A comb will allow you to gently pull away the spine clusters, and tweezers or lightweight pliers will help you remove any individual embedded spines. Another problematic spiny plant is the agave, or century plant. It consists of a rosette of fleshy leaves, each tipped with a rigid thorn containing a mild toxin. A headlong fall into either an agave or one of the more vicious kinds of cacti could easily make you swear off desert travel permanently. It's best to give these devilish plants as wide a berth as possible.

Ladybug on a cactus (see Hike 97, page 235)

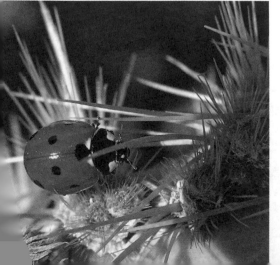

Rattlesnakes

Rattlesnakes are common everywhere in Southern California below an elevation of about 7,000 feet. Seldom seen in either cold or very hot weather, they favor temperatures in the 75°F–90°F range—spring and fall in the desert and coastal areas and summer in the mountains. Most rattlesnakes are as interested in avoiding contact with you as you are with them.

Watch carefully where you put your feet and especially your hands during the warmer months. In brushy or rocky areas where you cannot see as far, try to make your presence known. Tread with heavy footfalls, or bang a stick against rocks or bushes. Rattlesnakes will pick up the vibrations through their skin and will usually buzz (an unmistakable sound) before you get too close for comfort. Most bad encounters between rattlesnakes and hikers occur in April and May, when snakes are irritable and hungry after their long hibernation period.

Rattlesnakes will warn you to give them space.

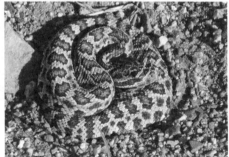

Mountain Lions

Mountain lion attacks, although statistically rare, have been increasing all over California in the past three decades. This trend may continue as the natural habitat for these carnivorous cats becomes more and more fragmented by suburban and rural development. Several attacks and many more incidents of threatening behavior by mountain lions toward humans have taken place in urban-edge park and national-forest lands, such as those covered in this book.

Here are some basic tips for dealing with this potential hazard:

- Hike with one or more companions.
- Keep children close at hand.
- Never run from a mountain lion. This may trigger an instinct to attack.
- Make yourself large: face the animal, maintain eye contact with it, shout, blow a whistle, and do not act fearful. Do anything you can to convince the animal that you are not its prey.

Ticks

Ticks can be the scourge of overgrown trails in the coastal foothills and lower mountain slopes, particularly during the first warm spells of the year, when they climb to the tips of shrub branches and lie in wait for warm-blooded hosts. If you can't avoid brushing against vegetation along the trail, be sure to check yourself for ticks frequently. Upon finding a host, a tick will usually crawl upward in search of a protected spot, where it will try to attach itself. If you are aware of the slightest irritation on your body, you'll usually intercept ticks long before they attempt to bite. Ticks would be of relatively minor concern here, except that tick-borne Lyme disease, which can have serious health effects, has been reported within Southern California.

Poison Oak

Poison oak grows profusely along many of the coastal and mountain canyons below 5,000 feet in elevation. It is often found on the banks of streamcourses in the form of a bush or vine, where it prefers semishady habitats. Quite often, it's seen beside or encroaching on

Poison oak leaves

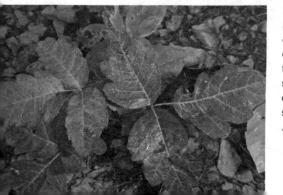

well-used trails. Learn to recognize its distinctive three-leafed structure, and avoid touching it with skin or clothing. Because poison oak retains some of the toxic oil in its stems when it loses its leaves during the winter months (and sometimes during summer and fall drought), it can be extra hazardous at that time because it is harder to identify and avoid. Midweight pants, like blue jeans, and a long-sleeve shirt will serve as a fair barrier against the toxic oil of the poison oak plant. Do, of course, remove these clothes as soon as the hike is over, and make sure they are washed carefully afterward.

Other Safety Concerns

Deer-hunting season in Southern California usually runs through the middle part of the autumn. Although conflicts between hunters and hikers are rare, you may want to confine your autumn explorations to state and county parks, as well as wilderness areas where hunting is prohibited.

There is always some risk in leaving a vehicle unattended at a trailhead. It may be worthwhile to disable your car's ignition or attach an anti-theft device to your steering wheel. Never leave valuable property visible in an automobile; this is an invitation for a break-in. Report all theft and vandalism of personal or public property to the local county sheriff or the appropriate park or forest agency.

Permits and Camping

SOME OF THE trails on national-forest lands (Angeles, San Bernardino, and Cleveland National Forests) are at present subject to the National Forest Adventure Pass program. This applies only to vehicles parked on national forest land and not to users who arrive on foot or by bicycle. Adventure Passes are available at all national-forest offices, ranger stations, and fire stations. They are also sold through commercial vendors—typically sports shops throughout the region, gas stations and markets near the principal national-forest entry roads, and small businesses within national-forest borders. They are not available at most trailheads, so you must plan ahead if you need a pass. Adventure Passes cost $5 per day or $30 for year. The Adventure Pass must be prominently displayed on your parked car—otherwise your car will likely be ticketed and fined.

In the 2014 *Fragosa et al. v. U.S. Forest Service* decision, the California Central District Court ruled that people who do not use facilities and services such as restrooms, picnic tables, and trash cans cannot be required to buy a pass to park in or enter a national forest. At any Adventure Pass trailhead, the Forest Service is required to allow free roadside parking within half a mile for visitors who are not using the facilities. The Forest Service generally does not inform the public about the existence of this free parking.

If you plan to visit national-forest territory more than two or three times a year, it is time-efficient at the very least to purchase the $30 yearly pass instead of worrying about obtaining one each day you come up for a visit. Another option is the $80 America the Beautiful Annual Pass, which also covers national parks and many other federal lands.

If you are planning an overnight trip of some type into the Southern California backcountry, be aware that camping in roadside campgrounds is not always a restful experience. Off-season camping (late fall through early spring) offers relief from crowds but not from chilly nighttime weather. Most national-forest campgrounds are less well supervised than those in state and county parks, which means that they sometimes attract a noisy crowd. In my experience, facilities with a campground host promise a quieter clientele and a better night's sleep.

The nice advantage of a developed campground is that you can always have a campfire there—unless the facility is closed. On trails where backpacking is allowed, fire regulations vary. Most jurisdictions prohibit campfires all or part of the year. Others permit fires, as long as you have the necessary free permit.

Some national forest areas allow remote, primitive-style camping: you are not always restricted to staying at a developed campground or designated trail camp. For sanitation

reasons, you must locate your camp well away from the nearest source of water. And, of course, you must observe the fire regulations stated earlier. Always check with the U.S. Forest Service to confirm these rules if you intend to do any remote camping.

Most federally managed wilderness areas around the state require special wilderness permits for entry. Many in Southern California have self-registering permits at trailheads; others require permits only for overnight visits. The San Gorgonio and San Jacinto Wildernesses are so popular that their managing agencies sometimes implement trailhead quotas.

Facilities

IN GENERAL, YOU can expect restrooms and picnic tables at trailheads with use fees but rarely at other trailheads. Any national-forest trailhead that requires you to post an Adventure Pass will have facilities. City, county, state, and national parks have restrooms at most trailheads, and facilities are usually available at visitor centers or museums near some trailheads.

Trail Courtesy

WHENEVER YOU TRAVEL the backcountry, you take on a burden of responsibility—to leave the wilderness as you found it. Aside from commonsense prohibitions against littering, vandalism, and inappropriate campfires, there are some less obvious guidelines every hiker should be aware of. We'll mention a few:

Never cut trail switchbacks. This practice breaks down the trail tread and hastens erosion. You may, however, improve designated trails by removing branches, rocks, or other debris from the path. Springtime growth can quite rapidly obscure pathways in the chaparral country, and funding for trail maintenance is often scarce, so try to do your part by joining a volunteer trail crew or by performing your own small maintenance tasks while walking the trails. Report any damage to trails or other facilities to the appropriate ranger office.

When backpacking, be a Leave No Trace camper. Leave your campsite as you found it or in an even more natural condition. Visit lnt.org /why/7-principles to learn the seven principles of minimum-impact camping and trail use.

Most jurisdictions prohibit the collection of minerals, plants, animals, and historical objects without a special permit. These regulations usually cover common things, such as pine cones, wildflowers, and lizards, too. Leave them for all visitors to enjoy. Limited collecting of items like pine cones may be allowed on some national-forest lands; check with the local agency first.

We have covered most of the general regulations associated with Southern California's public lands, but keep in mind that you, as a visitor, are responsible for knowing any additional rules as well.

Each hike described in this book includes a reference to the agency responsible for the area you'll be visiting. Phone numbers for those agencies appear in the back of this book.

Internet research is often helpful too. Using a search engine, enter keywords for the park or area in question to find an abundance of information. The quality of this information, however, varies, and it is important to note the date of its posting and the source itself.

Map Legend

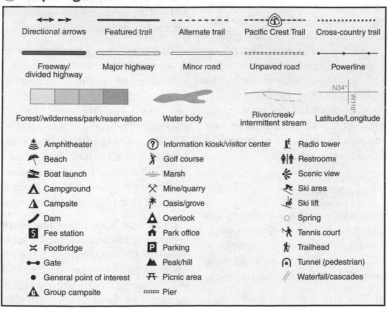

Using This Book

There are three principal ways to find hiking trips in this book that are suitable for you: You can check the overview map for all 101 hikes (pages x–xi) and focus your search on a specific geographic area; you can scan the hike overview table (pages xii–iv); or you can just leaf through the book, browsing hike summaries, route descriptions, and photos.

To get the most out of this guide, please take the time to read, below, about the key information that appears before each hike description.

Maps are provided for each hike. The hiker symbol on each map denotes the start point of the hike. The GPS coordinates for the trailhead are shown in decimal degrees. One-way (point-to-point) hikes have two hiker symbols—one at the beginning of the hike and one at the end. For nearly all of the hikes described in this book, the map we provide is adequate for basic navigation. For a few hikes, we recommend a specific detailed topographic map.

Key Information

EACH HIKE BEGINS with a summary that details its location, highlights, distance, elevation gain and loss, time required, optional or recommended maps, best times to go, managing agency, difficulty rating, and trail uses.

Location: This field states the general location of the hike: a well-known park, mountain range, or nearby city or town.

Highlights: One or two engaging features of the hike are mentioned here.

Distance & Configuration: The total distance is given. For hikes shorter than 6 miles, the distance is given to the nearest tenth of a mile. For hikes 6 miles and longer, the distance is rounded

to the nearest whole number. Out-and-back trips show the round-trip distance. This section also indicates what type of trip it is: out-and-back, point-to-point (one-way), or loop.

Elevation Gain: These are estimates of the sum of all the vertical gain segments along the total length of the route (both ways for out-and-back trips). This is often considerably more than the net difference in elevation between the high and low points of the hike. If the starting and ending elevations are substantially different, the trip may also list Elevation Loss.

Hiking Time: This figure states the time spent in motion for the average hiker. It *does not* include time for rest stops, lunch, and so on. Fast walkers could complete the routes in 30% less time, and slower hikers may take 50% longer. We assume the hiker is traveling with a light day pack. Hikers carrying heavy packs could easily take nearly twice as long, especially if traveling under adverse weather conditions. Remember, too, that the progress made by a group as a whole is limited by the pace of its slowest member.

Optional or Recommended Map(s): This section lists maps to use if you want a broader view than the one presented in this book. Tom Harrison publishes the best maps for Southern California's most popular hiking areas, including the Santa Monica, San Gabriel, San Bernardino, and San Jacinto Mountains and Joshua Tree National Park. Trails Illustrated maps are missing odd things, such as the most popular trails on Mount Baldy and Mount Waterman, but are often good enough and can be more economical because they cover larger areas. Both of these brands are available at ranger stations, at hiking stores such as REI, or from online retailers. Many county and city parks have decent maps available on government websites. This book used to recommend U.S. Geological Survey 7.5-minute topographic maps, but those have become outdated and less useful and are now only suggested when I haven't found a better alternative.

Electronic maps are becoming more popular, although if your phone runs out of charge, you may find yourself with neither a map nor a way to call for help. The FarOut app for Android and iOS phones and tablets includes a guide for this book as an in-app purchase. The guide includes live maps and elevation profiles showing your position on the trail. It also links to navigation apps for driving directions. To purchase this guide in the app, click on the Store icon, and search for "101 Hikes."

You can also download the tracks and waypoints for this book from eTrails.net in GPX format and display them on your favorite mapping app, such as Gaia. Another option is Avenza, which sells downloadable, high-resolution Tom Harrison and U.S. Forest Service maps and displays your position on the map.

Best Times: Due to the extreme heat, avoid strenuous desert trips during any period except the one recommended in this field. Trips elsewhere in Southern California are usually safe enough, though less rewarding, outside their best times.

Agency: This entity has jurisdiction over or manages the area being hiked and can provide more information about a particular hike and its current regulations. Contact information is listed on page 248.

Difficulty: This subjective, overall rating takes into account the length of the hike and the nature of the terrain. The following are general definitions of the five categories:

Easy Suitable for every member of the family.

Moderate Suitable for all physically fit people.

Moderately strenuous Long length, substantial elevation gain, and/or difficult terrain. Recommended for experienced hikers only.

Strenuous A full day's hike (or a backpack trip) over a long and/or challenging route. Suitable only for experienced hikers in excellent physical condition.

Very strenuous Long and rugged route in extremely remote area. Suitable only for experienced hikers or climbers in top physical condition. Only two hikes in this book—San Jacinto Peak: Hard Way (Hike 58) and Villager Peak (Hike 97)—get this rating.

Each higher level represents more or less a doubling of the difficulty.

Trail Use: This field, if listed, specifies whether dogs are allowed, whether the hike is appropriate for kids, and more.

Permit: This section lists any required entry fees or permits.

Google Maps: Enter this keyword into Google Maps for automated guidance to the trailhead on your smartphone. Note that these keywords sometimes change and are not standardized across apps; before driving, confirm that the app is guiding you to the right place.

HIKE 1   Paradise Falls

Location	Wildwood Park, City of Thousand Oaks
Highlights	Gem of a waterfall in a steep gorge
Distance & Configuration	2.7-mile loop
Elevation Gain	400'
Hiking Time	2 hours
Optional Map	cosf.org/files/maps/wildwood_trail_map.pdf
Best Times	All year
Agency	Conejo Recreation and Park District
Difficulty	Moderate
Trail Use	Dogs allowed, good for kids
Permit	None required
Google Maps	Wildwood Regional Park

Wildwood Park in Thousand Oaks is Ventura County's most scenic suburban park. The scenery here has been imprinted in the minds of many in the over-56 age group, as the area was once an outdoor set for Old Hollywood movies, as well as for TV's *Gunsmoke, The Rifleman,* and *Wagon Train.* The short but steep hike—down and then up—described here takes you to Wildwood Park's gem: the Arroyo Conejo gorge and Paradise Falls. The lovingly maintained park offers drinking fountains, picnic tables, interpretive signs, and shady rest spots along this fine loop.

To Reach the Trailhead: From the 101 Freeway at Exit 45 in Thousand Oaks, take Lynn Road north 2.5 miles to Avenida de los Arboles. Turn left and follow Avenida de los Arboles 1 mile west. At this point traffic goes sharply right on Big Sky Drive; you make a U-turn and park on the right at Wildwood Park's principal trailhead, open 8 a.m.–5 p.m. Nearby curbside parking is also available.

Description: Three trails radiate from the Avenida de los Arboles trailhead. Two are wide and relatively bland dirt roads. The third (the one you want), the narrow and scenic Moonridge Trail, descends sharply from the east side of the parking area. This is the left side of the parking area as you drive in. Right away you come to a T-intersection amid oak woods. Turn right, remaining on the Moonridge Trail. The

trail descends a sunny slope covered with aromatic sage-scrub vegetation and dappled with succulent live-forever plants that sprout white, comical-looking flower stalks. Beware of the prickly pear cactus flanking the trail. There's a brief passage across a shady ravine using wooden steps and a plank bridge. At 0.5 mile,

Exploring Indian Cave

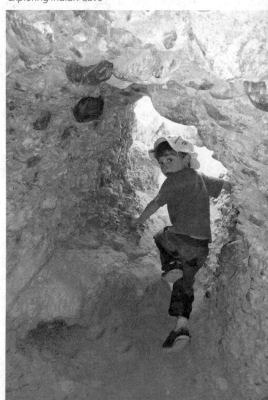

Paradise Falls

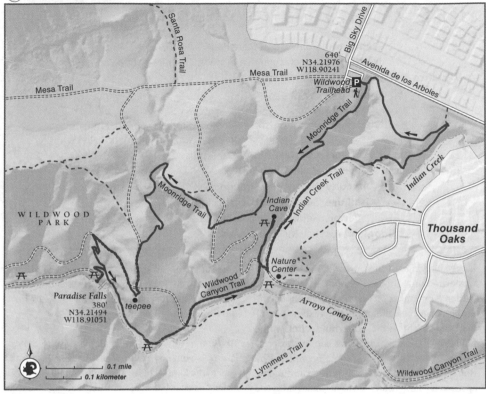

you cross over a dirt road and continue on the narrow Moonridge Trail.

Ahead, the trail curls around a deep ravine, edging into the crumbly sedimentary rock. At 1.4 miles you join another dirt road and use it to descend toward a large wooden teepee structure on a knoll just below. Make a right at the teepee, further descending into the Arroyo Conejo gorge. As you descend, watch for the narrow side trail on the left that will take you straight down to Paradise Falls—a beautiful, 30-foot-high cascade that makes its presence known by sound before sight. The high water table in the canyon bottom ensures a nearly year-round flow of water. Watch for poison oak, especially on the far side of the creek.

After you've admired the falls, continue by climbing back up the slope in the direction you came, and take the fenced, cliff-hanging trail around the left (east) side of the falls. Beyond that fenced stretch, the narrow trail descends a

little and sidles up alongside the creek, where large coast live oaks spread their shade. Soon, you continue on a path of dirt-road width. Stay with that path until you reach a major crossroads. It's worth a 0.1-mile detour straight ahead to walk through Indian Cave. Then, returning to the junction, cross the bridge. The small Wildwood Nature Center is just around the bend to the right, and your return route up along Indian Creek is to the left.

On the Indian Creek Trail, you pay your debt to gravity by ascending nearly 300 feet in about 0.7 mile. The beautifully tangled array of live oak and sycamore limbs along this trail keeps your mind off the climb. At one point, you can look down into a deep ravine where an inaccessible mini waterfall and pool lie practically hidden. When you finally reach Avenida de los Arboles, turn left and then return a short distance to the trailhead parking lot.

HIKE 2 La Jolla Valley Loop

Location	Point Mugu State Park
Highlights	Spectacular ocean views and rare native vegetation
Distance & Configuration	11-mile loop
Elevation Gain	1,950'
Hiking Time	6 hours
Optional Maps	Tom Harrison *Point Mugu State Park* or Trails Illustrated *Santa Monica Mountains National Recreation Area*
Best Times	October–June, 8 a.m.–sunset
Agency	Point Mugu State Park
Difficulty	Moderately strenuous
Trail Use	Suitable for backpacking
Permit	Required for overnight use; day-use parking fee
Google Maps	Ray Miller Trailhead

Lazily curving up the rumpled slopes of the western Santa Monica Mountains, the Ray Miller Trail takes in sweeping views of the Point Mugu coastline and the distant Channel Islands. This is the westernmost link in the Backbone Trail, which skims along the crest of the Santa Monicas for some 65 miles. The Ray Miller Trail offers a well-graded and scenic approach to the rounded ridge that divides the two largest canyons in Point Mugu State Park: La Jolla and Big Sycamore. The trail was named after California's first official State Park Campground Host, who served here from 1979 until his death in 1989.

The Ray Miller Trail is just the start of the big loop we're suggesting here: a comprehensive trek through the western quadrant of Point Mugu State Park. If this is too big a chunk to bite off for a single day, there are shortcuts, as our map suggests. You could also extend your trip by staying overnight at La Jolla Valley Walk-In Camp. For that, you must register with a park ranger across the highway at Thornhill Broome Beach Campground.

Note: The May 2013 Springs Fire, driven by unseasonably high temperatures, strong winds, and dry conditions, swept from Thousand Oaks to the Pacific and damaged the state park. The La Jolla Canyon Trail was washed away in subsequent flooding, and is currently closed and in awful condition, even for experienced hikers. Check with the park whether it has reopened. If

it has not, you can still do a loop by descending the Chumash Trail. This requires a 2-mile car or bicycle shuttle or carefully walking back on the shoulder of the highway.

To Reach the Trailhead: Point Mugu State Park lies some 32 miles west of Santa Monica via Pacific Coast Highway (Highway 1). Immediately west of the Thornhill Broome Beach Campground, turn north onto a poorly marked road, and follow it to the end for the Ray Miller Trailhead parking. If you haven't registered for

The Boney Mountains are an eroded volcanic mass.

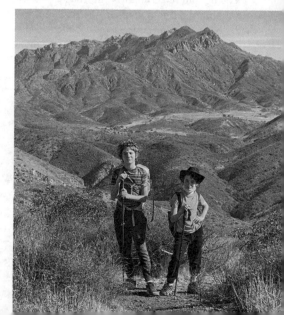

🐾 La Jolla Valley Loop

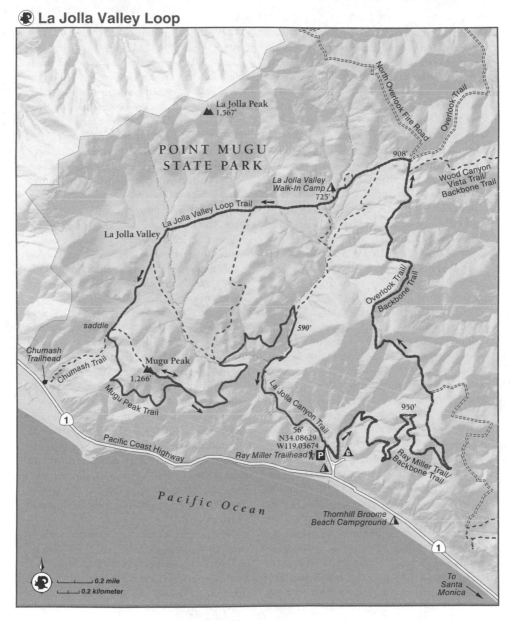

overnight camping, pay your day-use fee at the parking area.

Description: Two trails diverge from the parking lot. The wide one going up along the dry canyon bottom ahead is the La Jolla Canyon Trail, your return route. Look at the trailhead kiosk to see if La Jolla Canyon has reopened; otherwise, plan to descend Chumash. To begin, take the narrower Ray Miller Trail to your right. It doggedly climbs 2.7 miles to a junction with the Overlook Trail, a wide fire road. This is the major ascent along the loop—better to get it over with at the beginning. Ever-widening views of the ocean, along with fine springtime wildflower displays, keep your mind off the effort. This is a popular turnaround point for a shorter hike.

Turn left when you reach the Overlook Trail, and wend your way around several bumps on the undulating ridge. Enjoy the terrific views of Boney Mountain's eroded volcanic core to the east and La Jolla Valley's grassy fields to the west. When you arrive at a saddle where five wide trails diverge (4.5 miles from the start), take the trail to the left (west) that descends into the green- or flaxen-colored (depending on the season) La Jolla Valley.

The valley is managed by the state park as a natural preserve to protect the native bunchgrasses that flourish there. Because so much of California's coast ranges have been biologically disturbed by grazing for more than a century, opportunistic, nonnative grasses have taken over just about everywhere. The authentic California tallgrass prairie in parts of La Jolla Valley is a notable exception.

The La Jolla Valley Walk-In Camp ahead has an outhouse and oak-shaded picnic tables. Bring your own water if you plan to camp; the faucets are not operational at the time of this writing. The campground lost much of its charm after the fire and will take years to fully recover. Just south of there, beside a trail leading directly back to the Ray Miller Trailhead, you'll find a tule-fringed pond, seasonally dry in some years. Look for chocolate lilies on the slopes around it.

From the camp, continue west in the direction of a military radar installation on Laguna Peak. Stay right where marked trails diverge to the left, circling the perimeter of the La Jolla Valley grassland and rising sharply on the Chumash Trail to a saddle (7 miles) on the northwest shoulder of the Mugu Peak ridge. At that saddle you'll have a great view of the Pacific Ocean. The popping noises you may hear below are from a military shooting range near the Pacific Coast Highway. Up the coast is the Point Mugu Naval Air Station.

Beyond the saddle, the Chumash Trail descends sharply to the Pacific Coast Highway. If the La Jolla Canyon Trail is still closed, this is your exit route. Otherwise, you veer left on the Mugu Peak Trail and contour south and east around the south flank of Mugu Peak. (Alternatively, a steep trail on the left just before the saddle shortcuts directly to the peak.) You arrive at another saddle (8 miles) just east of Mugu's 1,266-foot summit. Five minutes of climbing on a steep path puts you on top, where there's a dizzying view of the east-west-oriented coastline. You can look down upon The Great Sand Dune (coastal dunes) and the Pacific Coast Highway where it squeezes past some coastal bluffs. On warm days there's a desertlike feel to this rocky and sparsely vegetated mountain, oddly juxtaposed with the sights and sounds of the surf below.

Return to the saddle east of the peak, and continue descending to a junction in a wooded recess of La Jolla Canyon. Turn right, proceed east along a hillside, and then hook up with the La Jolla Canyon Trail, where you turn right.

There's an exciting stretch through a rock-walled section of La Jolla Canyon where giant coreopsis bloom in spring. Quite common in the Channel Islands, this plant is found only in scattered coastal locales, from far western Los Angeles County to San Luis Obispo County. Some coreopsis plants have forked stems towering as high as 10 feet. The massed, yellow, daisylike flowers are an unforgettable sight in March and April.

Descending toward the canyon's mouth, you'll pass a little grove of native walnut trees and a small seasonal waterfall. After a final descent, join a dirt road that was built to haul stone out of the area for the construction of the coast highway, and arrive a few minutes later at the trailhead.

HIKE 3   Sandstone Peak

Location	Circle X Ranch (Santa Monica Mountains National Recreation Area)
Highlights	Most expansive view in the Santa Monicas, volcanic rock formations
Distance & Configuration	6-mile loop

Elevation Gain	1,400'
Hiking Time	3.5 hours
Optional Maps	Tom Harrison *Point Mugu State Park* or Trails Illustrated *Santa Monica Mountains National Recreation Area*
Best Times	October–June
Agency	Santa Monica Mountains National Recreation Area
Difficulty	Moderately strenuous
Trail Use	Dogs allowed
Permit	None required
Google Maps	Sandstone Peak Trailhead

Sandstone Peak is the quintessential destination for peak baggers in the Santa Monica Mountains. The 3,111-foot summit can be efficiently climbed from the east via the Backbone Trail in a mere 1.5 miles, but the far more scenic way to go is the loop outlined below. Take a picnic lunch, and plan to make a half day of it. Try to come on a crystalline day in late fall or winter to get the best skyline views. Or, if it's wildflowers you most enjoy, come in April or May, when the native vegetation blooms most profusely at these middle elevations. In addition to blue-flowering stands of ceanothus, the early- to mid-spring floral bloom includes monkey flower, nightshade, Chinese houses, wild peony, wild hyacinth, morning glory, and phacelia. Delicate, orangish Humboldt lilies unfold by June. The 2018 Woolsey fire scorched parts of this loop, but the native vegetation is adapted to fire and is returning quickly.

Sandstone Peak lies within Circle X Ranch, formerly owned by the Boy Scouts of America and now a federally managed unit of the Santa Monica Mountains National Recreation Area. The National Park Service generously provides free trail maps at the trailhead.

To Reach the Trailhead: The Sandstone Peak Trailhead is located near the western end of the Santa Monica Mountains, a few miles (by crow's flight) south of Thousand Oaks. From the Pacific Coast Highway near mile marker 1 VEN 1.00, turn north onto Yerba Buena Road and proceed 6.4 miles.

Or from the 101 Freeway in Thousand Oaks, take Highway 23 south for 7.2 miles. Turn right (west) on Mulholland Highway, then in

🔊 Sandstone Peak

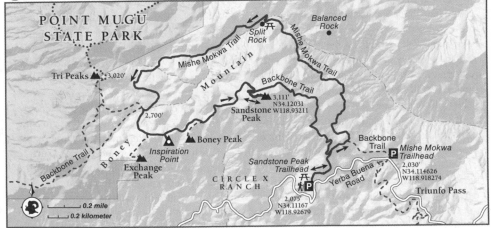

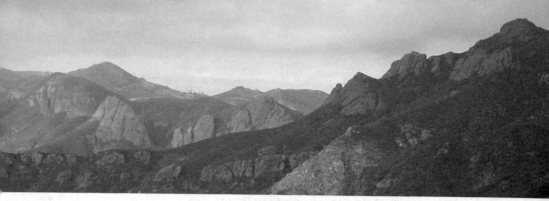

Sandstone Peak is actually a volcanic outcrop.

0.4 mile turn right again onto Little Sycamore Canyon, which soon becomes Yerba Buena Road and reaches the trailhead in 4.5 miles. On either approach, you face a white-knuckle drive on paved but narrow and curvy roads.

Description: Start hiking at the large parking lot on the north side of Yerba Buena Road, 1.1 miles east of the Circle X Ranch park office. Proceed on foot past a gate and up a fire road 0.3 mile, then veer right onto the marked Mishe Mokwa Trail. Shortly thereafter, pass a spur on the right descending to the Mishe Mokwa Trailhead, but stay left.

The hand-tooled route is delightfully primitive, but it requires frequent maintenance to keep the chaparral from knitting together across the path. One of the notable and attractive shrubs is red shanks (also known as ribbonwood), which is identified by its wispy foliage and perpetually peeling, rust-colored bark. It is found only around here in the Santa Monica Mountains and in the Peninsular Ranges south of San Jacinto. After about half an hour on the Mishe Mokwa Trail, keep an eye out for Balanced Rock, which rests precariously on the opposite wall of the canyon. You'll likely see rock climbers on the Echo Cliffs of Carlisle Canyon below.

By 1.7 miles from the start, you will have worked your way around to the north flank of Sandstone Peak, where you suddenly come upon a picnic table shaded beneath glorious oaks beside Split Rock, a fractured volcanic boulder with a gap wide enough to walk through (please do so to maintain the Scouts' tradition). A climbers' trail on the right leads to Balanced

Rock, but you continue on the vestiges of an old dirt road that crosses the canyon and turns west (upstream). You pass beneath some hefty volcanic outcrops, and at 3.1 miles come to a signed junction and turn left onto the Backbone Trail toward Sandstone Peak.

Pass some water tanks on the right and an unsigned service road up to the tanks. Shortly thereafter, a spur on the right takes you about 50 yards to the top of a rock outcrop called Inspiration Point. The direction-finder there indicates local features as well as very distant points such as Mount San Antonio (Old Baldy), Santa Catalina Island, and San Clemente Island.

Press on with your ascent. At a point just past two closely spaced hairpin turns in the wide Backbone Trail, make your way up a slippery path to Sandstone Peak's windswept top. The plaque on the summit block honors W. Herbert Allen, a longtime benefactor of the Scouts and Circle X Ranch. To the Scouts this mountain is Mount Allen, although cartographers have, so far, not accepted that name. In any event, the peak's real name is misleading. It, along with Boney Mountain and most of the western crest of the Santa Monicas, consists of beige- and rust-colored volcanic rock, not unlike sandstone when seen from a distance.

On a clear day the view is truly amazing from here, with distant mountain ranges, the hazy LA Basin, and the island-dimpled surface of the ocean occupying all 360 degrees of the horizon. To complete the loop, return to the Backbone Trail and resume your travel eastward. Descend a twisting 1.5 miles to return to the trailhead.

The Grotto

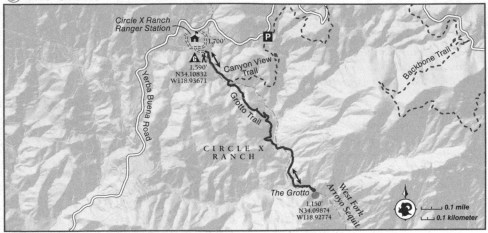

HIKE 4   The Grotto

Location	Circle X Ranch (Santa Monica Mountains National Recreation Area)
Highlights	Spooky rock formations and live oak groves
Distance & Configuration	2.8-mile out-and-back
Elevation Gain	650'
Hiking Time	2 hours
Optional Maps	Tom Harrison *Point Mugu State Park* or Trails Illustrated *Santa Monica Mountains National Recreation Area*
Best Times	All year
Agency	Santa Monica Mountains National Recreation Area
Difficulty	Moderate
Trail Use	Dogs allowed, good for kids
Permit	None required
Google Maps	Circle X Ranch

The 1,655-acre Circle X Ranch, formerly run by the Boy Scouts of America but now administered by the National Park Service, is positively riddled with Tom Sawyer–esque hiking paths. Chief among those is the Grotto Trail, perfect for young or young-in-thought adventurers. This hike is almost entirely downhill on the way in and uphill on the way back. Plan accordingly and bring enough drinking water.

To Reach the Trailhead: The Circle X Ranch Ranger Station is located near the western end

of the Santa Monica Mountains, a few miles (by crow's flight) south of Thousand Oaks. From the Pacific Coast Highway near mile marker 1 VEN 1.00, turn north onto Yerba Buena Road and proceed 5.4 miles.

Or from US 101 in Thousand Oaks, take Highway 23 south for 7.2 miles. Turn right (west) onto Mulholland Highway, and then in 0.4 mile turn right again onto Little Sycamore Canyon, which soon becomes Yerba Buena Road and reaches the trailhead in 5.5 miles. On either approach, you face a white-knuckle drive on paved but very narrow and curvy roads.

You may park at the ranger station or drive 0.1 mile down a dirt road behind the ranger station to signed day-use parking. The trailhead is 0.1 mile farther down at the bottom of the road beside the Circle X Ranch Group Campground (camping by reservation only).

Description: Start hiking at the Circle X Ranch park office. Walk down to the group campground, where you find and follow the Grotto Trail heading south down along a shady seasonal creek. Keep going downhill as you pass the Canyon View Trail intersecting on the left. Shortly afterward, you cross the creek at a point immediately above a 30-foot drop, which becomes a trickling waterfall in winter and spring. You then go uphill, gaining about 50 feet of elevation, and cross an open meadow offering fine views of both Boney Mountain above and a deep-cut gorge (the west fork of Arroyo Sequit) below. Maintain your descent, which becomes sharper as you get closer to the bottom of the gorge.

When you come upon an old roadbed at the bottom, stay left, cross the creek, and continue downstream on a narrowing trail along the shaded east bank. Curve left when you reach a grove of fantastically twisted live oaks at the confluence of two stream forks. On the edge of this grove, an overflow pipe coming out of a tank discharges tepid spring water. Continue another 200 yards down along the now-lively brook to the trail's abrupt end at The Grotto, a narrow, spooky constriction flanked by sheer volcanic-rock walls. If your sense of balance is good, you can clamber over gray rock ledges and massive boulders that have fallen from the canyon walls—just as thousands of Boy Scouts have done in the past. At one spot you can peer cautiously into a gloomy cavern, where you more easily hear than see the subterranean stream. Watermarks on the boulders above are evidence that this part of the gorge probably supports a two-tier stream in times of flood.

When you've had your fill of adventuring, return by the same route, uphill almost the whole way.

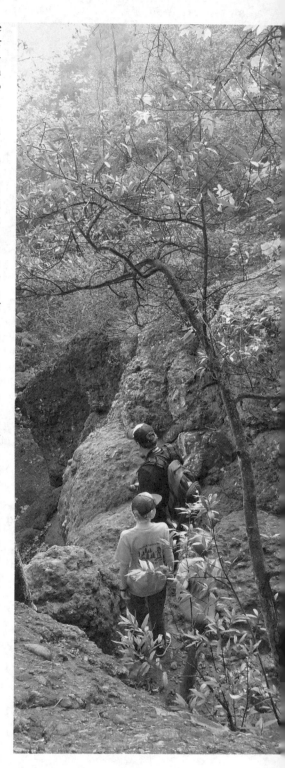

Rock-hopping in the Grotto

℗ Zuma Canyon

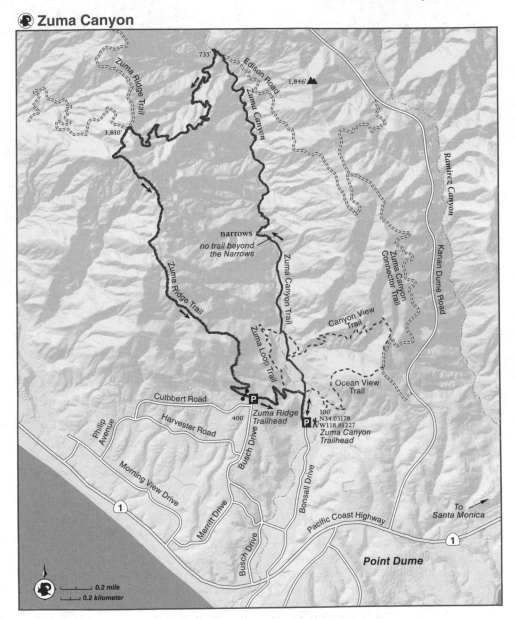

Zuma Ridge Trail

735'

Edison Road

1,846' ▲

Zuma Canyon

1,810'

Ramirez Canyon

narrows
*no trail beyond
the Narrows*

Zuma Ridge Trail

Zuma Canyon Trail

Zuma Canyon
Connector Trail

Canyon View
Trail

Kanan Dume Road

Zuma Loop Trail

Ocean View
Trail

Cuthbert Road

Zuma Ridge
Trailhead

Harvester Road

400'

100'
N34.03178
W118.81227
*Zuma Canyon
Trailhead*

Philip
Avenue

Busch Drive

Morning View Drive

Bonsall Drive

To
Santa Monica

Merritt Drive

Pacific Coast Highway

Busch Drive

Point Dume

1

1

0.2 mile
0.2 kilometer

HIKE 5   Zuma Canyon

Location	Santa Monica Mountains
Highlights	Spectacular, wild canyon trek, ocean views on the return
Distance & Configuration	9-mile loop
Elevation Gain	1,700'
Hiking Time	6 hours
Optional Maps	Tom Harrison *Zuma-Trancas Canyons* or Trails Illustrated *Santa Monica Mountains National Recreation Area*

Best Times October–June, 8 a.m.–sunset
Agency Santa Monica Mountains National Recreation Area
Difficulty Strenuous
Permit None required
Google Maps Zuma Canyon Trailhead

Although it slices only 6 miles inland from the Pacific shoreline, Zuma Canyon harbors one of the deepest gorges in the Santa Monica Mountains. Easily on a par with nearby Malibu and Topanga Canyons in scenic wealth but much less known, Zuma Canyon holds the further distinction of never having suffered the invasion of a major road. *Zuma* comes from the Chumash word for abundance. Under cover of junglelike growths of willow, sycamore, oak, and bay, the canyon's small stream cascades over sculpted sandstone boulders and gathers in limpid pools adorned with ferns. These natural treasures yield their secrets begrudgingly, as they should, only to those willing to scramble over boulders, plow through sucking mud and cattails, and thrash through scratchy undergrowth.

On this challenging trek, you'll proceed straight up the canyon's scenic midsection, climb out of the canyon depths via a powerline service road, and loop back to your starting point on the ridge-running Zuma Ridge Trail (a fire road). The roads are shadeless, yet they offer great vistas of the canyon, the ocean, and the seemingly interminable east–west sweep of the Santa Monica Mountains.

Hiking the canyon bottom is least problematic in the fall season, before the heavy rains set in. The stream may have shrunk to isolated pools by then, and you'll step mostly on dry rocks with good traction. Winter flooding can render the canyon impassable, but such episodes are rare and short-lived. During spring, the stream flows heartily and there's plenty of greenery and wildflowers; at the same time there's an increased threat of exposure to poison oak (which grows in fair abundance along the banks), and you're likely to surprise a rattlesnake. Summer days are usually too oppressively warm and humid for such a difficult hike. Whatever the season, take along plenty

of water; the water in the canyon is not potable. Expect to get your feet wet, and bring sandals or a change of socks.

To Reach the Trailhead: Start at the Zuma Canyon Trailhead at the north end of Bonsall Drive, in the Point Dume area of Malibu. From the intersection of Kanan Dume Road and Pacific Coast Highway (Highway 1) at mile marker 001 LA 54.00, drive 0.9 mile west on the highway to Bonsall Drive. Turn right and continue 1 mile to where Bonsall Drive ends at the trailhead.

Description: From the trailhead, walk north on the Zuma Canyon Trail, following the canyon's winter-wet, summer-dry creek. Several trails branch off along either side, but stay on the main trail up the canyon bottom. You pass statuesque sycamores, tall laurel sumac bushes, and scattered wildflowers in season. This is a promising area for spotting wildlife anytime—squirrels, rabbits, and coyotes are commonly seen, deer and bobcats less so.

After a mile's walk along the creek or dry canyon bottom, the canyon walls close in tighter, oaks appear in greater numbers, and you notice a small grove of eucalyptus trees on a little terrace. The path abruptly ends at a pile of sandstone boulders, 1.3 miles from the start. During the dry months, surface water may get only this far down the canyon. Often, however, the water trickles or tumbles past here, disappearing at some point downstream into the porous substrate of the canyon floor.

Now you begin a nearly 2-mile stretch of boulder-hopping (and possibly wading)—2 or 3 hours' worth depending on the conditions. Other than a few rusting pieces of pipeline from an old dam and irrigation system, you may find that the canyon is completely litter-free; please keep it that way.

The great variety of rocks that have been washed down the stream or have fallen from the canyon walls says a lot about the geologic complexity of the Santa Monicas. You'll scramble over fine-grained siltstones and sandstones, conglomerates that look like poorly mixed aggregate concrete, and volcanic rocks of the sort that make up Saddle Rock (a local landmark near the head of Zuma Canyon) and the Goat Buttes of nearby Malibu Creek State Park. Some of the larger boulders attain the dimensions of midsize trucks, presenting an obstacle course that you must negotiate by moderate climbing with your hands and feet.

Pass directly under a set of high-voltage transmission lines—so high they're hard to spot. These lines, plus the graded road built to give access to the towers, represent the major incursion of civilization into Zuma Canyon. If you can ignore them, however, it's easy to imagine what all the large canyons in the Santa Monicas were like a century ago.

When you finally reach the Zuma Edison Road, turn left and follow it to the top of the west ridge, 5.2 miles from the start. From there, turn left on the Zuma Ridge Trail (another dirt road) and follow its lazily curving, downhill course toward the coastal plain, enjoying clear-air vistas of the vast Pacific Ocean much of the way. On a fine day, you can see all the way from San Jacinto, Santiago Peak, and the Palos Verdes Hills to Catalina, San Clemente, Anacapa, and Santa Cruz Islands. This and many other utility service roads in the Santa Monicas are closed to unauthorized motorized vehicles and are popular among hikers and mountain bikers.

When you reach the bottom of the Zuma Ridge Trail in 7.8 miles, where Busch Drive and Cuthbert Road meet, take the path across the hillside to your left (east). You lose about 300 feet as you zigzag down to the bottom of the Zuma Canyon floodplain. Turn right when you reach the main Zuma Canyon Trail (8.4 miles), and walk the final short stretch over to where you began your hike.

Pool in Zuma Canyon

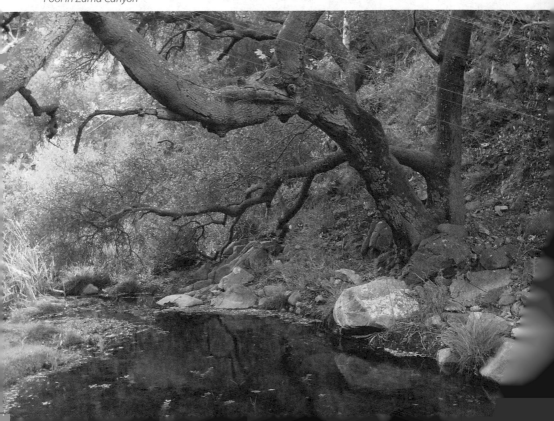

HIKE 6   Point Dume to Paradise Cove

Location	Malibu coast
Highlights	Panoramic ocean vistas and superb intertidal exploration
Distance & Configuration	2.1-mile point-to-point
Elevation Gain	200'
Hiking Time	1.5 hours
Optional Maps	Tom Harrison *Zuma-Trancas Canyons* or Trails Illustrated *Santa Monica Mountains National Recreation Area*
Best Times	All year (passable during low tide)
Agency	Santa Monica Mountains National Recreation Area
Difficulty	Moderate
Trail Use	Good for kids
Permit	None required
Google Maps	Westward Beach

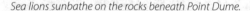

Like the armored bow of an icebreaker, flat-topped Point Dume juts into the Pacific about 20 miles west of Santa Monica. Just east of the point itself, an unbroken cliff wall shelters a secluded beach from the sights and sounds of the civilized world. Below the sometimes-narrow stretch of sand east of the point, a strip of rocky coastline harbors tidepools and a mind-boggling array of plant and animal life.

A pleasant walk anytime the tide is low, this trip is doubly rewarding when the tide dips as low as negative 2 feet. Some of the tidepool inhabitants include limpets, periwinkles, chitons, tube snails, sandcastle worms, sculpins, mussels, shore and hermit crabs, green and aggregating anemones, three kinds of barnacles, and two kinds of sea stars. Extremely low tides occur during the afternoon two or

Sea lions sunbathe on the rocks beneath Point Dume.

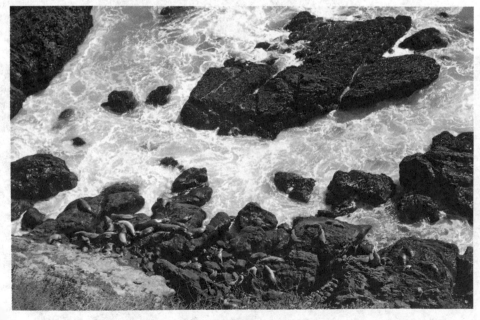

🐾 Point Dume to Paradise Cove

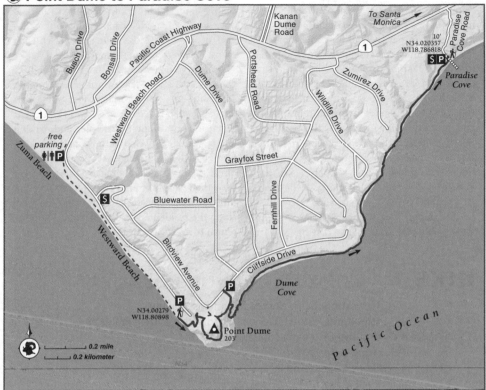

three times each month from October through March. During the summer, you'll have to get up early to catch the rare negative tides. Consult tide tables to find out exactly when.

To Reach the Trailhead: From the Pacific Coast Highway (Highway 1) on Malibu's west side, 0.4 mile west of mile marker 001 LA 54.5, turn south onto Westward Beach Road. Drive down Westward Beach Road to the road's end at Westward Beach (which is open daylight hours and charges a parking fee). Alternatively, you may park for free along the roadside before reaching the pay station and then stroll 0.7 mile southeast along the beach to Point Dume.

Description: Starting out at Westward Beach, you have a choice between two routes: over the top of the point or around the end of the point at sea level. The shorter, much easier route (and the only practical alternative during all but extremely low tides) is the first one, the trail slanting left up the cliff. On top is an area popular for sighting gray whales during their southward migration in winter and a state historic monument. Point Dume, you'll learn, was named by Royal Navy officer and explorer George Vancouver in 1793 in honor of Padre Francisco Dumetz of Mission San Buenaventura (the name was misspelled on Vancouver's map).

As you stand on Point Dume's apex, note the marked contrast between the lighter sedimentary rock exposed on cliff faces to the east and west and the darker volcanic rock just below. This unusually tough mass of volcanic rock has thus far resisted the onslaught of the ocean swells. After you descend from the apex, some metal stairs will take you down to crescent-shaped Dume Cove.

The alternate route is for skilled climbers only (and definitely inappropriate for small children). During the very lowest tides, you round the point itself, making your way by hand-and-toe climbing in a couple of spots over huge, angular shards of volcanic rock along the base of the cliffs. The tidepools here and to the east along Dume Cove's shoreline have some of the best displays of intertidal marine life in Southern California. This visual feast will remain for others to enjoy if you refrain from taking or disturbing in any way the organisms that live there. (*Warning:* Exploring the lower intertidal zones can be hazardous. Be very cautious when traveling over slippery rocks, and always be aware of the incoming swells. Don't let a rogue wave catch you by surprise.)

The going is easy once you're on Dume Cove's ribbon of sand. Signs posted here warn against nude bathing and sunning. This was once a popular nude beach, much to the chagrin of some of those living in the cliffside mansions overlooking the area.

When you reach the northeast end of Dume Cove, swing left around a lesser point, and continue another mile over a somewhat wider beach to Paradise Cove, site of an elegant beachside restaurant, private pier, and parking lot (the public is welcome for a hefty parking fee unless they spend at least $20 at the restaurant). If you've parked a bicycle or second car here, then your hike ends here. Otherwise, you can return the way you came or wend your way along the residential streets of Point Dume to return to Westward Beach.

HIKE 7   Solstice Canyon Park

Location	Santa Monica Mountains (Malibu)
Highlights	Superb oak woodland and lessons in fire ecology
Distance & Configuration	2.4-mile out-and-back
Elevation Gain	350'
Hiking Time	1.5 hours
Optional Maps	Tom Harrison *Malibu Creek State Park* or Trails Illustrated *Santa Monica Mountains National Recreation Area*
Best Times	All year
Agency	Santa Monica Mountains National Recreation Area
Difficulty	Easy
Trail Use	Dogs allowed, good for kids
Permit	None required
Google Maps	Solstice Canyon

The easygoing but scenic Solstice Canyon Trail takes you through the grounds of the former Robert's Ranch—now Solstice Canyon Park, a site administered by the National Park Service. The canyon once hosted a private zoo where giraffes, camels, deer, and exotic birds roamed. At trail's end you come to Tropical Terrace, the site of an architecturally notable grand home that burned in a 1982 wildfire.

To Reach the Trailhead: From Highway 1 in Malibu, 0.3 mile west of mile marker 001 LA 50.0, turn north onto Corral Canyon Road. In 0.2 mile turn left into the park. There's overflow parking for several cars at the entrance,

and a more spacious lot 0.3 mile farther inside at the main trailhead. Parking is free. Carpooling is encouraged since parking space is limited. Posted park hours are 8 a.m.–sunset. The trail description begins from the inside parking lot.

Description: Starting at the main trailhead, pass through a gate and continue upstream alongside the canyon's melodious creek. The path is paved for much of the way. You travel through a fantastic woodland of alder, sycamore, bay, and live oak—the latter with trunks up to 18 feet in circumference. In 0.7 mile, you pass an 1865 stone cottage on the right that is thought to be the oldest existing stone building in Malibu.

Solstice Canyon Park

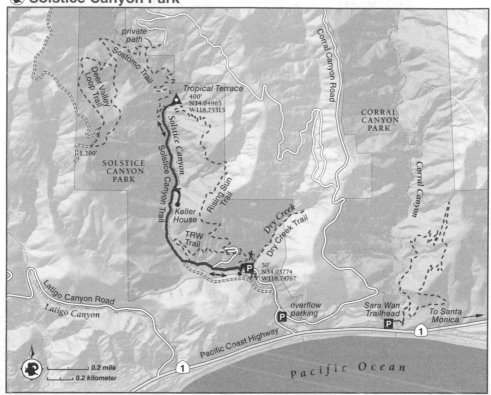

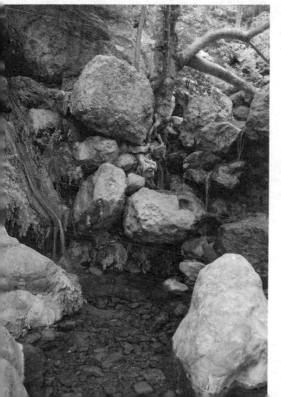

At 1.2 miles, you arrive at the remains of Tropical Terrace. In a setting of palms and giant birds-of-paradise, curved flagstone steps sweep toward the roofless remains of what was for 26 years one of Malibu's grand homes. Beyond the house, crumbling stone steps and pathways lead to what used to be elaborately decorated rock grottoes, as well as a waterfall on Solstice Canyon's creek. Hidden among the Tropical Terrace ruins are the remains of a concrete bomb shelter. For all its perfectly natural setting, Tropical Terrace's destiny was that of a temporary paradise, wiped out by both fire and flood. Take the easy trail back to the trailhead.

VARIATIONS

The steep and rugged Sostomo Trail continues up the canyon, eventually joining the Deer Valley Loop for those who want a longer trip. A beautiful but strenuous option for a loop hike

Fairies might come to dance by the creek by Tropical Terrace.

is to return via the Rising Sun Trail, which adds 500 feet of climbing onto the canyon wall but offers fantastic coastline views stretching from the Palos Verdes Peninsula to Point Dume.

Back at the trailhead parking lot, you may want to check out the Dry Creek Trail, which goes northeast up an oak-shaded ravine for about 0.6 mile before entering private property. An outrageously cantilevered "Darth Vader" house overlooks the ravine as well as a 150-foot-high precipice that infrequently becomes a spectacular waterfall.

HIKE 8   Malibu Creek State Park

Location	Santa Monica Mountains
Highlights	Lakes, rock formations, oaks, wildflowers, *M*A*S*H* site
Distance & Configuration	5-mile out-and-back
Elevation Gain	300'
Hiking Time	3 hours
Optional Maps	Tom Harrison *Malibu Creek State Park* or Trails Illustrated *Santa Monica Mountains National Recreation Area*
Best Times	October–May
Agency	Malibu Creek State Park
Difficulty	Easy
Permit	Parking fee
Google Maps	Malibu Creek State Park Trailhead

Popular Malibu Creek State Park is full of interesting surprises. This hike samples many of the highlights, including rolling hills with oaks and outstanding spring wildflowers, Rock Pool and Century Lake Dam at the Goat Rocks, and the set where the television show *M*A*S*H* was filmed. The park is still used for television and movie backdrops, so don't be surprised if you spot a film crew. The 2018 Woolsey Fire swept through this area, but the park quickly reopened and the trails remain attractive.

To Reach the Trailhead: From the 101 Freeway in Calabasas, take Exit 32 for southbound Las Virgenes Road. Drive 3 miles south to Mulholland Highway, and continue on Las Virgenes 0.2 mile farther to the Malibu Creek State Park entrance, on the right. Pay the day-use fee and drive 0.4 mile to the hikers' parking lot, open 8 a.m.–10 p.m.

Description: From the trailhead kiosk just west of the hikers' parking lot, walk west on unpaved Crags Road and immediately make a concrete-ford crossing of Malibu Creek. In 0.3 mile come to an unsigned fork—the High Road stays right, but you veer left down across the creek on Crags Road. At 0.4 mile, you'll come to a second fork where Mott Road veers left—stay right on Crags Road, taking the most direct route to the visitor center.

The visitor center is housed in a grand old home once occupied by a member of Crags Country Club and later by the groundskeeper for 20th Century Fox. Even if the center isn't open, you can peruse the interpretive panels set up outside beneath the oaks.

From the visitor center, cross Malibu Creek on a sturdy bridge. Turn left onto the unsigned Gorge Trail, a narrow and rocky but short trail leading past a picnic area and pockmarked crags popular with rock climbers. In a few minutes you'll come upon the Rock Pool, a placid stretch of water framed by volcanic cliffs. This wild-looking site has served as a backdrop for outdoor sequences filmed for *Swiss Family Robinson,* the 1930s *Tarzan* movies, and many other productions. Although you're also likely to see young cliff jumpers, be aware that cliff jumping here is illegal (the rangers issue citations), the

Malibu Creek State Park

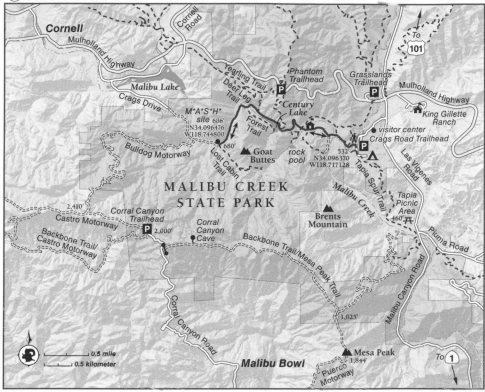

water depth is highly variable, and the creek is heavily contaminated with coliform bacteria. Malibu Search and Rescue responds to accidents here several times a month.

Return to Crags Road and follow it up the hill, a trudge on a hot day. When you reach the crest, look for an unsigned trail descending left. In a minute or two, you'll reach the shady east shoreline of Century Lake, created in 1901 by damming Malibu Creek with a tall concrete structure. Subsequent silting-in has allowed a freshwater marsh to overtake much of what was previously open water. Ducks, coots, and herons frequent the lake, their squallings and callings reverberating off the weathered, honeycombed volcanic cliffs rising from the reservoir's far shore. Redwing blackbirds flit among the cattails and rushes.

Return to Crags Road again and follow it past various side trails, crossing Malibu Creek for the third time. The road turns sharply left and follows a lonely, remote-feeling canyon that

burned heavily in the Woolsey Fire. Soon you reach clearing where the TV series *M*A*S*H* was filmed. The set was removed after the final season in 1982, but volunteers have restored the site with a picnic area, vehicles, and show memorabilia. When you've enjoyed a break and checked out the sights, return via Crags Road to the starting point.

VARIATION

For a grand tour of the park, you could loop back along the backbone of the Santa Monica Mountains. This strenuous hike is 14 miles long with 3,000 feet of elevation gain. Continue on Crags Road to Bulldog Road and up to Castro Peak Road, where you meet the Backbone Trail. Turn left and follow the trail past the Castro Crest sandstone formations and Mesa Peak all the way to Malibu Canyon Road. A maze of trails on the west side of the road leads back to your parking area, but it may be less confusing to simply walk back along the side of the road.

HIKE 9   Topanga Overlook

Location	Santa Monica Mountains (Pacific Palisades)
Highlights	Unsurpassed views of Santa Monica Bay, lush canyon
Distance & Configuration	7-mile out-and-back
Elevation Gain	1,700'
Hiking Time	4 hours
Optional Maps	Tom Harrison *Topanga State Park* or Trails Illustrated *Santa Monica Mountains National Recreation Area*
Best Times	All year
Agency	Topanga State Park
Difficulty	Moderate
Permit	None required
Google Maps	Los Leones Trailhead

From the perch known as Topanga Overlook, Parker Mesa Overlook, or simply the Overlook, you get a bird's-eye view of surfers off Topanga Beach, the crescent-shaped shoreline of Santa Monica Bay, Los Angeles' west-side cityscape—and much, much more if the air is really transparent. On a clear day, you'll find no better ocean viewpoint in Southern California. This trip is especially rewarding when done early on certain fall or winter mornings, when tendrils of fog fill the canyons, leaving the mountains to rise above a cottony sea. It's also excellent as a sunset or night hike. For a special treat, do it on any clear, full-moon evening between May and August. In the fading twilight, you'll watch the moon's pumpkinlike disk silently materialize in the east or southeast, hovering over a million glittering lights. The Los Leones Trail section

The Overlook is a romantic spot to picnic above Santa Monica Bay.

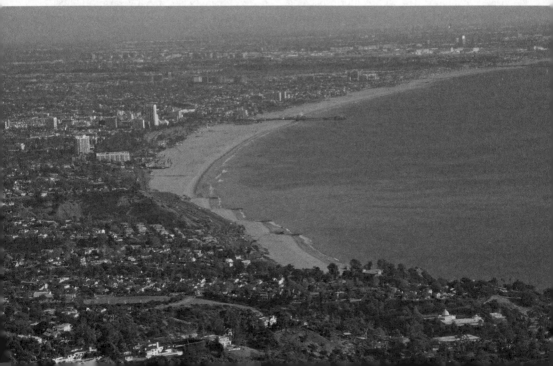

🅟 Topanga Overlook

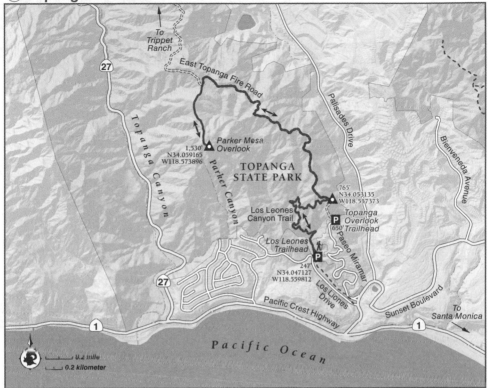

is shady and enjoyable anytime, but avoid the sunbaked upper fire road on a hot day.

To Reach the Trailhead: From Pacific Coast Highway (Highway 1) in Pacific Palisades 0.3 mile west of mile marker 001 LA 39.0, take Sunset Boulevard north 0.3 mile to Los Liones Drive on the left. Go 0.5 mile to the end. Park on the street, observing parking restrictions.

Description: Start on the signed Los Leones Trail. (The name is Spanish for "the lions," after the mountain lions that still roam the Santa Monica Mountains. Some signage misspells it as Los Liones Trail.) You'll immediately pass an unmaintained trail on the left to a hilltop cross, and a spur trail on the right paralleling Los Liones Drive. The well-graded trail climbs a lush canyon shaded by canyon live oak, California black walnut, lemonade berry, laurel sumac, ceanothus, and other tall chaparral. Topanga is

an excellent place for spring wildflowers, and the cliff aster, monkey flower, nightshade, and buckwheat persist into the summer.

At 1.3 miles, reach a broad dirt road coming up from the top of Paseo Miramar (an alternate and shorter starting point, but with poor parking). Here you can take a break on a bench with an outstanding ocean view. The remainder of the hike is on a fire road. Farther ahead you briefly traverse a cool, north-facing slope overlooking Santa Ynez Canyon and neighboring ridges. You arrive at a road junction (3.2 miles) with views of Topanga Canyon to the west. Turn south and walk out along the bald ridge to Topanga Overlook. Down below are Parker and Castellammare Mesas, parts of a striking marine-terrace structure that continues east into Pacific Palisades. This is a great spot to enjoy a picnic while savoring the fabulous views. When it's time to go back, return the way you came.

HIKE 10   Temescal Canyon

Location	Santa Monica Mountains (Pacific Palisades)
Highlights	Pseudoaerial coastline views, shady riparian and oak woodland
Distance & Configuration	2.8-mile loop
Elevation Gain	850'
Hiking Time	1.5 hours
Optional Maps	Tom Harrison *Topanga State Park* or Trails Illustrated *Santa Monica Mountains National Recreation Area*
Best Times	All year
Agency	Santa Monica Mountains National Recreation Area
Difficulty	Moderate
Trail Use	Good for kids
Permit	Parking fee
Google Maps	Temescal Gateway Park

Spring lingers long on the coastal slopes of the Santa Monica Mountains, which are frequently bathed from May until July in the sopping-wet breath of the marine layer. This is quintessential coastal sage-scrub and chaparral country, a particular habitat that is fast succumbing to urban development all over Southern California. All through spring and early summer, you can enjoy the scents of sage and wildflowers on the trails of Temescal Canyon, part of the Santa Monica Mountains National Recreation Area and Topanga State Park. With an early start on a foggy morning, you may find yourself punching right through the mist as you ascend into the bright, sunny world above.

To Reach the Trailhead: Begin at Temescal Gateway Park, just north of the intersection of Sunset Boulevard and Temescal Canyon Road in Pacific Palisades, 1 mile north of Pacific Coast Highway by way of Temescal Canyon Road. Park for a fee inside the park from sunrise to sunset. Pets are allowed on the short paths in Temescal Gateway Park, but they are prohibited on the outlying trails ahead, which enter Topanga State Park.

Description: This hike traverses the Temescal loop clockwise, climbing the scrubby west wall of Temescal Canyon on the way up and then making a nice, easy descent down through

Temescal Ridge has good city views.

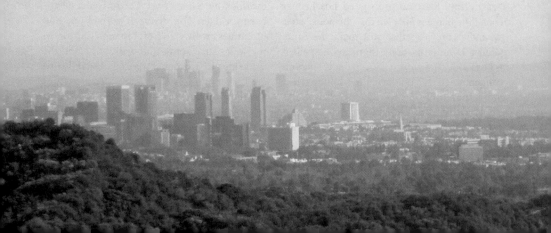

◉ Temescal Canyon

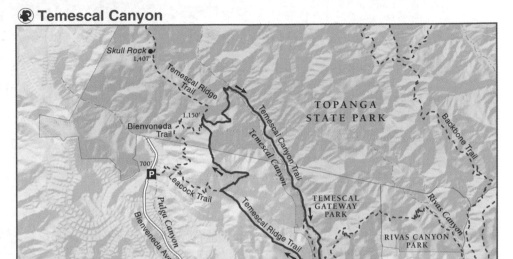

the canyon. To do this, head north up the road past several buildings that comprise the former Presbyterian conference grounds. Stay left onto a dirt path and climb to a signed junction where you can pick up the Temescal Ridge Trail on the left. The narrow trail immediately starts a vigorous ascent up the scrubby canyon slope to the west. After several twists and turns, the trail gains a moderately ascending crest and sticks to it. Pause often so you can turn around and look at the ever-widening view of the coastline curving from Santa Monica Bay to Malibu.

Ahead, two short trails (the Leacock and Bienveneda Trails) strike off to the left toward the end of Bienveneda Avenue. Ignore those paths and continue to a junction (1.3 miles from the start) with the Temescal Canyon Trail on the right. At this juncture you have

the option of making a side trip north 0.4 mile to a wind-carved sandstone outcrop known as Skull Rock. To stay on the loop route, turn right and follow the Temescal Canyon Trail into the shady bottom of Temescal Canyon.

At the bottom you cross Temescal Canyon's creek on a footbridge. Above and below that bridge are small, trickling waterfalls and shallow, limpid pools. You can poke around the creek a bit for a look at its typical denizens: water striders and newts. When you've finished sightseeing, continue down the canyon trail back to the conference buildings, a mile away. That final stretch follows the canyon bottom and then contours along a slope behind the buildings. Lots of live oak, sycamore, willow, and bay trees, their woodsy scents commingling on the ocean breeze, highlight your return.

HIKE 11   Will Rogers Park

Location	Santa Monica Mountains (Pacific Palisades)
Highlights	City, ocean, and mountain views from a single stance
Distance & Configuration	2.0-mile loop
Elevation Gain	350'
Hiking Time	1 hour
Optional Maps	Tom Harrison *Topanga State Park* or Trails Illustrated *Santa Monica Mountains National Recreation Area*
Best Times	All year, especially on weekdays or early on weekend mornings
Agency	Will Rogers State Historic Park
Difficulty	Easy
Trail Use	Suitable for mountain biking, dogs allowed, good for kids
Permit	Parking fee
Google Maps	Will Rogers State Historic Park

Drive up a short mile from the speedway known as Sunset Boulevard toward Will Rogers State Historic Park, and you'll instantly leave the rat race behind. This quiet spot is perfect for getting some exercise and taking advantage of multimillion-dollar views of Santa Monica, West LA, and downtown LA.

Newspaperman, radio commentator, movie star, and pop philosopher Will Rogers purchased this 182-acre property in 1922 and lived here with his family from 1928 until his death in 1935. Historic only by Southern California standards, his 31-room mansion is nevertheless interesting to tour. Your main goal, however, is

Santa Monica Bay

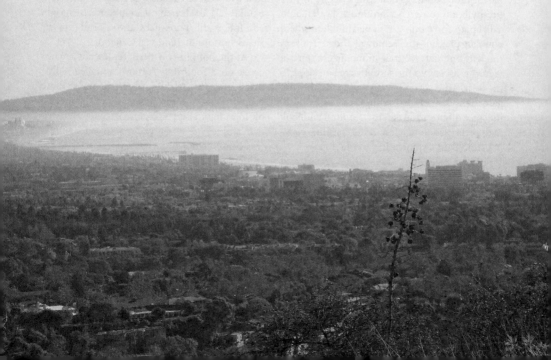

🐾 Will Rogers Park

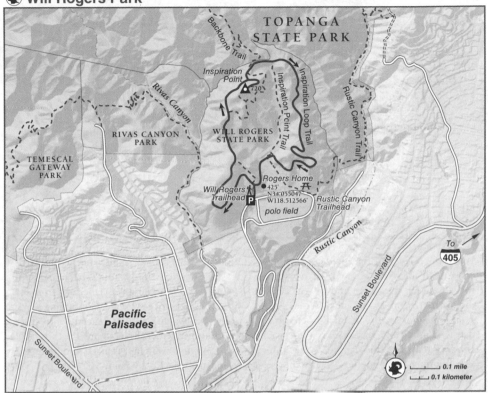

to reach Inspiration Point, a flat-topped bump on a ridge overlooking the entire spread.

To Reach the Trailhead: Drive 1.5 miles east on Sunset Boulevard from the commercial district of Pacific Palisades (Sunset Boulevard and Temescal Canyon Road) to reach the Will Rogers Park entrance road. Or take Sunset Boulevard 4 miles west from I-405 to reach the same entrance. The park is open daily (except certain holidays), 8 a.m.–sunset, and charges a parking fee.

Description: You may want to obtain a copy of the detailed hikers' map, available at the gift shop in a wing of the home. Printed on the map is one of Rogers's memorable (if not apropos) aphorisms: "If your time is worth anything, travel by air. If not, you might just as well walk." To reach Inspiration Point, follow the main,

wide riding and hiking trail that makes a 2-mile loop, starting at the north end of the big lawn adjoining the Rogers home. Or use any of several shorter, more direct paths (mountain bikes and leashed pets are allowed only on the main, looping trail).

Relaxing on the benches at the top on a clear day, you can admire true-as-advertised, inspiring vistas stretching east to the front range of the San Gabriel Mountains and southeast to the Santa Ana Mountains. South past the swelling Palos Verdes Peninsula you can sometimes spot Santa Catalina Island rising in ethereal majesty from the shining surface of the sea.

Will Rogers Park serves as the east terminus of the Backbone Trail, which skims some 65 miles along the crest of the Santa Monica Mountains. Its west end lies in Point Mugu State Park (described in Hike 2).

HIKE 12   Malaga Cove to Bluff Cove

Location	Palos Verdes Peninsula
Highlights	Boulder-hopping beneath sea cliffs and past small tidepools
Distance & Configuration	2.0-mile loop
Elevation Gain	200'
Hiking Time	2 hours
Optional Map	USGS 7.5-minute *Redondo Beach*
Best Times	All year
Agency	Palos Verdes Estates Shoreline Preserve
Difficulty	Moderate
Trail Use	Good for kids
Permit	None required
Google Maps	Roessler Point

When the tide is not too high, curious hikers can thread their way along a narrow strip of rocks between the ocean and the sea cliffs at the northern end of the Palos Verdes Peninsula. Watch for sea life in small tidepools and debris from an old shipwreck. While young children may love this trip, folks uncomfortable hopping along slippery rocks will prefer exploring elsewhere.

To Reach the Trailhead: From the 110 Freeway, exit west on the Pacific Coast Highway (Highway 1). In 0.6 mile, turn left on Normandie. Then in 0.5 mile, veer right onto Palos Verdes Drive North. Follow this scenic, winding road for 6.7 miles, then keep left onto Palos Verdes Drive West. In 0.2 mile, turn right onto Via Almar. In 0.5 mile, turn right again onto Via Arroyo, and in 0.1 mile, turn right yet again onto Paseo del Mar, where you will find a large parking area.

Description: Walk to the east end of the parking area, where you will see a trail just beyond a gazebo at Roessler Point overlooking the Pacific. Follow the trail down to Malaga Cove. This hike leads left (southwest) along the rocks beneath the sea cliffs. If the tide looks too high or the surf is excessive, consider diverting right instead and taking a stroll along Torrance Beach.

Otherwise, pick a path over the sedimentary rocks. Surfers flock to the cove to test their skills on the waves. Look carefully for

small sea anemones, snails, and hermit crabs in the tidepools. In 0.3 mile, watch and sniff for a natural mineral spring emerging from the rocks near the ocean's edge. Continuing along the rocks, watch for rusted metal debris from an unknown wreck. The famous 1961 wreck of the *Dominator* freighter is located south on the peninsula near Rocky Point.

Near Bluff Cove

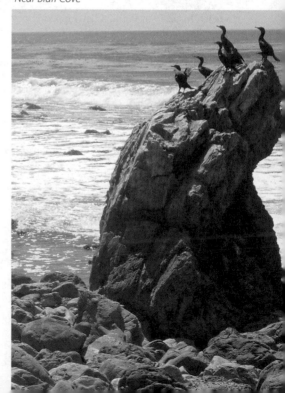

Malaga Cove to Bluff Cove

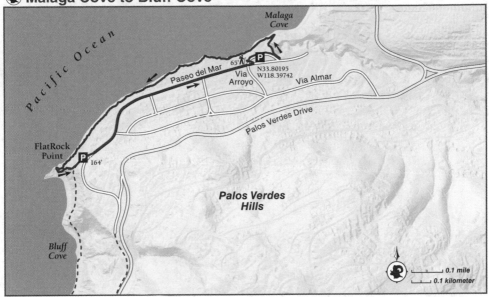

After a slow mile of picking your way through the rocks, reach Flat Rock Point, another popular spot to view tidepools. Bluff Cove lies on the far side of the point. Your goal is to reach Paseo del Mar above. An extremely steep and potentially hazardous trail leads straight up from Flat Rock Point. A safer choice is to continue along the cove to find a graded path on the left. In either event, once you reach Paseo del Mar, turn left and walk a half mile back to your vehicle, enjoying the elaborately landscaped mansions along the way.

HIKE 13 Cheeseboro and Palo Comado Canyons

Location	Simi Hills (east of Thousand Oaks)
Highlights	Classic green or golden California grassland dotted with oaks
Distance & Configuration	10-mile loop
Elevation Gain	1,200'
Hiking Time	5 hours
Optional Maps	Tom Harrison *Cheeseboro-Palo Comado Canyons* or Trails Illustrated *Santa Monica Mountains National Recreation Area*
Best Times	October–June
Agency	Santa Monica Mountains National Recreation Area
Difficulty	Moderately strenuous
Trail Use	Suitable for mountain biking, dogs allowed
Permit	None required
Google Maps	Chesebro (sic) Canyon Trailhead

To China Flat

Sheep Corral Trail

sheep corral

1,530'

1,640'

1,720'

Dead Cow Trail

CHEESEBORO CANYON PARK

Sulphur Springs

Cheeseboro Ridge Trail

Las Virgenes Canyon

Upper Las Virgenes Canyon Trail

1,929'
Baleen Wall

PALO COMADO CANYON PARK

Palo Comado Canyon Trail

Cheeseboro Canyon Trail

Doubletree Road

Ranch Center Connector

1,170'

Cheeseboro Canyon

1,120'

Smoketree Avenue

Palo Comado Connector

1,290'

1,060'

Cheeseboro Ridge Trail

Las Virgenes Canyon Trailhead

880'

P

Palo Comado Canyon

Modelo Trail

Cheeseboro Canyon Trail

Chesebro Road

Modelo Spur Trail

Canyon View Trail

P

Morrison Ranch Trail

Las Virgenes Road

1,020'
N34.15650
W118.73087

P

Driver Avenue

P

LIBERTY CANYON OPEN SPACE

Agoura Hills

101

Palo Comado Canyon Road

Ventura Freeway

101

Agoura Road

Calabasas

0.2 mile

0.2 kilometer

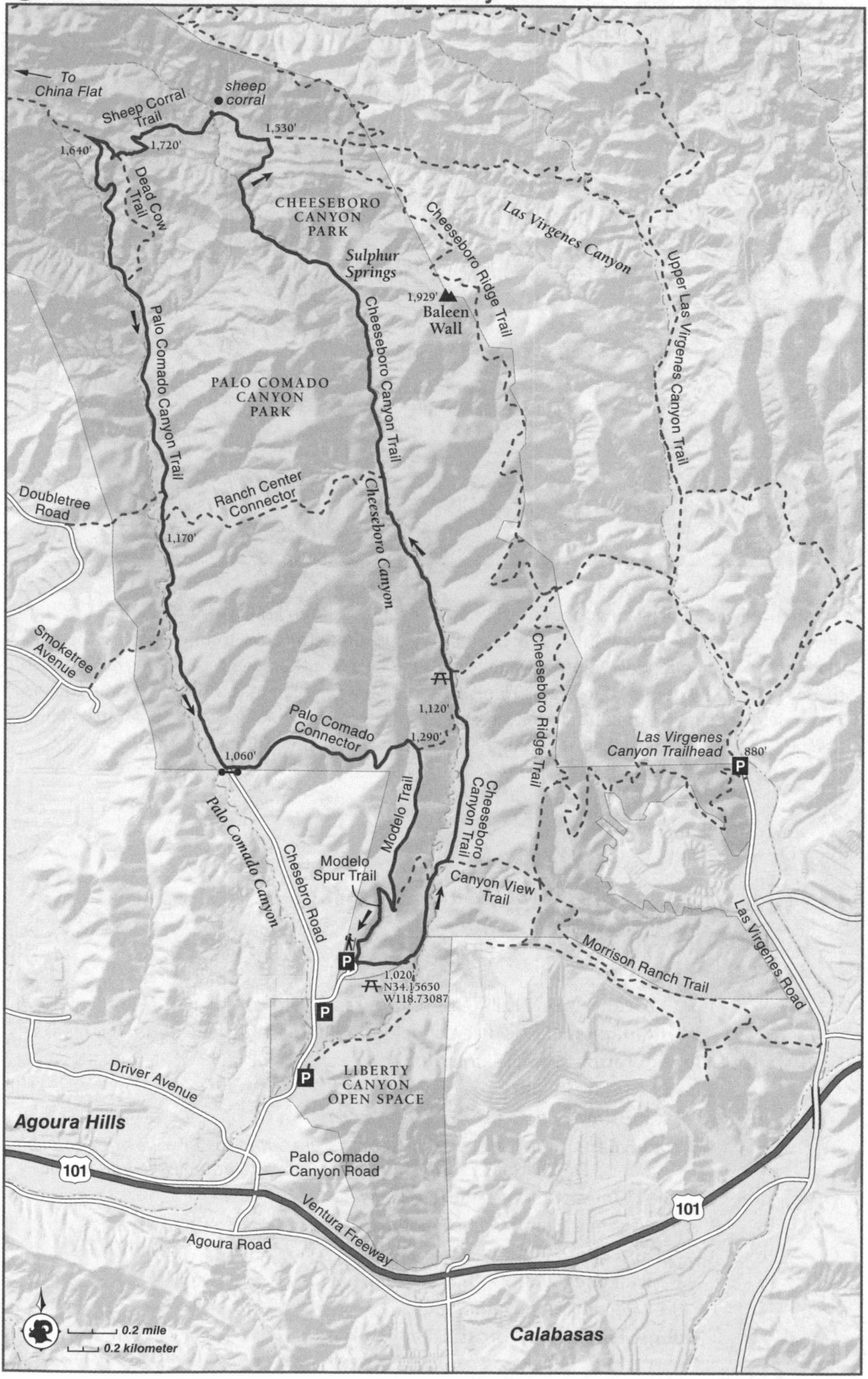

The Cheeseboro and Palo Comado Canyons park site, a unit of the Santa Monica Mountains National Recreation Area, serves as an important wildlife corridor between the interior Transverse Ranges in the north and the Santa Monica Mountains to the south. Travelers by the thousands have discovered the place, but there's plenty of room for visitors to spread out. The long, leisurely loop route described here visits the two canyons, both surprisingly serene and pristine despite extensive suburban development in the surrounding region. Deer, bobcats, coyotes, rabbits, owls, and various birds of prey can be spotted in both canyons, especially in the early morning.

Without question, the period between the emergence of tender green grass (December or January) and the shift from green to gold (April or May) is the very best time to visit Cheeseboro and Palo Comado Canyons. July, August, and September bring midday temperatures in the 90s, making this area unpleasant for all but perhaps mountain bikers, who may enjoy the benefit of evaporative cooling if they move fast enough.

To Reach the Trailhead: From US 101 at Exit 35 in Agoura Hills, take the Chesebro (sic) Road exit, go north about 200 yards on what is signed Palo Comado Canyon Road, and then turn right on Chesebro Road. Drive 0.7 mile north to the main entrance to the Cheeseboro and Palo Comado Canyons site, on the right. Gates to the trailhead parking lot swing open at 8 a.m.—often earlier on weekends, when volunteers sometimes staff a National Park Service information booth here. A fenced trail into Cheeseboro Canyon bypasses the parking area, and hikers, bikers, and equestrians use it even when the gates are shut. Be aware that soggy trail conditions may close the park.

Description: From the trailhead parking lot, follow the wide Cheeseboro Canyon Trail, which goes briefly east and then bends north up along the wide, nearly flat canyon floor. Stay on the broad main path, disregarding narrow trails branching off either side. Two kinds of oak trees dominate the Cheeseboro landscape: evergreen coast live oaks cluster along the canyon bottoms, while widely spaced deciduous

Cheeseboro Canyon is notable for its magnificent valley oaks.

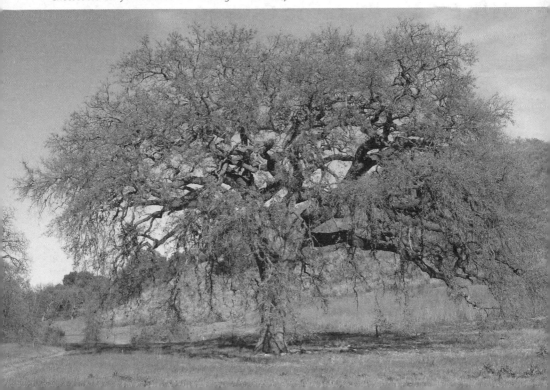

valley oaks strike statuesque poses in the meadows and on the hillsides. It looks like typical California cattle-grazing land, and indeed it was for a period of about 150 years. Now that the cattle have been removed, oak seedlings are taking root in increasing numbers, and native spring wildflowers are returning, creating splashes of color across the grassy hillsides.

At 1.6 miles on Cheeseboro Canyon Trail, near the Palo Comado Connector joining from the west, you come upon a pleasant trailside picnic area. Stay on the main, wide trail going north through the canyon bottom. At 3.0 miles you pass Sulphur Springs. Let your nose be your guide for locating the springs. There's not much to see—mere seeps if they are flowing at all.

As you continue, the oaks clustering along the canyon bottom thin out, and you can gaze upward, to your right, at the whitish sedimentary outcrop known as the Baleen Wall. The trail narrows and becomes rocky in places. At 4.1 miles, reach a T-junction at Shepherds Flat. Pause here for a picnic, perhaps, before resuming your trip.

From the corral continue west on the narrow Sheep Corral Trail through the brush.

This is a segment of the Juan Bautista de Anza National Historic Trail, a 1,200-mile trail commemorating the Spanish captain's famed 1775 expedition leading 240 people across the desert to found San Francisco. You pass over a saddle and briefly descend to meet the graded-dirt Palo Comado Canyon Trail (5.2 miles). Turn left now, and commence a short mile of crooked descent on the wide dirt road. You look down on a lovely tapestry of canyon-bottom woods and slopes adorned with dense patches of chaparral and sandstone outcrops. Soon you are amid those woods, which are mostly live oaks and sycamores. The going is easy for another 2 miles as you proceed almost imperceptibly downhill along the canyon bottom.

At 8.2 miles, there's a forced left turn out of the canyon (off-limits private land lies ahead) and onto the Palo Comado Connector. You meander uphill and across two minor canyons for 1.0 mile to a rounded ridge, where you meet the Modelo Trail on the right. This trail, which connects with the Modelo Spur Trail, is the most expeditious route back to the trailhead.

HIKE 14   Placerita Canyon

Location	Santa Clarita
Highlights	Wooded ravines, waterfall, historically interesting features
Distance & Configuration	5-mile out-and-back
Elevation Gain	700'
Hiking Time	2.5 hours
Optional Map	Tom Harrison *Angeles Front Country*
Best Times	October–June
Agency	Placerita Canyon State Park (operated by the county)
Difficulty	Moderate
Trail Use	Dogs allowed, good for kids
Permit	None required
Google Maps	Placerita Canyon Nature Center

Note: The Waterfall Trail was damaged in the 2016 Sand Fire and has not reopened at the time of this writing. If it is not yet open when you visit, you will still enjoy the 3.6-mile out-and-back to Walker Campground.

Barely 10 minutes' drive from northern San Fernando Valley and the sprawling suburban city of Santa Clarita, Placerita Canyon Park nestles comfortably at the foot of one of the more verdant slopes of the San Gabriel Mountains.

℗ Placerita Canyon

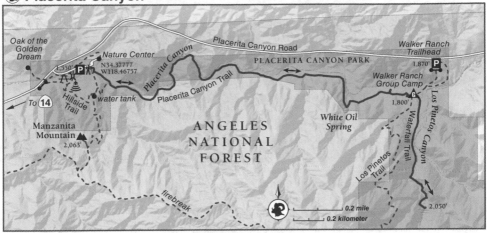

A very civilized nature center housing exhibits on local history, prehistory, geology, plants, and wildlife complements the park's wild backcountry sector (the subject of this hike).

Placerita Canyon's fascinating history is highlighted by the discovery of gold there in 1842. That event, which touched off California's first (and relatively trivial) gold rush, predated by six years John Marshall's famous discovery of gold at Sutter's Mill in Northern California. By the 1950s, Placerita Canyon had become one of the more popular generic Western site locations used by Hollywood's moviemakers and early television producers. First the state and then the county eventually acquired the canyon as parkland.

To Reach the Trailhead: Take Exit 3 for Placerita Canyon from Antelope Valley Freeway (Highway 14) at Newhall, and drive east 1.5 miles to reach the park's main gate, which is open from sunrise to sunset. Nearby lie the nature center and the Oak of the Golden Dream, the exact site (according to legend) where in 1842 a herdsman pulling up wild onions for his after-siesta meal discovered gold.

Description: This trip begins at the signed trailhead near the nature center and parking lot. Go straight ahead, and then veer left onto the signed Canyon Trail. Pass an unsigned junction on the right leading to a water tank, and continue east up Placerita Canyon. The canyon

burned in the 2016 Sand Fire, and then the trail washed out in subsequent flooding, but it was rebuilt in 2020 and is even better than before.

The canyon's melodious creek flows decently about half the year (winter and spring), caressing the ears with white noise that echoes off the canyon walls. During the fall, when the creek may be bone dry, you make your own noise instead by crunching through the crispy leaf litter of sycamore and live oak. Down by the grassy banks are wild blackberry vines, lots of willows, and occasionally cottonwood and alder trees.

Soaring canyon walls ahead tell the story of thousands of years of natural erosion, as well as the destructive effects of hydraulic mining, which involved aiming high-pressure water hoses at hillsides to loosen and wash away ores. Used extensively in Northern California during the big gold rush, hydraulic mining was finally banned in 1884 after catastrophic damages to waterways and farms downstream. At Placerita Canyon, several hundred thousand dollars' worth of gold was ultimately recovered, but at considerable cost, effort, and general messiness. Oil was also found here in 1900, and the trail passes an unusual spring of bubbling white oil, naturally filtered through the underlaying rock.

In 1.8 miles, you reach Walker Ranch Group Campground, where Frank Walker, his wife, and their 12 children built their ranch in the early 20th century. Water faucets are available here. Call the park in advance for camping reservations.

Our way lies ahead, along the Waterfall Trail, which leads 0.5 mile into Los Pinetos Canyon. Don't confuse this trail with the Los Pinetos Trail on the right. The Waterfall Trail momentarily slants upward along the canyon's steep west wall and then drops onto the canyon's sunny floodplain. Presently you bear right into a narrow ravine (Los Pinetos Canyon), avoiding a wider tributary bending left (east).

Continue past and sometimes over water-polished metamorphic rock. Live oaks and big-cone Douglas-firs cling to the slopes above, and a few big-leaf maples grace the canyon bottom. Beware of the poison oak that abounds along the trail and near the waterfall, especially in the winter when its bare twigs are difficult to recognize. About 0.2 mile after the first fork in the canyon, there's a second fork.

Stay right at a second fork and continue 50 yards to a small waterfall and a sublime little grotto, cool and dark except when the sun passes almost straight overhead. As you listen to water dashing or dribbling down the chute, enjoy the serenity of this private place and contemplate that it lies only a few miles—but a world away—from the creeping boundary of the LA metropolis. Return the way you came.

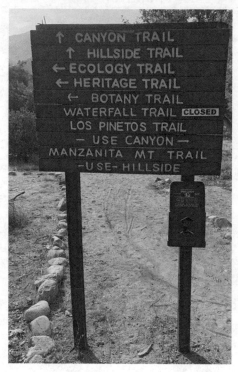

Many trails lead from the Placerita Canyon Nature Center.

HIKE 15   HOLLYWOOD Sign via Cahuenga Peak

Location	Griffith Park
Highlights	HOLLYWOOD sign
Distance & Configuration	2.8-mile out-and-back
Elevation Gain	1,000'
Hiking Time	2 hours
Optional Map	laparks.org/sites/default/files/griffith/pdf/griffithparkmap.pdf
Best Times	October–May
Agency	Los Angeles Department of Recreation and Parks
Difficulty	Moderate
Trail Use	Dogs allowed, good for kids
Permit	None required
Google Maps	Wonder View Trail Head

Tourists from around the world flock to see the HOLLYWOOD sign, one of the world's most recognized landmarks. Excellent views of the sign abound from Griffith Observatory and the neighborhoods below (see Hike 16), but this is the most direct route to actually reach the sign

HOLLYWOOD Sign via Cahuenga Peak

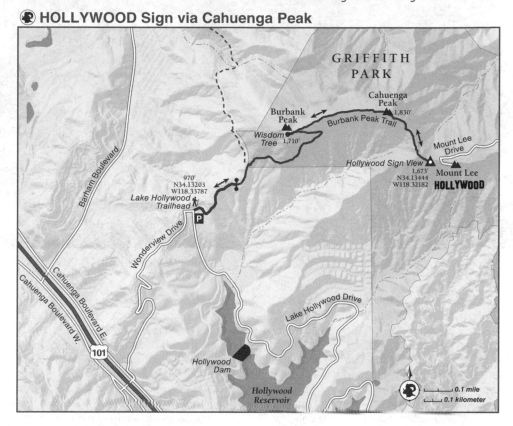

itself. The Hollyridge Trail from Beachwood Drive was even more direct, but it was closed in 2017 after a lawsuit from the Sunset Ranch Hollywood Stables, which disliked the heavy hiker traffic on Beachwood.

This short but rugged hike follows the ridge over Burbank and Cahuenga Peaks to the HOLLYWOOD sign overlook on Mount Lee. The mountain is named for Don Lee, a TV pioneer who built the early W6AXO broadcast tower here in the 1930s. (Don't mix up this summit with nearby Mount Hollywood, which is not the site of the eponymous sign.) The ridge was part of a 138-acre parcel purchased in 1940 by Howard Hughes and rezoned in 2008 for luxury estate development. The Trust for Public Land acquired the parcel in 2010, and it is now protected as part of Griffith Park. Tens of thousands of people rallied and donated to purchase the land, with major gifts from Steven Spielberg, George Lucas, Hugh Hefner, Aileen Getty, and the Tiffany & Co. Foundation.

Cahuenga Peak takes its name from a nearby Tongva village called Kawengna, or "place of the mountain."

The trail is open sunrise–sunset. Griffith Park's famous resident mountain lion, P-22, favors these hills and has been spotted here after dark. As a young male, P-22 apparently left the Santa Monica Mountains, crossed two major freeways, and made his way through Beverly Hills to reach Griffith Park, where he was photographed beneath the HOLLYWOOD sign in 2013. At the time of this writing, construction was about to begin for a wildlife bridge over the 101 Freeway, enabling P-22 and other animals to cross the 10-lane road in search of food and mates.

To Reach the Trailhead: From the 101 Freeway, take Exit 11A for Barham Boulevard. Follow the Cahuenga Boulevard frontage road north for 0.5 mile; then turn right on Barham Boulevard. In 0.3 mile turn right again

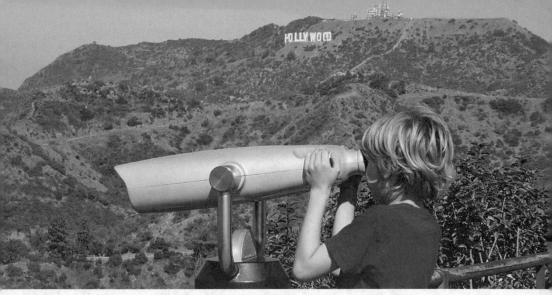

The HOLLYWOOD sign, visible from Griffith Observatory, is a Southern California icon.

onto Lake Hollywood Drive, and proceed 0.5 mile to its junction with Wonder View Drive. Park on Lake Hollywood Drive south of the intersection.

Description: Begin your hike by walking east up Wonder View Drive. Pass through a gate onto a dirt road, and soon join the narrow Burbank Peak Trail at a high-voltage transmission-line tower. Climb steeply to the 1,690-foot summit, where you'll find the solitary Wisdom Tree. According to legend, the pine was originally a Christmas tree and was replanted on the mountaintop by a man who wanted to honor his mother. Look for a box with the musings of countless visitors.

The path, now signed as the Aileen Getty Ridge Trail, continues east to the 1,820-foot summit of Cahuenga Peak, the highest summit in Griffith Park, from which you can enjoy splendid views over the Los Angeles Basin. Turning clockwise on a clear day, your views encompass Griffith Park, Mounts Baldy and Wilson, Burbank, the Hollywood Hills, Santa Monica Bay, Hollywood, and downtown Los Angeles.

Continue east to the end of paved Mount Lee Drive, a service road reaching the antennas above the HOLLYWOOD sign. A formidable fence divides the topmost part of Mount Lee from the sheer slope below, which precariously supports the spindly looking whitewashed letters of the famous sign.

HIKE 16　Mount Hollywood Loop

Location	Griffith Park
Highlights	Griffith Observatory, panoramic views
Distance & Configuration	5-mile loop
Elevation Gain	1,000'
Hiking Time	2 hours
Optional Map	laparks.org/sites/default/files/griffith/pdf/griffithparkmap.pdf
Best Times	October–May
Agency	Los Angeles Department of Recreation and Parks
Difficulty	Moderate
Trail Use	Dogs allowed, good for kids
Permit	None required
Google Maps	Fern Dell Nature Trail

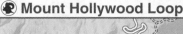 Mount Hollywood Loop

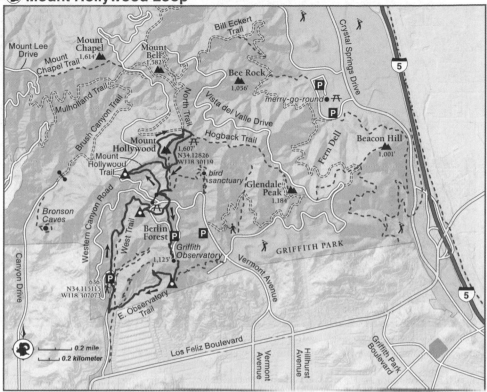

The bald, flattish 1,625-foot summit of Mount Hollywood would scarcely be something to write home about except for its strategic location overlooking just about everything. Hikers approach from all directions, but the most popular starting point is the overcrowded observatory parking lot. On the somewhat longer trek described here, you'll start out below the observatory so you can enjoy the exotically landscaped Fern Dell area too. The dell features picnic tables, a year-round brook (a part of the observatory's cooling system, but appealing nonetheless), plenty of succulent plants, and shade trees.

To Reach the Trailhead: From I-5, take Exit 141 for Los Feliz Boulevard. Go west 2.5 miles, then turn right onto Fern Dell Drive into Griffith Park. Find a parking spot in the lot 0.7 mile north or along the street nearby.

From Fern Dell's main parking lot, walk across the lowermost horseshoe curve on Western Canyon Road, and continue on the wide dirt fire road heading uphill (north) into sunny chaparral country. Dry and a bit trampled at first, the landscape improves as you climb. Along the trail are larger shrubs such as toyon, elderberry, laurel sumac, sugar bush, and ceanothus, and smaller ones such as black sage, buckwheat, and fuchsia-flowered gooseberry—all are very typical of the drier south- and west-facing slopes in the park. Here, too, are common noxious invasive plants such as fennel, tree tobacco, and castor bean. Planted eucalyptus and pine trees stand high on the nearby slopes, while a handful of native live oaks tucked into the bigger creases on the sun-seared slopes draw just enough moisture from the soil to survive.

After passing under a couple of shade-giving oaks, the trail curves left and crosses the west observatory road. Soon you're on the ridgeline south of Mount Hollywood, passing high over a road tunnel. Listen for horns blaring as cars barrel through below.

A couple of long, lazy switchback legs up the Charlie Turner Trail take you to a trail junction

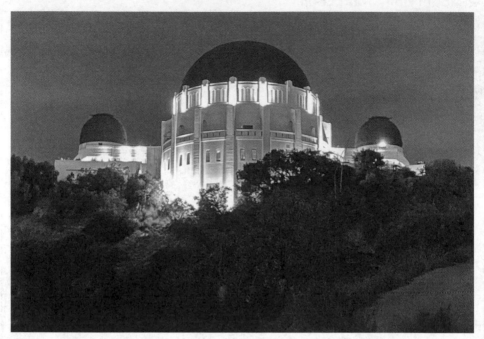

Griffith Observatory is lit up at sunset.

not far below Mount Hollywood's summit. Make a sharp left, pass the Captain's Roost picnic area (drinking water here), and continue to a wide trail junction just north of the summit. Make a hard right here and walk over to the picnic tables on the top. Your gaze takes in (among many other things) the downtown LA skyline and the antenna-topped Mount Lee with its famous HOLLYWOOD sign facing south over Tinseltown. Just beyond Mount Lee is the top of Cahuenga Peak (1,820'), the highest summit in this corner of the Santa Monica Mountains (see previous hike).

On your return, backtrack to the wide junction and go right, circling Mount Hollywood's east side. Retrace your steps on the two switchback segments, or follow a steeper trail straight south; then keep south along the ridgeline after you reach the top of the tunnel. Walk across the observatory parking lot toward the monumental, three-domed building that houses a state-of-the-art planetarium and museum, a massive antique Zeiss refractor telescope, and various solar instruments. Swing around the back side of the building

to discover observation decks offering commanding views of the LA Basin.

For the final leg of the trip, follow the trail that descends the slope just east of the observatory. It starts from the left side of the building as you face its grand entrance. After 0.2 mile, swing sharply right on the Observatory Trail. Go either way at the next junction where the trail divides into West Observatory Trail and East Observatory Trail. The two branches meet down below at Fern Dell. After winding past golden-blossomed silk oak trees, you arrive at Fern Dell's bubbling brook. Your starting point is just up the road to the right.

VARIATION

For a grand tour of Griffith Park's most famous attractions, continue to the top of the HOLLYWOOD sign from the summit of Mount Hollywood via the Three Mile Trail, Mount Hollywood Drive, the Mulholland Trail, and Mount Lee Drive. Return on Mount Hollywood Drive to Griffith Observatory rather than climbing over Mount Hollywood again. This trip is 10 miles with 2,000 feet of elevation gain.

HIKE 17   Verdugo Mountains: South End Loop

Location Glendale
Highlights Incomparable city and regional views
Distance & Configuration 6-mile loop
Elevation Gain 1,500'
Hiking Time 3.5 hours
Optional Maps Tom Harrison *Verdugo Mountains* or *Angeles Front Country*
Best Times November–May
Agency Glendale Parks and Recreation
Difficulty Moderately strenuous
Trail Use Suitable for mountain biking, dogs allowed
Permit None required
Google Maps Beaudry Loop Trail

The Verdugo Mountains stand as a remarkable island of undeveloped land—a haven for wildlife such as deer and coyotes—completely encircled by an urbanized domain. Public access to the network of trails and fire roads on the mountain is by foot, horse, or mountain

Verdugo Mountains: South End Loop

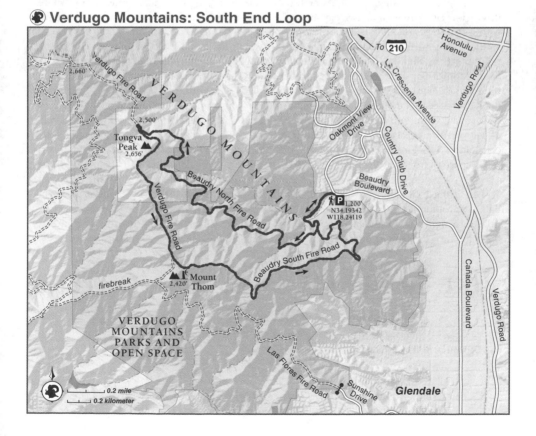

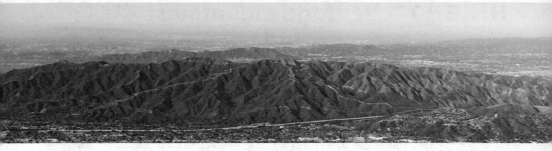

The Verdugo Hills from Mount Lukens

bike—great news if you're looking for a quick escape from the ubiquitous automobile and the pressures of city life.

Along the south crest of the Verdugos, your gaze takes in the San Gabriel Mountains, much of the LA megalopolis, and even the ocean on occasion. Do this trip late in the day if you want to enjoy both a spectacular sunset and a blaze of lights after twilight fades. At best, try this on any cloud-free, smog-free day that falls within two weeks on either side of the winter solstice (December 21). During that period, the sun sets on the flat ocean horizon behind Santa Monica Bay at around 5 p.m. At other times of year, the sun's sinking path is likely to intersect the coastal mountains. The seemingly strange fact of the sun setting over land most of the year is a consequence of the east–west orientation of California's coastline in the first miles up-coast from Los Angeles.

To Reach the Trailhead: From I-210 in Glendale, exit south on La Crescenta Avenue. In 1 mile, turn right onto Oakmont View Drive. In 0.2 mile, turn left (south) onto Country Club Drive. In 0.7 mile, turn right onto Beaudry Boulevard, and proceed 0.4 mile to the trailhead where the road veers right. Park on the street.

Description: From Beaudry Boulevard, walk up a paved segment of fire road, bypass a vehicle gate, and continue on dirt past a debris basin to where the fire road splits (0.3 mile). Choose the shadier right branch, Beaudry North Fire Road. You'll return to this junction by way of the left branch, the Beaudry South Fire Road, which has better views. About halfway up the north road you come to a trickling spring and a water tank nestled in a shady ravine, a good place for a breather.

When you reach the summit ridge (2.3 miles), turn sharply left on Verdugo Fire Road, and continue climbing toward a cluster of brightly painted radio towers atop a 2,656-foot bump, the highest point along this hike (2.7 miles). From the towers, continue south along the ridge to a road junction at 2,420 feet (3.3 miles). The right branch descends to Sunshine Drive in Glendale; take the left branch, and return along an east ridge to the split just above the debris basin.

HIKE 18 Mount Lukens: Grizzly Flat Loop

Location	San Gabriel Mountains, Big Tujunga
Highlights	Urban, mountain, and ocean vistas
Distance & Configuration	13-mile loop
Elevation Gain	3,400'
Hiking Time	8 hours
Recommended Maps	Tom Harrison *Angeles Front Country* or Trails Illustrated *Angeles National Forest (811)*

Best Times	October–May
Agency	Angeles National Forest/Los Angeles Gateway District
Difficulty	Strenuous
Trail Use	Dogs allowed
Permit	Adventure Pass
Google Maps	Stonyvale Picnic Site

This all-day adventure lets you walk on the wild side of the Tujunga canyon-and-peak country. After a grueling climb up the north slope from Big Tujunga Canyon, circle back by way of a long, gradually descending route that passes through secluded Grizzly Flats. The hike feels best on a cool day, but beware of periods following heavy rain: the trip begins and ends with crossings of Big Tujunga Creek, which can be hazardous in high water. This is a wild hike, with steep, narrow sections of lightly maintained trail, but is highly rewarding for those who wish to escape the crowds.

Mount Lukens is named for Theodore Lukens, who supervised the San Gabriel and San Bernardino Forest Reserves and served as mayor of Pasadena. Grizzly Flats is named for the grizzly bear, which is California's state mammal and is featured on the flag. Some 10,000 grizzlies roamed the state at their peak in the early 19th century. Many were shot for sport, but many others were killed when they threatened humans and livestock. In 1916, Cornelius Johnson, a Big Tujunga fruit rancher, killed the last known grizzly bear in Southern California, after the bear spent three nights

Mount Lukens: Grizzly Flat Loop

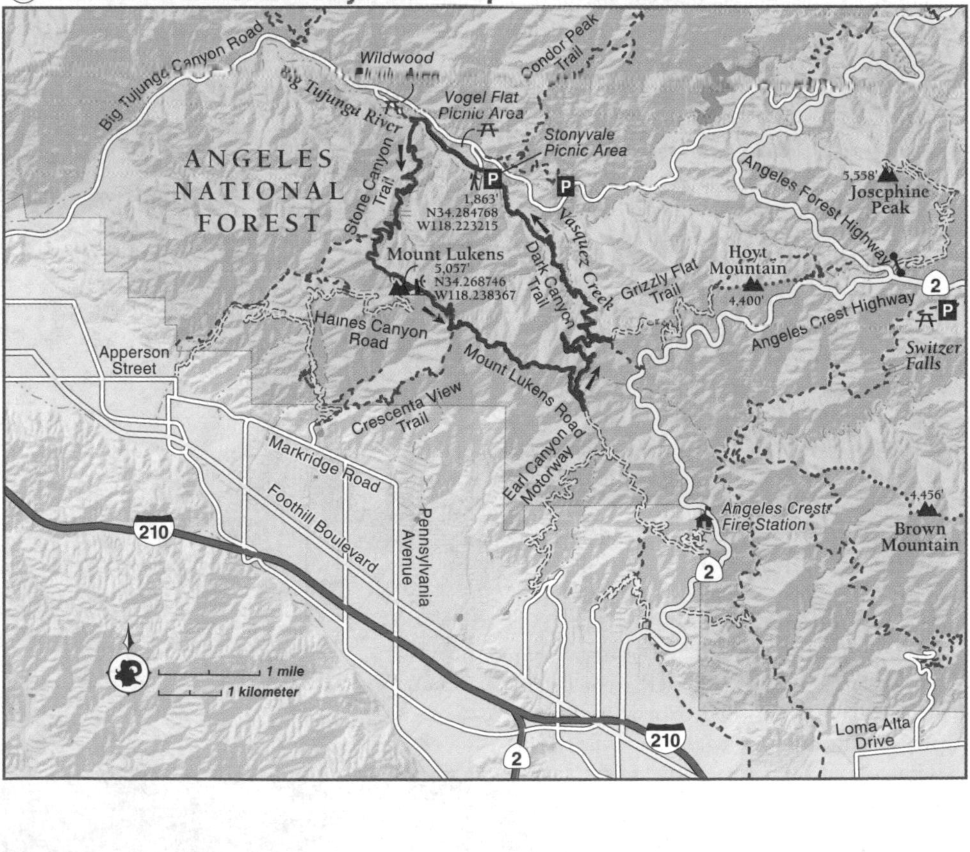

ransacking his orchard. By 1924, the grizzly was extinct in California.

To Reach the Trailhead: From the 210 Freeway in Sunland, take Exit 11 for Sunland Boulevard. Go east for 0.7 mile, as the road name changes to Foothill Boulevard; then turn left onto Oro Vista Avenue. Proceed 7.7 miles as the road name changes to Big Tujunga Canyon Road. Turn right onto Vogel Flat Road; then veer left at the bottom of the hill onto Stonyvale Road, and go 0.2 mile to its end at the Stonyvale Picnic Area.

Description: On foot, head west on Stonyvale Road 0.3 mile to the Vogel Flat Picnic Area, and continue down the narrow, paved road (private, but with public easement) through the cabin community of Stonyvale. When the pavement ends after 0.7 mile, continue on dirt for another quarter mile or so, staying close to the crumbling cliff and avoiding the streamside thickets. After a narrow stretch, you can scramble down to Big Tujunga Creek at a good ford. On the far side, turn left onto the Stone Canyon Trail, which switchbacks south and becomes clearly defined as it leaves the creek. From afar you can spot this trail going straight up the sloping terrace just left (east) of Stone Canyon's wide, boulder-filled mouth. Settle into a pace that will allow you to persevere up 20 switchbacks over the next 3 miles and 3,200 feet of vertical ascent.

From the vantage point of the second switchback, you can look down on the thousands of storm-tossed granitic boulders filling Stone Canyon from wall to wall. Although the boulders are frozen in place, you can almost sense their movement over geologic time. Indeed, floods continue to reshape this canyon and many others in the San Gabriels during every major deluge.

Ahead, you turn along precipitous slopes covered in sage scrub and chaparral—buckwheat, thick-leaf yerba santa, black sage, chamise, yucca, ceanothus, sugar bush, and scrub oak. At or near ground level, a profusion of ferns, mosses, and herbaceous plants forms its own pygmy understory. The dizzying view encompasses a long, linear stretch of Big Tujunga Canyon. This segment of the canyon is underlain by the San Gabriel Fault and its offshoot, the Sierra Madre Fault. The latter fault splits from the former near Vogel Flat and continues southeast past Grizzly Flat, following a course roughly coincident with the final leg of this loop hike. According to current understanding, the San Gabriel Fault is inactive and not likely to be the cause of major movement or earthquakes in the near future. The depth of Big Tujunga Canyon and the steepness of its walls are due primarily to stream-cutting following uplift of the whole mountain range.

The trail climbs above an unnamed canyon to the east that is nearly equal in drainage to Stone Canyon but very steep and narrow. During the wet season, you may glimpse a waterfall from the fifth switchback, at 2.4 miles, and another at 3 miles. At 3.2 miles, step across a ravine with a seasonal spring-fed creek.

Long and short switchback segments take you rapidly higher to a steep, bulldozed track leading to the bald summit ridge of Mount Lukens. Go 0.5 mile farther, connecting with

Crossing Big Tujunga Creek during low flow. During high flow, the rocks are submerged.

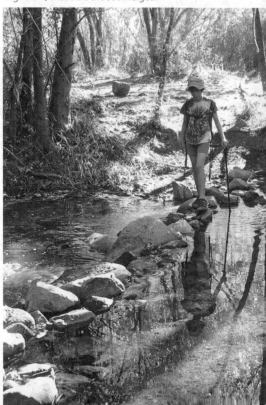

Mount Lukens Road along the way, to reach the 5,075-foot highest point on the ridge (5.1 miles), which is occupied by several antenna structures. Lukens's summit technically lies within the city limits of Los Angeles and is the highest point in any incorporated city in the county; Glendale almost claims this honor, as its corporate limit reaches within 300 yards of the summit. Both cities encompass parts of the Angeles National Forest, of course. The view can be fabulous on a clear day.

The remaining two-thirds of the hike is almost entirely downhill—a little monotonous, but mostly easy on the knees. Follow Mount Lukens Road southeast down the main ridge. At 6.1 miles stay left at a junction with an abandoned road that descends to Deukmejian Wilderness Park. At 8.1 miles stay left again at a junction with a service road leading 4 miles down to the Angeles Crest Fire Station. Notice how the sides of the trail are infested with invasive Spanish broom. At 10.1 miles reach a four-way junction at a saddle—the Upper Dark Canyon Trail, on the right, descends to Highway 2, and the abandoned fire road ahead also continues to the Grizzly Flat Trailhead on Highway 2. Our trip turns left onto 2N80, now deteriorated to a trail, and descends on a zig-zag course to Grizzly Flats (11.3 miles) near a ravine called Vasquez Creek.

The trees that once graced this area are mostly gone after the Station Fire, as are a maze of roads and trails, including the old Dark Canyon Trail from Angeles Crest Highway to Big Tujunga Canyon—roughly the escape route used by the outlaw Tiburcio Vasquez and his unsuccessful pursuers during a hot chase more than a century ago.

Follow the trail through lush vegetation, descend sharply down a ridge overlooking the pitlike gorge of Silver Creek, and finally reach a wildflower-dotted bench along Big Tujunga Creek. Watch for signs of former homesteads. Head downstream, crossing the creek five times in the next mile, to reach your car at Stonyvale Picnic Area.

HIKE 19 Mount Wilson

Location	San Gabriel Mountains above Pasadena
Highlights	Prominent summit, historic trail, great views
Distance & Configuration	15-mile out-and-back
Elevation Gain	4,800'
Hiking Time	9 hours
Optional Maps	Tom Harrison *Angeles Front Country* or Trails Illustrated *Angeles National Forest*
Best Times	October–May
Agency	Angeles National Forest/Los Angeles Gateway Ranger District
Difficulty	Strenuous
Trail Use	Dogs allowed
Google Maps	Mt. Wilson Trailhead

Note: The upper reaches of this hike are in the 2020 Bobcat Fire burn zone. The lower portion of the trail sometimes closes during periods of extreme fire danger. Check with the U.S. Forest Service to avoid disappointment. The road to the summit is generally open from April 1 to November 30, 10 a.m.–5 p.m., weather permitting. Guided tours of the Mount Wilson Observatory generally run on weekends at 1 p.m. when the road is open.

Mount Wilson (5,710') is the most prominent peak in the San Gabriel Front Range overlooking Pasadena. The mountain was named for Benjamin David Wilson, who, in 1864, turned an old American Indian footpath into the first modern trail into the San Gabriels.

ANGELES
NATIONAL
FOREST

Barley Flats

Upper
Big Tujunga
Road

Silver Moccasin Trail

Shortcut Saddle
4,780'

Mount
Lawlor
5,957'

2

Angeles Crest Highway

2

Red Box
Station

Rincon-
Red Box
Road

Valley Forge
Campground
3,467'

West Fork
San Gabriel River

Shortcut Canyon

Silver Moccasin Trail

West Fork
Campground
3,040'

De Vore
Camp

Mount
Deception
5,994'

San Gabriel
Peak
6,161'

Gabrielino Trail

Valley Forge Trail

Falls Canyon

Kenyon
DeVore
Trail

Sevajns
Canyon

Mount Wilson Road

Rincon-Red Box Road

Rim Trail

Newcomb
Pass
4,100'

Mount
Disappointment

Markham Saddle
5,110'

Mount
Markham
5,742'

Eaton
Saddle

Mount Wilson

Mount Lowe
Fire Road

Mount Lowe
5,603'

Eaton Canyon

Mount Lowe Camp
4,480'

Inspiration
Point

Idlehour Trail

Mount Wilson
Observatory
5,710'
5,660'
N34.22298
W118.06287

Sturtevant
Trail

Sturtevant
Camp
3,200'

Spruce Grove
Trail Camp

Gabrielino Trail

Cascade
Picnic Area

Muir
Peak
4,714'

Idlehour
Trail Camp
2,600'

Mount
Harvard
5,441'
4,960'

Winter Creek

Winter Creek
Trail

Mount Zion Trail

Mount
Zion
3,575'

Sturtevant
Falls
2,100'

Hoegee's
Trail Camp
2,500'

Mount Wilson
Toll Road

Mount
Yale
3,140'

Mount Wilson Trail

Orchard
Camp
2,961'

Santa Anita Ridge

Little Santa Anita Canyon

Upper Winter
Creek Trail

1,780'

Chantry Flat

San Olene
Fire Road
2,170'

Pinecrest
Drive

Visitor
Center
2,510'

Henninger
Flats

Bailey Canyon

Jones
Peak
3,375'

First
Water
1,944'

Bastard Ridge

3,400'

Altadena Drive

EATON CANYON
NATURAL AREA

Eaton Canyon
1,350'

980'

Eaton Canyon
Nature Center

New York Drive

1,100'

BAILEY
CANYON
PARK

Mira Monte
Avenue

970'
N34.16968
W118.04920

Allen Avenue

Pasadena

Sierra Madre

Sierra Madre Boulevard

Baldwin Avenue

Arcadia

Santa Anita Avenue

Big Santa Anita Canyon

Monrovia

210

Foothill Boulevard

210

0.5 mile
0.5 kilometer

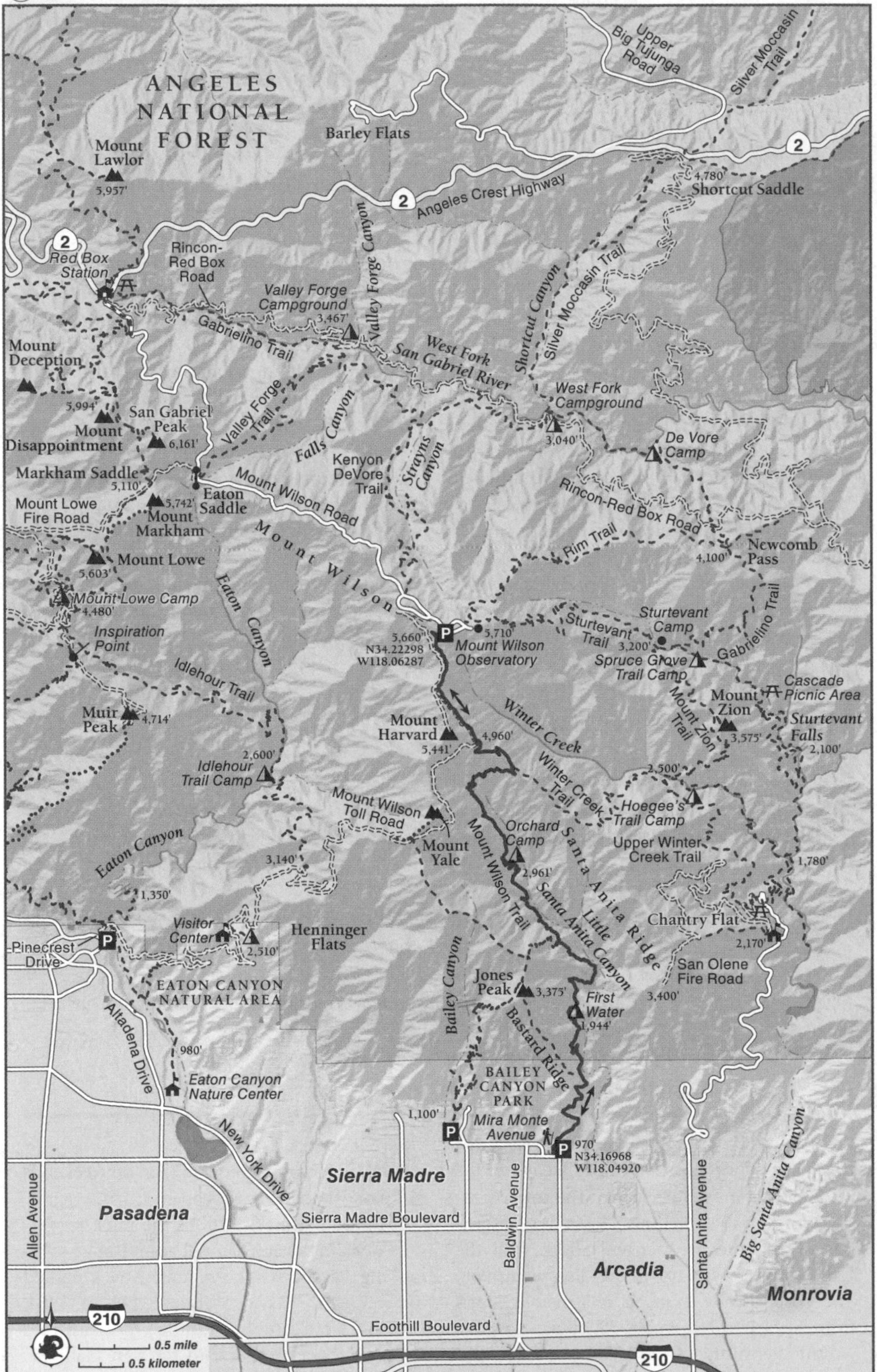

Although his logging venture failed, the trail became popular in the 1880s for the newly emerging sport of recreational hiking. In the area's great hiking era (1895–1938), hundreds would disembark from the red Pacific Electric trollies in Sierra Madre each Saturday, intent on a weekend at the mountain resorts.

Before the turn of the century, a massive telescope was hauled up the trail piece by piece, and Mount Wilson soon became home to the world's leading observatory of the era. Light pollution in the Los Angeles Basin now limits its capabilities. Eventually, the Mount Wilson Toll Road from Henninger Flats became the preferred route for vehicle traffic to the summit, and Frank Benedict set the automotive speed record of 22 minutes in 1922.

Mount Wilson has more trails than any other peak in the San Gabriel Mountains. This hike follows Benjamin Wilson's original route. Although it is described as an out-and-back, you could arrange a car or bicycle shuttle to do it as a one-way trip either up or down, or you could link to the Winter Creek Trail, Sturtevant Trail, or old Mount Wilson Toll Road to find an alternative descent (with a shuttle).

To Reach the Trailhead: From I-210 in Arcadia, exit north on Baldwin Avenue. In 1.5 miles, turn right on Mira Monte Avenue. The trailhead is on the left in two blocks.

If you wish to station a vehicle at the summit, return to I-210 and follow it west to the Angeles Crest Highway (Highway 2), which leads 13.5 miles north and east up to Red Box Station. Turn right on Mount Wilson Road and proceed 4 miles to the Skyline Park parking area at the end of the road. The drive between trailheads takes about 50 minutes.

Description: The signed route, initially a road, detours left onto a trail around private property, rejoins the road in a quarter mile, and soon narrows to a trail again. Only the dedicated work of many volunteers keeps this trail on the steep wall of Little Santa Anita Canyon from collapsing.

At 1.8 miles, pass a branch to the canyon bottom (First Water), then make a steep climb through the chaparral. Eventually, the grade relaxes in a grove of oaks. At 2.0 miles, watch for a trail on the left leading up to the ridge by Jones Peak. At 3.6 miles, reach the shady streamside ruins of Orchard Camp. In its heyday of 1911, 40,000 hikers and equestrians signed the camp register, but now only foundations remain. Wilson originally established a construction camp at this spot and called it Halfway House because it marks the midpoint

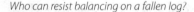
Who can resist balancing on a fallen log?

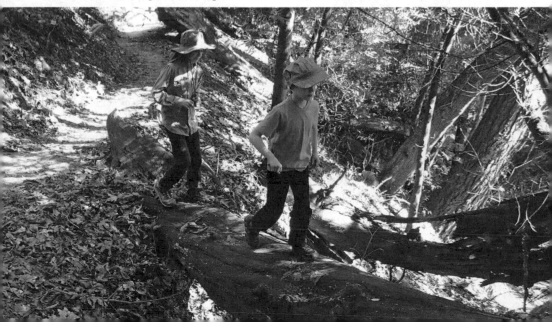

of the route. Here you can find the last dependable water of the trip. The huge canyon oak here is one of the largest and oldest in the San Gabriels; it is estimated to be 1,500 years old.

The Mount Wilson Trail now kicks off an earnest climb with a set of switchbacks, eventually reaching a ridgeline (5.3 miles), where it meets the Winter Creek Trail on the right. Your path turns left up the ridge. At 5.9 miles, meet the dirt roadbed of the Mount Wilson Toll Road just east of Mount Harvard. Follow this road north to a point north of Mount Harvard where you can veer right onto trail again (6.5 miles). The trail climbs directly to Mount Wilson's flat summit.

The domes here are part of the Mount Wilson Observatory. The radio antennas to the northwest include most of the major television stations of Los Angeles, along with much of the basin's emergency communications network.

HIKE 20   Down the Arroyo Seco

Location	San Gabriel Mountains above Pasadena
Highlights	Sylvan glens, sparkling stream
Distance & Configuration	10-mile point-to-point
Elevation Gain/Loss	450'/2,600'
Hiking Time	5 hours
Optional Maps	Tom Harrison *Angeles Front Country* or Trails Illustrated *Angeles National Forest*
Best Times	October–June
Agency	Angeles National Forest/Los Angeles Gateway Ranger District
Difficulty	Moderately strenuous
Trail Use	Suitable for backpacking
Permit	Adventure Pass
Google Maps	Switzer Picnic Area

The Spanish colonists who christened Arroyo Seco (meaning "dry creek") evidently observed only its lower end—a hot, boulder-strewn wash emptying into the Los Angeles River. Upstream, inside the confines of the San Gabriels, Arroyo Seco is a scenic treasure—all the more astounding when you consider that its exquisite sylvan glens and sparkling brook lie just 12–15 miles from LA's city center. If you haven't yet been freed from the notion that Los Angeles is nothing but a seething megalopolis, a walk down the canyon of the Arroyo Seco will convince you otherwise.

The 2009 Station Fire ravaged much of the canyon, which did not reopen until 2018. Although the fire killed many of the splendid trees in the canyon, many others remain standing, and wildflowers flourish after fire. A quick census one spring day before the fire (in a dry year, no less) yielded the following blooming plants: golden yarrow, prickly phlox, western wallflower, Indian pink, live-forever, wild pea, deerweed, bush lupine, Spanish broom, baby blue eyes, yerba santa, phacelia, chia, black sage, bush poppy, California buckwheat, shooting star, western clematis, Indian paintbrush, sticky monkey flower, scarlet bugler, and purple nightshade. Beware of the extensive stands of poison oak that impinge upon the trail.

To Reach the Trailheads: This trip requires a 15-mile car shuttle or ride-sharing trip, or a friend who will drop you off and pick you up. Leave your getaway vehicle at the south end of the hike: From the 210 Freeway in Pasadena, take Exit 22B for northbound Windsor Avenue. In 0.8 mile park at a busy lot on the left, where Windsor meets Ventura Street. To reach the north end, return to the 210 and go west to Highway 2, then 10 miles north to the turnoff

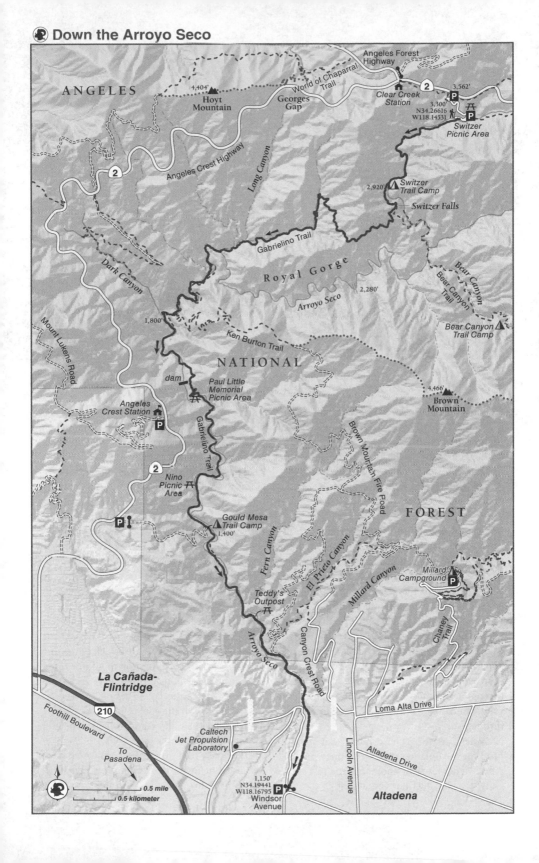

ANGELES

Angeles Forest Highway

World of Chaparral Trail

Clear Creek Station

2

3,562'

3,300'
N34.26616
W118.14531

Switzer Picnic Area

4,404'
Hoyt Mountain

Georges Gap

Long Canyon

2

2,920'
Switzer Trail Camp

Switzer Falls

Angeles Crest Highway

Dark Canyon

Gabrielino Trail

Royal Gorge

Bear Canyon Trail

2,280'

Arroyo Seco

Bear Canyon Trail Camp

Mount Lukens Road

1,800'

Ken Burton Trail

NATIONAL

dam

Paul Little Memorial Picnic Area

4,466'
Brown Mountain

Angeles Crest Station

P

Gabrielino Trail

Brown Mountain Fire Road

2

Nino Picnic Area

FOREST

P

Gould Mesa Trail Camp

1,400'

Fern Canyon

El Prieto Canyon

Millard Canyon

Millard Campground

P

Teddy's Outpost

Chaney Trail

Arroyo Seco

Canyon Crest Road

La Cañada-Flintridge

210

Foothill Boulevard

Loma Alta Drive

Caltech Jet Propulsion Laboratory

Lincoln Avenue

Altadena Drive

To Pasadena

1,150'
N34.19441
W118.16795

P

Windsor Avenue

Altadena

0.5 mile

0.5 kilometer

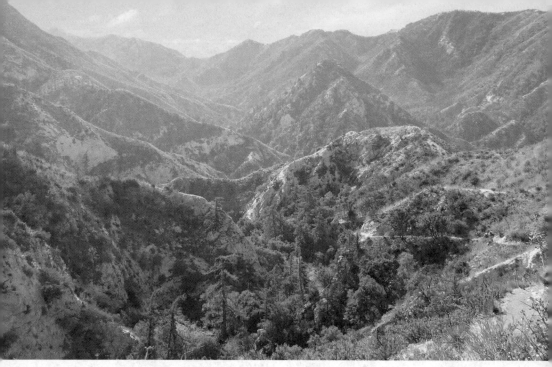

Arroyo Seco Creek cuts through the rugged Royal Gorge.

for Switzer Picnic Area, on the right (mile marker 2 LA 34.2). Continue 0.5 mile down the paved access road to the parking lot next to the picnic area. (If the lot is full or the access road happens to be closed and gated, you can park at the top and walk down into the picnic area—250 feet of elevation loss in a half mile.)

Description: You'll be traveling the western-most leg of the Gabrielino Trail, one of four routes in Angeles National Forest specially designated as National Recreation Trails. The trip is a testament to the San Gabriel Mountains' awesome powers to wipe themselves clean of humankind's imprint through fire, flood, and avalanche. In the early 1900s, many tourist camps and cabins were erected along the canyon. Virtually all the structures were either destroyed by flooding in 1938 or removed through condemnation proceedings (based on water and flood-control needs) in the 1920s through the 1940s.

Note: Carry whatever drinking water you'll need for the duration of the trip; there may be piped water at one or another of the rest stops along the way, but don't count on it.

For the easier, downhill direction suggested here, you start hiking from the west end of Switzer Picnic Area on the Gabrielino Trail. Make your way across the bridge and along a road past outlying picnic tables, and then down along the alder-shaded stream. Soon nothing but the clear-flowing stream and rustling leaves disturbs the silence. Remnants of an old paved road will occasionally appear underfoot. In a couple of spots you ford the stream by boulder-hopping—easy except after heavy rain.

One mile down the canyon, you come upon the foundation remnants of Switzer's Camp—now occupied by a trail campground. Established in 1884, the camp became the San Gabriels' premier wilderness resort in the early 1900s, patronized by Hollywood celebrities and anyone who had the gumption to hike or ride a burro up the tortuous Arroyo Seco Trail from Pasadena. After the construction of Angeles Crest Highway in the early 1930s and a severe flood in the 1938, the resort lost its appeal. It was finally razed in the late 1950s.

The main trail crosses to the west side of the creek at Switzer's Camp. Don't be lured onto one of the use trails continuing down the east side to some crumbling cliffs above Switzer Falls, where many have fallen to their death.

Walk down to a fork in the trail at 1.2 miles. You will probably hear, if not clearly see, the 50-foot cascade known as Switzer Falls, to the east. Your way continues on the right fork (Gabrielino Trail), which now begins a mile-long traverse through burned chaparral. This stretch avoids a narrow, twisting trench called Royal Gorge, through which Arroyo Seco tumbles and sometimes abruptly drops.

At 2.3 miles the trail joins a shady tributary of Long Canyon, and later Long Canyon itself, replete with a trickling stream. The trail mostly clings to a narrow ledge cut at great effort into the east wall of the canyon. Alongside the trail you'll discover at least five kinds of ferns, plus mosses, miner's lettuce, poison oak, and Humboldt lilies (in bloom during early summer).

At 3.4 miles, the waters of Long Canyon swish down through a sculpted grotto to join Arroyo Seco. The trail descends to Arroyo Seco canyon's narrow floor and vanishes. The portions once cut into the east wall have mostly collapsed or become overgrown, and the trail on the floor has been washed away. Pick the best route down the canyon, crossing the creek many times over the next few miles. In the springtime, expect to get your feet wet. The fire killed most of the gorgeous oaks, maples, and alders that once filled the canyon. At 4.5 miles look for a tributary on the right where Camp Oak Wilde stood from 1911 until its destruction by flood in 1938. The Oakwilde Picnic Area was rebuilt in the same place, but the Station Fire wiped it out.

The canyon widens a bit. At 5.5 miles, the large Brown Canyon Debris Dam abruptly blocks your way. Built in the 1940s to reduce the flow of detritus into Pasadena, it has completely filled up and no longer serves its purpose, but it remains as a scar on the canyon that will take nature many more years to demolish. Look for a faint trail bypassing the dam high on the east wall of the canyon. Backtrack 0.2 mile and look for an obscure cairn marking the start of the trail, which climbs sharply and then descends steeply to reach the canyon bottom at a sign for the Paul Little Memorial Picnic Area.

The hardest work is over, and a decent path takes you down the remainder of the gently sloping canyon. The trail gradually improves into a road and crosses several bridges in varying states of repair. At 7.5 miles, pass the Gould Mesa Campground, named for Will Gould, a homesteader who lived here in the 1890s. Reaching the south end of the burn area, watch for a gauging station on the right and some U.S. Forest Service residences on the left. Since the last segment of the trail is paved, you are likely to run into cyclists, joggers, parents pushing strollers, and even skateboarders. Pass the imposing complex of Caltech's Jet Propulsion Laboratory on the right, and eventually emerge at the Arroyo Boulevard Trailhead.

HIKE 21   Mount Lowe

Location	San Gabriel Mountains above Pasadena
Highlights	Mountain, city, and ocean views
Distance & Configuration	3.2-mile out-and-back
Elevation Gain	500'
Hiking Time	1.5 hours
Optional Maps	Tom Harrison *Angeles Front Country* or Trails Illustrated *Angeles National Fores*t
Best Times	All year
Agency	Angeles National Forest/Los Angeles Gateway Ranger District
Difficulty	Moderate
Trail Use	Dogs allowed, good for kids
Google Maps	Eaton Saddle Trailhead

◉ Mount Lowe

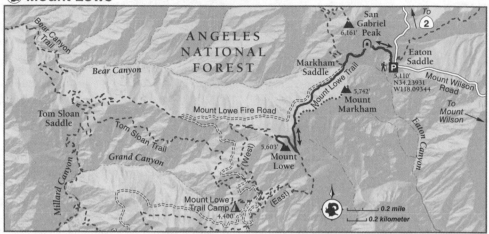

Late in the year, when the smog lightens but temperatures still hover within a moderate register, come up to Mount Lowe to toast the setting sun. You can sit on an old bench, pour some champagne, and watch Old Sol sink into Santa Monica Bay.

To Reach the Trailhead: To reach the starting point from I-210 at La Cañada-Flintridge, drive up Angeles Crest Highway (Highway 2) for 14 miles to Red Box Divide, and turn right on Mount Wilson Road. Proceed 2.4 miles to a large roadside parking area at unmarked Eaton Saddle.

Description: Walk past the gate on the west side, and proceed up Mount Lowe Fire Road, a dirt road that carves its way under the precipitous south face of San Gabriel Peak. The dramatic peak ahead to the west is Mount Markham. As you approach a short tunnel (0.3 mile) dating from 1942, look for the remnants of a former cliff-hanging trail to the left of the tunnel's east entrance.

At Markham Saddle (0.5 mile), reach the edge of the burn area from the vast 2009 Station Fire. Don't continue on the road. Instead, find the unmarked Mount Lowe Trail on the left (south). On it, you contour southwest above the fire road and then cross a saddle between Lowe and Markham and start climbing south across the east flank of Mount Lowe (1.1 miles).

At 1.3 miles, make a sharp right turn at a sign for Mount Lowe. At 1.5 miles, go left on a short

spur trail to Mount Lowe's summit, where a small grove of live oaks miraculously survived the fire. Mount Lowe was the proposed upper terminus for Professor Thaddeus Lowe's famed scenic railway (see Hike 22). Funding ran out, however, and tracks were never laid higher than Ye Alpine

Mount Markham from the Mount Lowe Fire Road

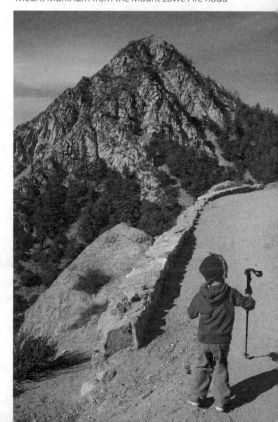

Tavern, 1,200 feet below. During the railway's heyday in the early 1900s, thousands disembarked at the tavern and tramped Mount Lowe's east- and west-side trails for world-class views of the basin and the surrounding mountains. Some reminders of that era remain on the summit of Mount Lowe and along some of the trails: volunteers have repainted, relettered, and returned to their proper places some of the many sighting tubes that helped the early tourists familiarize themselves with the surrounding geography.

VARIATIONS

Peak baggers can amplify their fun by visiting Mount Markham and/or San Gabriel Peak on the way back. Markham is a 1-mile round-trip with 400 feet of elevation gain via a climber's path from the saddle between Lowe and Markham. San Gabriel Peak, the highest point in the vicinity, is 2 miles round-trip with 1,000 feet of elevation gain via a good trail from Markham Saddle.

HIKE 22   Mount Lowe Railway

Location	San Gabriel Mountains, above Pasadena
Highlights	Grand vistas and historically interesting
Distance & Configuration	11-mile loop
Elevation Gain	2,800'
Hiking Time	6 hours
Optional Maps	Tom Harrison *Angeles Front Country* or Trails Illustrated *Angeles National Forest*
Best Times	October–May
Agency	Angeles National Forest/Los Angeles Gateway Ranger District
Difficulty	Moderately strenuous
Trail Use	Suitable for backpacking, dogs allowed
Permit	None required
Google Maps	Sam Merrill Trailhead

An engineering marvel when it was built in the 1890s, the Mount Lowe Railway has lived a checkered past full of both glory and destruction. Before its last run in 1937, the line carried more than 3 million passengers—virtually all of them tourists. Unheard of by millions of Southland newcomers today, the railway was for many years the most popular outdoor attraction in Southern California.

Today hikers are taking a new interest in the old roadbed; the Rails-to-Trails Conservancy (which promotes the conversion of former rail corridors into recreation trails) ranked the Mount Lowe Railway as one of the nation's 12 most scenic and historically significant recycled rail lines.

The line consisted of three stages, of which almost nothing remains today. Passengers rode a trolley from Altadena into lower Rubio Canyon and then boarded a steeply inclined cable railway that took them 1,300 feet higher to Echo Mountain, where two hotels, a number of small tourist attractions, and an observatory stood. At Echo Mountain, non-acrophobic passengers hopped onto the third phase, a mountain trolley that climbed another 1,200 vertical feet along airy slopes to the end of the line—Ye Alpine Tavern (later Mount Lowe Tavern, on whose ruins stands today's Mount Lowe Trail Camp). The U.S. Forest Service and volunteers have put together a self-guided trail, featuring 10 markers fashioned from railroad rails, along the route of the mountain trolley.

To Reach the Trailhead: The Sam Merrill Trailhead lies on the grounds of the long-demolished Cobb Estate, at the intersection of Lake Avenue and Loma Alta Drive in Altadena.

Ⓡ Mount Lowe Railway

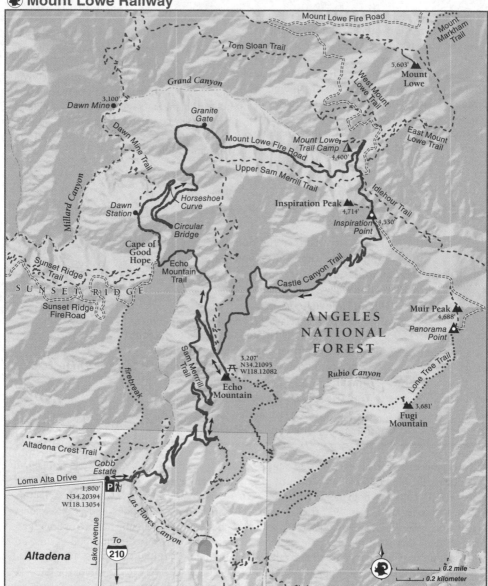

Take the Lake Avenue exit from I-210 in Pasadena, and drive 3.6 miles north to where Lake Avenue turns left (west) and becomes Loma Alta Drive. Park on the street (no National Forest Adventure Pass needed).

Description: Walk east past the stone pillars at the Cobb Estate entrance, and continue 150 yards on a narrow, blacktop driveway.

The driveway bends left, but you keep walking straight (east). Soon you come to a water fountain on the rim of Las Flores Canyon and a sign indicating the start of the Sam Merrill Trail. This trail goes left over the top of a small debris dam and begins a switchbacking ascent of Las Flores Canyon's precipitous east wall, while another trail (the Altadena Crest equestrian trail) veers to the right, down the canyon.

Inspired by the fabulous views (assuming you're doing this early on one of LA's clear winter days), the 2.5 miles of steady ascent on the Sam Merrill Trail may seem to go rather quickly. Turn right at the top of the trail, and walk south over to Echo Mountain, which is more like the shoulder of a ridge. There you'll find a historical plaque and some picnic tables near a grove of incense-cedars and big-leaf maples. Poke around and you'll find many foundation ruins and piles of concrete rubble. An old bullwheel and cables for the incline railway were thoughtfully left behind after the U.S. Forest Service cleared away what remained of the buildings here in the 1950s and '60s. After visiting Echo Mountain, go north on the signed Echo Mountain Trail, where you walk over railroad ties still embedded in the ground.

The railbed is now marked with a series of interpretive signs highlighted on the following pages. Numbers in parentheses refer to hiking mileage starting from Echo Mountain.

Station 1 (0.0), Echo Mountain. This area was known as the White City during its brief heyday in the late 1890s, but most of its tourist facilities were destroyed by fire or windstorms in the first decade of the 1900s. The mountain remained a transfer point for passengers until the mid-1930s.

Station 2 (0.5), View of Circular Bridge. You can't see it from here, but passengers at this point first noticed the 400-foot-diameter circular bridge (Station 6) jutting from the slope above. As you walk on, you'll notice the many concrete footings that supported trestles bridging the side ravines of Las Flores Canyon.

Station 3 (0.8), Cape of Good Hope. You're now at the junction of the Echo Mountain Trail and Sunset Ridge Fire Road, where the route crosses from Las Flores to Millard Canyon. The tracks swung in a 200-degree arc around the rocky promontory just west, the Cape of Good Hope. (Walk around the cape, if you like, to get a feel for the experience.) North of this dizzying passage, riders were treated to the longest stretch of straight track—only 225 feet long. The entire original line from Echo Mountain to Ye Alpine Tavern had 127 curves and 114 straight sections. The Cape of Good Hope also marks the edge of the vast burn area from the 2009 Station Fire. (*Note:* Plenty of mountain bikers use this section of the old railroad grade. They mostly arrive by way of the Sunset Ridge Fire Road.)

Station 4 (1.0), Dawn Station and Devil's Slide. Gold-bearing ore, packed up by mules from Dawn Mine in the bottom of Millard Canyon, was loaded onto the train here. Ahead lay a treacherous stretch of crumbling granite, the Devil's Slide, which was eventually bridged by a trestle. (The current fire road has been shored up with much new concrete, and cement-lined spillways seem to do a good job of carrying away flood debris.)

Station 5 (1.2), Horseshoe Curve. Just beyond this station, Horseshoe Curve enabled the

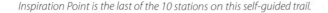

Inspiration Point is the last of the 10 stations on this self-guided trail.

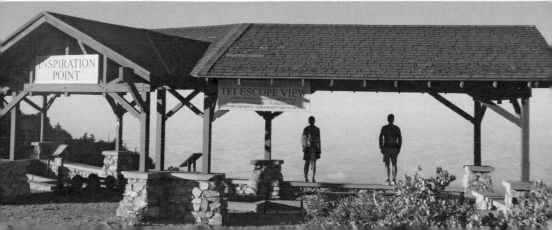

railway to gain elevation above Millard Canyon. The grade just beyond Horseshoe Curve was 7%, the steepest on the mountain segment of the line.

Station 6 (1.6), Circular Bridge. An engineering accomplishment of worldwide fame, the Circular Bridge carried startled passengers into midair over the upper walls of Las Flores Canyon. Look for the concrete supports of this bridge down along the chaparral-covered slopes to the right.

Station 7 (2.0), Horseshoe Curve Overview. Passengers here looked down on Horseshoe Curve and could also see all three levels of steep, twisting track climbing the east wall of Millard Canyon.

Station 8 (2.4), Granite Gate. A narrow slot carefully blasted out of solid granite on a sheer north-facing slope, Granite Gate took eight months to cut. Look for the electric wire support dangling from the rock above.

Station 9 (3.4), Ye Alpine Tavern. The tavern, which later became a fancy hotel, was located at Crystal Springs, the source that still provides seasonal water (requires purification) for backpackers staying overnight at Mount Lowe Trail Camp in a splendid forest of oak and big-cone Douglas-fir. The railway never got farther than here, although the hope was that it would one day reach the summit of Mount Lowe, 1,200 feet higher.

Station 10 (3.9), Inspiration Point. From Ye Alpine Tavern, tourists could saunter over to Inspiration Point along part of the never-finished rail extension to Mount Lowe. Sighting tubes (still in place there) helped visitors locate places of interest below.

Inspiration Point is the last station on the self-guided trail. The fastest and easiest way to return is by way of the Castle Canyon Trail, which descends directly below Inspiration Point. After 2 miles you arrive back on the old railway grade just north of Echo Mountain. Retrace your steps on the Sam Merrill Trail.

HIKE 23   Eaton Canyon Falls

Location	Altadena (Pasadena)
Highlights	Lessons in fire ecology, waterfall
Distance & Configuration	3.4-mile out-and-back
Elevation Gain	400'
Hiking Time	1.5 hours
Optional Maps	Tom Harrison *Angeles Front Country* or Trails Illustrated *Angeles National Forest*
Best Times	All year
Agency	Eaton Canyon Natural Area
Difficulty	Moderate
Trail Use	Dogs allowed, good for kids
Permit	None required
Google Maps	Eaton Canyon Nature Center

Eaton Canyon Natural Area is a well-known gem at the foot of the San Gabriel Mountains. On a pleasant spring weekend, hundreds of people gather at the busy trailhead for a stroll. The canyon burned to ash in the 1993 Altadena Fire but has completely recovered. The rebuilt Nature Center is staffed with knowledgeable volunteers who will share their passion for the outdoors with you.

Upstream from the 190-acre park, where the waters of Eaton Canyon have carved a raw groove in the San Gabriel Mountains, you'll discover Eaton Canyon Falls. Impressive only during the wetter half of the year, the falls possess, as

🅡 Eaton Canyon Falls

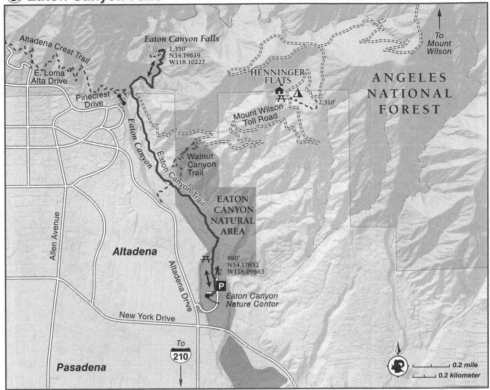

John Muir once put it, "a low sweet voice, singing like a bird." The falls are well worth visiting, especially in the aftermath of a winter storm, if only to witness the power of large (by Southern California standards) volumes of falling water.

To Reach the Trailhead: From I-210 at Exit 29A, take Sierra Madre Boulevard north. In 0.3 mile, turn left on Orange Grove Boulevard. In 0.2 mile, turn right on Altadena Drive. Proceed 1.3 miles to Eaton Canyon Natural Area on the right. If the parking lot is full, follow signs to the overflow area.

If you prefer, you can shorten the walk to the falls by starting from the lower gate of Mount Wilson Toll Road on Pinecrest Drive in Altadena. Be sure to obey any signs about parking restrictions in that neighborhood.

Description: The Eaton Canyon Trail splits near the trailhead. Both branches run in parallel and rejoin before crossing to the east side of the canyon; the west branch has a picnic area. Pass many splits along the way, but stay on the wide dirt track. After crossing the canyon's cobbled bottom, the trail sticks to an elevated stream terrace, passing some beautiful live-oak woods.

At 1.1 miles you rise to meet the Mount Wilson Toll Road bridge over Eaton Canyon. Just before it, veer left onto a narrower track at a sign for Eaton Canyon Falls. The rough path leads up the canyon, crossing the creek eight times. Expect plenty of boulder-hopping, and prepare to get your feet wet if the stream is lively. (This is not a place to be when the creek is flooding.) Except for a line of alders along part of the stream and some live oaks on benches just above the reach of floods, the canyon bottom and the precipitous walls are desolate and desertlike. After a half mile of canyon-bottom travel, you come to the falls, where the water slides and then free-falls for a total of about 35 feet down a narrow chute in the bedrock.

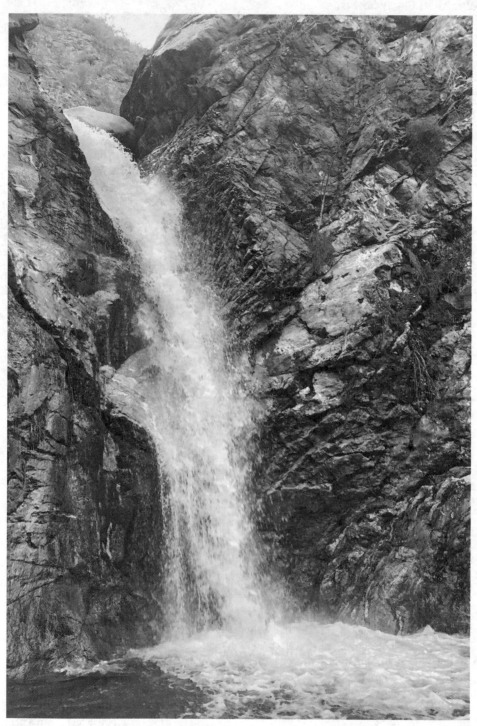

Eaton Falls (see previous page)

HIKE 24   Santa Anita Canyon Loop

Location	San Gabriel Mountains above Arcadia
Highlights	Sparkling streams, botanical and historical interest
Distance & Configuration	9-mile loop
Elevation Gain	2,300'
Hiking Time	5 hours
Optional Maps	Tom Harrison *Angeles Front Country* or Trails Illustrated *Angeles National Forest*
Best Times	October–June
Agency	Angeles National Forest/Los Angeles Gateway Ranger District
Difficulty	Moderately strenuous
Trail Use	Suitable for backpacking, dogs allowed
Permit	National Forest Adventure Pass required at Chantry Flat lot (but not along roadside)
Google Maps	Chantry Flat

Note: This area was within the 2020 Bobcat Fire burn zone.

In the lush, shady recesses of Santa Anita Canyon and its tributary, Winter Creek, you can easily lose all sight and sense of the hundreds of square miles of dense metropolis and the millions of people that lie just over the ridge to the south. With easy access from the San Gabriel Valley by city street and mountain road, you can be strolling along a fern-lined path less than half an hour after leaving the freeway traffic behind.

To Reach the Trailhead: From I-210 in Arcadia, follow Santa Anita Avenue north. Continue to the edge of the city, pass a sturdy gate (open 6 a.m.–8 p.m.), and ascend along a curling and precipitous ribbon of asphalt to your destination at the end of the road: Chantry Flat. Here you'll find spacious but often inadequate parking lots (Adventure Pass required), a picnic ground, and a mom-and-pop concession stand. If you don't arrive early, expect to backtrack in search of roadside parking.

Chantry Flat also features an old-fashioned freight business—the last pack station operating year-round in California. Almost every day, horses, mules, and burros carry supplies and building materials from the Adams Pack Station down into the canyon bottom, where an anachronistic cabin community has survived since the early 1900s.

Backpackers can stay at the free first-come, first-served Hoegee's or Spruce Grove Trail Camp. With reservations, you can stay in a historic cabin at Sturtevant Camp (sturtevantcamp.com) and even have a pack train carry in your gear.

Sturtevant Falls   Kiby McDaniel

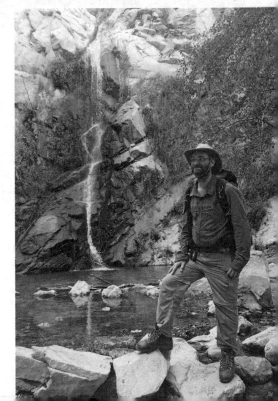

🚶 Santa Anita Canyon Loop

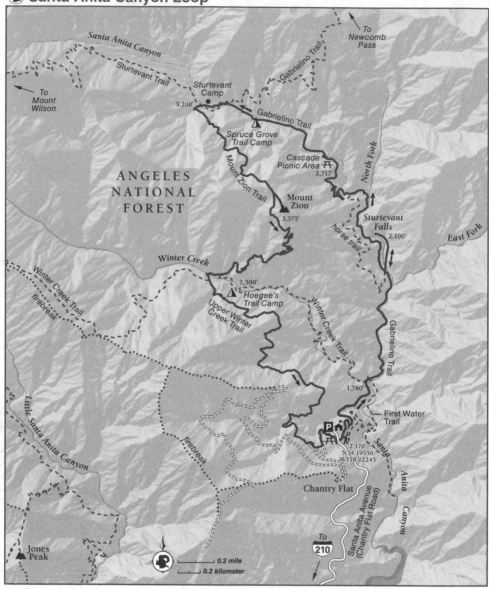

Description: In this scenic loop trip from Chantry Flat, you'll climb by way of the Gabrielino Trail to historic Sturtevant Camp and return by way of the Mount Zion and Upper Winter Creek Trails. Do it in a day, or take your time on an overnight backpacking trip, with a stay at Spruce Grove Trail Camp. The camp is popular, so plan to get there early to secure a spot on the weekend, or go on a weekday. Be sure you can recognize poison oak because it grows beside many parts of the trail.

From the south edge of the lower parking lot at Chantry Flat, hike the first, paved segment of the Gabrielino Trail down to the confluence of Winter Creek and Santa Anita Canyon at 0.6 mile. The pavement ends at a metal bridge spanning Winter Creek. Pass the restrooms and continue up alder-lined Santa Anita Canyon on a wide roadbed following the left bank. Edging alongside a number of small cabins, the deteriorating road soon assumes the proportions of a foot trail. Seventeen of the 80 historic cabins in the canyon burned in the 2020 Bobcat Fire.

At 1.4 miles, amid a beautiful oak woodland, you come to a four-way junction of trails. The right branch goes upcanyon to the base of 50-foot-high Sturtevant Falls, a worthy 0.6-mile round-trip detour during the wet season. The middle and left branches join again a mile upstream. The left, upper trail is recommended for horses. Take the middle (lower) trail—the more scenic and exciting alternative—unless you dislike heights. The lower trail slices across a sheer wall above the falls and continues through a veritable fairyland of miniature cascades and crystalline pools with giant chain ferns.

A half mile past the reconvergence of the upper and lower trails and at 2.8 miles from the trailhead, you come upon Cascade Picnic Area, which has tables and restrooms and is named for a smooth chute in the stream bottom just below. Press on past a hulking crib dam (flood-check dam) to reach Spruce Grove Trail Camp at 3.5 miles; it's named for the bigcone Douglas-fir (big-cone spruce) trees that attain truly inspiring proportions on the surrounding hillsides.

Reach a junction at 3.7 miles, and turn left onto the signed Sturtevant Trail. After only 0.1 mile, Sturtevant Camp comes into view. This is both the oldest (1893) and the only remaining resort in the Santa Anita drainage, accessible only by foot trail. All supplies are packed in from Chantry Flat on the backs of pack animals, not unlike a century ago.

At the camp, cross to the opposite side of the creek, and pick up the Mount Zion Trail on the left at 3.9 miles. This restored version of the original trail to Sturtevant Camp (reconstructed in the late 1970s and early '80s) winds delightfully upward across a ravine and then along timber-shaded, north-facing slopes.

When the trail crests at a notch just northwest of Mount Zion, take the short side path up through manzanita and scrub oak to the summit (5.0 miles), which has a broad, if somewhat unremarkable, view of surrounding ridges and a small slice of the San Gabriel Valley. You can see the telescope on Mount Wilson to the northwest.

Return to the main trail, and begin a long, switchbacking descent down the dry north canyon wall of Winter Creek—a sweaty affair if the day is sunny and warm. At the foot of this stretch you reach the cool canyon bottom and a T-intersection with the Winter Creek Trail at 6.4 miles, just above Hoegee's Trail Camp. Turn right, going upstream momentarily; follow the trail across the creek; and climb to the next trail junction at 6.6 miles. Bear left on the Upper Winter Creek Trail, which briefly climbs and then gradually descends through the cool woods overlooking Winter Creek. Upon reaching the paved service road at 8.9 miles, follow it down 0.3 mile past a water tank and the picnic grounds to reach the signed Winter Creek Trailhead at the upper Chantry Flat parking area.

HIKE 25   Strawberry Peak

Location	Central San Gabriel Mountains
Highlight	Rock scrambling on dramatic peak
Distance & Configuration	7-mile out-and-back
Elevation Gain	2,700'
Hiking Time	6 hours
Optional Maps	Tom Harrison *Angeles Front Country* or Trails Illustrated *Angeles National Forest*
Best Times	October–June

Agency	Angeles National Forest/San Gabriel Mountains National Monument
Difficulty	Strenuous
Permit	None required
Google Maps	Colby Canyon Trail

A well-worn trail followed the crest of one of the several ridges that radiate from the peak, and brought me to the base of an apparently perpendicular cliff a couple of hundred feet high and forming the last stage to the summit. A close scanning of the cliff's broken face showed plainly that the only way up was to scale it as best I could; so, holding on by fingers and toes, and carefully testing the stability of the jutting rocks, root-ends, and clinging bushes which served me as pegs to climb by, I got on pretty well.

—Charles Francis Saunders,
The Southern Sierras of California, 1923

Strawberry Peak's 6,164-foot summit beats by a smidgen 6,161-foot San Gabriel Peak, thus claiming the honor of being the highest peak in the Front Range, as well as the most fun. Although its profile appears rounded as seen from most places, in reality its flanks fall away sharply on three sides, leaving only one relatively easy route to the top. The peak was named by guests at Switzer's Camp, who felt its profile resembled a strawberry. Switzer himself would lead his guests on a favorite hike up Strawberry by way of the airy ridge in the 1880s. He carried a Winchester rifle on his saddle to defend against grizzly bears.

In March 1909, Strawberry Peak garnered national attention when a gas balloon and gondola carrying six passengers over Tournament Park in Pasadena was swept by violent gusts into storm clouds over the San Gabriel Mountains. After being tossed to as high as 14,000 feet, the balloon descended in whiteout conditions and crash-landed just below Strawberry's snow-covered summit—its gondola coming to rest just 10 feet from a vertical precipice. Nearly three days later, a telephone call from Switzer's Camp brought news to the world below that the riders had survived.

This hike takes the most fun route to the summit by way of Colby Canyon and the steep west ridge. It is not the easiest route (see the variation below) and is not recommended for hikers who are uncomfortable with heights

or scrambling. Long pants are recommended because of the sharp vegetation. You'll be traveling mostly along hot, south-facing slopes and open ridges exposed to the sun, so an early-morning start is best in the warmer months.

To Reach the Trailhead: Exit the 210 Freeway at Angeles Crest Highway (Highway 2) in La Cañada-Flintridge. Drive 10.2 miles north to the Colby Canyon Trailhead, at an unpaved turnout on the left at mile marker 34.55.

Description: The lower Colby Canyon Trail is masterfully designed, leading through a gorgeous canyon with year-round water, then along narrow ridges and across a cliff face. This scenic stretch eventually gives way to switchbacks climbing through the chaparral to reach Josephine Saddle at 2.1 miles.

From the saddle, trails depart west toward Josephine Peak and north toward Strawberry Potrero. Head north about 20 yards, then look for a prominent climbers' trail on the right that follows a ridge directly to Strawberry Peak. Take this route, which is generally in good condition because of heavy use. At 2.3 miles, reach the first obstacle: a steep step of decomposing granite. The trail may be vague here, but it's worth finding because getting off route takes you across dangerous crumbling rock. Beyond this step, dodge prickly Whipple

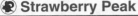 Strawberry Peak

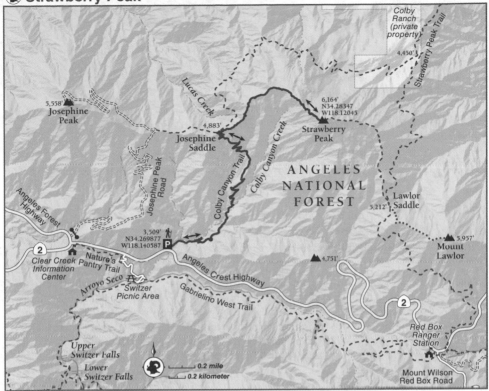

yuccas (also known as chaparral yuccas) on an easy ridge, then pick a path across a talus field to the steep ridge at 3.0 miles, where the climbing gets fun.

Start just right of the crest and look for faded painted arrows or flagging marking the route. The climbing is Class 2–3—fun but nowhere near as difficult as Saunders described—so long as you stay on the easiest route. However, straying from the route quickly leads you to sheer cliffs, and deaths and rescues have occurred here. Pay close attention so you can retrace your route on the descent.

Near the summit, scattered Coulter pines and big-cone Douglas-firs struggle for existence, their windblown limbs swept back in gestures that seem defiant. The view from the top is panoramic, but not as exciting as that from peaks such as Mount Lowe or Mount Lukens. On the other hand, Strawberry often basks in clean air, while the basin-bordering ramparts are wreathed in smog.

VARIATIONS

One could avoid descending the steep rocks and could make a loop around the mountain by descending the trail on the east side to the saddle between Lawlor and Strawberry, then turning north and circling back to Josephine Saddle. A flat beneath the north face has great views and camping beneath a surviving stand of Coulter pines. This loop is 12 miles with 3,500 feet of elevation gain.

Enthusiastic hikers can make a side trip to Josephine Peak from Josephine Saddle. This adds 4 miles out-and-back.

Strawberry Peak can also be climbed from Red Box Gap by way of the saddle between Lawlor and Strawberry. This trail is in good condition all the way and is substantially easier but not nearly as fun. The out-and-back trip is 7 miles with 1,700 feet of elevation gain.

HIKE 26   Cooper Canyon Falls

Location	Central San Gabriel Mountains
Highlight	Beautiful hidden waterfall
Distance & Configuration	3.2-mile out-and-back
Elevation Gain	800'
Hiking Time	1.5 hours
Optional Maps	Tom Harrison *Angeles High Country* or Trails Illustrated *Angeles National Forest*
Best Times	April–November, especially spring
Agency	Angeles National Forest/San Gabriel Mountains National Monument
Difficulty	Moderate
Trail Use	Dogs allowed, good for kids
Permit	National Forest Adventure Pass
Google Maps	Burkhart Trail to Cooper Canyon Falls

Note: This area was within the 2020 Bobcat Fire burn zone but was lightly impacted.

Cooper Canyon Falls roars with the melting snows of early spring and then settles down to a quiet whisper by June or July. You can cool off in the spray of the 25-foot cascade, or at least sit on a water-smoothed log and soak your feet in the chilly, alder-shaded pool just below the base of the falls. In the right season (April or May most years), these falls are one of the best unheralded attractions of the San Gabriel Mountains. The area has very little water by early fall, but the chilly ravines offer outstanding displays of autumn color.

The Burkhart Trail takes you quickly to the falls, downhill all the way, and then uphill all the way back. The forest traversed by the trail is dense enough to give you plenty of cool shade for most of the unrelenting climb back up.

To Reach the Trailhead: From I-210 in La Cañada-Flintridge, drive 34 miles up Angeles Crest Highway (Highway 2) to the Buckhorn Campground entrance road at mile marker 2 LA 58.25. Continue all the way through the campground to the far (northeast) end, where a short stub of dirt road leads to the Burkhart Trailhead. You must display an Adventure Pass in your car to park here.

Description: The Burkhart Trail takes off down the west wall of an unnamed, usually wet canyon garnished by two waterfalls. The first, a little gem of a cascade dropping 10 feet into a rock grotto, is easy to reach by descending from the trailside. The second, some 30 feet high, is dangerous to approach from above, but you can reach it from below by scrambling up the canyon bottom from Cooper Canyon.

At 1.2 miles, the trail bends to the east to follow the south bank of Cooper Canyon.

Cooper Canyon Falls

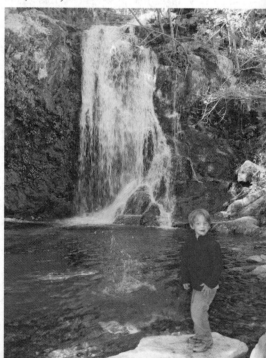

Cooper Canyon Falls

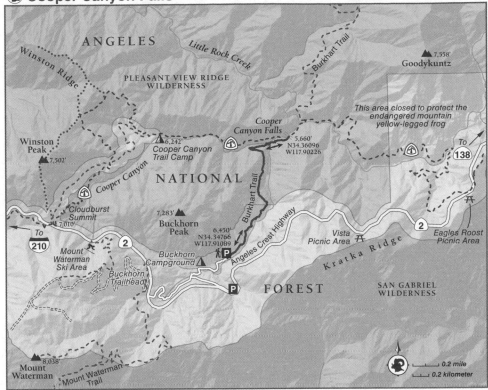

Continue down past the junction with the Pacific Crest Trail, which doubles back to follow the canyon's north bank upstream. At 1.5 miles, look and listen for water plunging over the rocky declivity to the left. A rough pathway leads down off the trail to the alder-fringed pool below. The bottom of the path is steep and slippery and might have a rope that you can use to steady yourself—inspect it before trusting it.

HIKE 27   Mount Waterman Trail

Location	Central San Gabriel Mountains
Highlights	Vistas of yawning canyons, possible bighorn sheep sightings
Distance & Configuration	8-mile point-to-point
Elevation Gain/Loss	1,400'/2,250'
Hiking Time	4.5 hours
Optional Map	Tom Harrison *Angeles High Country*
Best Times	May–November
Agency	Angeles National Forest/San Gabriel Mountains National Monument
Difficulty	Moderately strenuous
Trail Use	Suitable for backpacking, dogs allowed
Permit	None required
Google Maps	Waterman Hiking Trailhead

⊕ Mount Waterman Trail

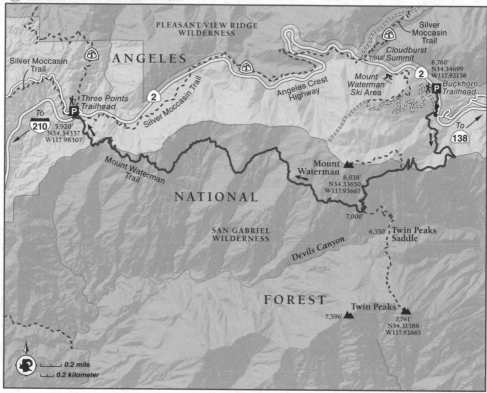

Note: This area was within the 2020 Bobcat Fire burn zone but was lightly impacted.

The Mount Waterman Trail across the north rim of San Gabriel Wilderness provides almost constant views of statuesque pines; yawning chasms; and distant, hazy ridges. You start near the entrance to Buckhorn Campground, and you end up half-circling broad-shouldered Waterman Mountain by the time you arrive at Three Points, 5 miles away by car. Snow can linger on the easternmost mile of the trail until May, but it tends to disappear much earlier on the remaining (mostly south-facing) parts of the trail. This is one of the most popular high-country summer hikes—one heartily recommended for all but the warmest days.

To Reach the Trailhead: This trip requires a 5-mile car or bicycle shuttle between the Three Points and Mount Waterman Trailheads. To reach the Three Points Trailhead from I-210 in

La Cañada-Flintridge, drive 29 miles up Angeles Crest Highway (Highway 2) to an unmarked turnout on the left near mile marker 2 LA 52.66, where you'll leave a getaway vehicle. The Pacific Crest Trail crosses the highway just beyond, but the small signs are easy to miss while driving. If you reach the Sulphur Springs and Santa Clara Divide Road, you've gone 0.1 mile too far. To reach the Mount Waterman Trailhead, continue 5 miles up to a large turnout on the left at mile marker 2 LA 58.02 across the road from the signed trailhead.

If you would prefer to use a bicycle for your shuttle, it is more enjoyable to do the hike in reverse, leaving your bike at the Mount Waterman Trailhead so that your return is mostly downhill. This approach adds 850 feet of elevation gain to the trip. If you don't want to set up a shuttle, try the enjoyable out-and-back (5.5 miles, 1,300′ elevation gain) to Mount Waterman from the Waterman Trailhead.

Description: From the Buckhorn end, follow the well-graded Mount Waterman Trail—not the old roadbed paralleling the trail at first—along a shady slope. Soon, cross another dirt service road. After 1.0 mile of easy ascent through gorgeous mixed-conifer forest, you come to a saddle overlooking Bear Creek. The trail turns west, follows a view-filled ridge, and then ascends on six long switchbacks to a trail junction at 2.1 miles. The trail on your right to Waterman Mountain's flat summit is a worthy side trip (see below). The main trip stays left and contours west, then zigzags south down to a second junction at 3.0 miles. Twin Peaks Saddle, a spacious spot suitable for camping, lies below to the left. If you're day-hiking this stretch, stay right (west).

The remaining 5 miles take you gradually downhill (steeper at the very end) along a generally south-facing slope. You wind in and out of broad ravines, either shaded by huge incense-cedars and vanilla-scented Jeffrey pines or exposed to the warm sunshine on chaparral-covered slopes. The older cedar trees are gnarled veterans of past fires. Portions of this area burned again in the massive 2009 Station Fire, and the last 2 miles of the trail were nearly incinerated.

The rugged topography of San Gabriel Wilderness below conceals herds of Nelson bighorn sheep. This area and another to the east, Sheep Mountain Wilderness, were classified as statutory wilderness areas, in part to preserve the habitat of these magnificent animals. The last 2 miles of the trip join the Pacific Crest Trail, which leads down to your vehicle at the Angeles Crest Highway near Three Points.

VARIATIONS

An excellent way to extend and embellish this hike is to visit the summits of Waterman Mountain and Twin Peaks. Waterman Mountain is an easy 1.6-mile round-trip that adds 400 feet of climbing from the trail junction. Shortly before you reach the summit, watch for an unmarked junction; stay left on the main path that leads up to the summit.

A bit more involved, visiting Twin Peaks adds 4 miles and 1,800 feet of climbing. Take

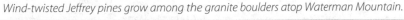

Wind-twisted Jeffrey pines grow among the granite boulders atop Waterman Mountain.

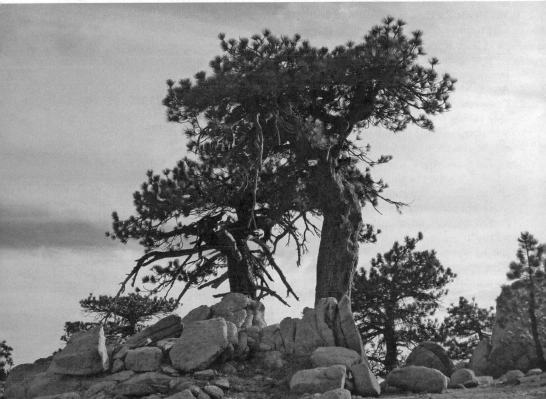

the trail that switchbacks down to Twin Peaks Saddle. A good climber's trail continues south, circling a bump to reach another minor saddle. It then steeply switchbacks up the north face of the peak. Upon reaching the ridgeline, it leads left to the taller and more accessible east summit of Twin Peaks. There, on rock outcrops just below the summit, you will have a dizzying view of the canyons below. Quite often you can look out over a low-lying blanket of smog in the Los Angeles Basin and see Santa Catalina Island floating out at sea beyond the hazy dome of Palos Verdes. The Santa Ana Mountains, Palomar Mountain, the Santa Rosa Mountains, San Jacinto Peak, and Old Baldy arc around the horizon from south to east.

HIKE 28   Devil's Punchbowl

Location	San Gabriel Mountains, north slope
Highlight	Spectacular geological formations
Distance & Configuration	1.4-mile loop
Elevation Gain	300'
Hiking Time	30 minutes
Optional Map	Tom Harrison *Angeles High Country*
Best Times	Sunrise–sunset, all year
Agency	Los Angeles County Parks & Recreation
Difficulty	Easy
Trail Use	Dogs allowed, good for kids
Permit	None required
Google Maps	Devils Punchbowl Natural Area

Note: This area burned in the 2020 Bobcat Fire. The Devil's Punchbowl Natural Area is closed until further notice. Call 661-944-2743 or visit parks.lacounty.gov for updates.

Tens of millions of years in the making, Devil's Punchbowl is without a doubt Los Angeles County's most spectacular geological showplace. Looking down into this 300-foot-deep chasm, you immediately sense the enormity of the forces that produced the tilted and tangled collection of beige sandstone slabs.

The Punchbowl is caught between two active faults—the main San Andreas Fault and an offshoot, the Punchbowl Fault—along which old sedimentary formations have been pushed upward and crumpled downward, as well as transported horizontally. Weathering and erosion have put the final touches on the scene, roughing out the bowl-shaped gorge of Punchbowl Canyon and carving, in a host of unique ways, the rocks exposed at the surface.

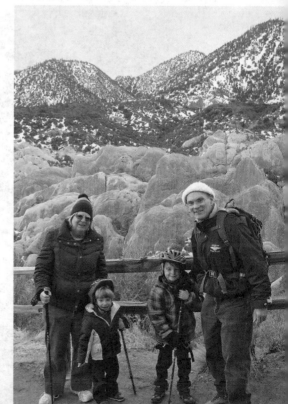

Devil's Punchbowl

Devil's Punchbowl

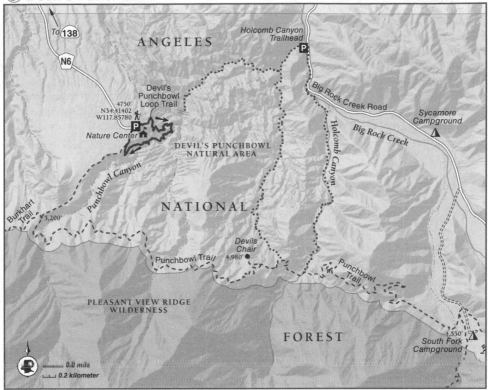

Devil's Punchbowl Natural Area lies in the pinyon-juniper transition zone between the Mojave Desert and the richly forested slopes of the higher San Gabriels. The park features a couple of short nature walks (including the loop trail described here), and the Punchbowl Trail—a part of the High Desert National Recreation Trail. South of the Punchbowl are long-distance trails leading through Angeles National Forest to the high country along Angeles Crest Highway.

To Reach the Trailhead: To reach Devil's Punchbowl from most parts of LA, exit Antelope Valley Freeway (Highway 14) at Pearblossom Highway (Highway 138), and follow it east through the town of Littlerock to Pearblossom. At Pearblossom, turn right (south) on Longview Road (County Road N6), and follow signs for the park, 8 miles ahead. The park is open daily from sunrise to sunset, with no admission charge.

Description: The 1-mile Loop Trail is a perfect introduction to the Punchbowl area. It begins just behind the nature center, zigzags down off the rim to touch the seasonal creek in Punchbowl Canyon, and then climbs back out of the canyon opposite some of the tallest upright rock formations in the park. Near the start of the trail is a side path, the 0.3-mile Piñon Pathway, a self-guided nature trail that loops through the pinyon-juniper forest along the Punchbowl rim.

During winter, occasional snowfalls dust the Punchbowl, leaving a lingering, thicker mantle of white on the pine-dotted slopes above it. At these times the Loop Trail can become muddy and slippery and is, therefore, unsuitable for small children.

VARIATION

Peripatetic walkers may wish to undertake the 6.4-mile round-trip trek via the Punchbowl Trail to the Devil's Chair, which perches on the upper rim of the canyon complex that generally encompasses the Punchbowl. From the parking area, head southwest up a broad path for 0.8 mile to a junction with a trail variously called the Burkhart Trail, the Devil's Chair Trail, the Punchbowl Trail, or the High Desert National Recreation Trail. The Pacific Crest Trail detours through here as well, to protect the endangered mountain yellow-legged frogs near Williamson Rock.

Turn left and proceed east, crossing Punchbowl Creek, climbing, and then undulating. At 3.2 miles, turn left at a signed junction leading to the Devil's Chair. At the fenced viewpoint there, you can peer over what looks like frozen chaos—a vast assemblage of sandstone chunks and slabs tipped at odd angles, bent, seemingly pulled apart here, compressed there. There's a reason for this chaos: Devil's Chair sits astride the crush zone of the Punchbowl Fault.

HIKE 29   Mount Williamson

Location	San Gabriel Mountains
Highlights	Views
Distance & Configuration	4.4-mile out-and-back
Elevation Gain	1,600'
Hiking Time	2.5 hours
Optional Maps	Tom Harrison *Angeles High Country* or Trails Illustrated *Angeles National Forest*
Best Times	May–November
Agency	Angeles National Forest/San Gabriel Mountains National Monument
Difficulty	Moderate
Trail Use	Suitable for backpacking, dogs allowed
Permit	National Forest Adventure Pass
Google Maps	Islip Saddle

Note: This area was within the 2020 Bobcat Fire burn zone.

Mount Williamson—named for US Army lieutenant Robert Stockton Williamson, who explored the northern San Gabriel Mountains in 1853 for the Pacific Railroad Survey—may not be as tall as its brethren on the opposite side of the Angeles Crest Highway, but it is nevertheless one of the most prominent and noteworthy mountains because of its commanding position overlooking the Mojave Desert. This popular hike via the Pacific Crest Trail (PCT) offers excellent views from the trail and summit.

The PCT is closed at Eagles Roost, 4 miles west of Islip Saddle, to protect the endangered mountain yellow-legged frog. You may see detour signs directing PCT hikers down the South Fork Trail, but the detour does not impact this hike.

To Reach the Trailhead: The trail begins at Islip Saddle on the Angeles Crest Highway (Highway 2) at its intersection with Highway 39. Your Adventure Pass must be displayed.

Description: Two trails depart from the north side of the parking lot. This trip takes the one on the left, the official PCT, which climbs steeply. Don't get lured onto the South Fork Trail, which may be marked as the PCT detour route. The trail climbs through a conifer forest, heading to a small saddle and then continuing to wind upward to a point on the south ridge of Mount Williamson, 1.6 miles from the start.

Veer right on an unmaintained but heavily used climber's trail leading up the ridge to Mount Williamson. The huge formation to the west above Little Rock Creek is Williamson Rock, which was a major Southern California sport-climbing destination before it was closed

Mount Williamson

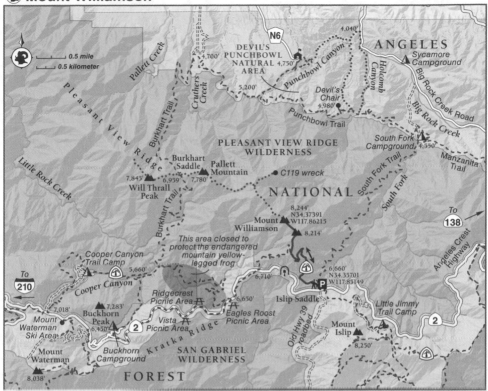

to protect the frogs. Pass a false summit on the right before reaching Mount Williamson's slightly higher true summit at 2.2 miles. A third summit just beyond is about the same height.

From here, you can clearly identify the linear rifts formed by the San Andreas and Punchbowl Faults. On a particularly clear day, you can look across tens of thousands of square miles of desert to see the Southern Sierra Nevada and Telescope Peak above Death Valley. For those

so inclined, there is adequate space to pitch a tent and enjoy exceptional stargazing.

VARIATION

To the north, you may see the metallic glint of wreckage on the northeast ridge of Pallett Mountain. A C-119 Flying Boxcar from March Air Force Base crashed in 1966, scattering aluminum on both sides of the ridge. The 1.5-mile ridge walk to the site is fairly strenuous.

Twin Peaks and Mount Waterman from Mount Williamson

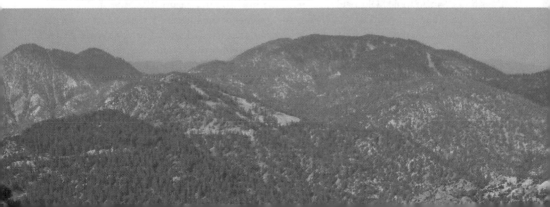

HIKE 30   Mount Baden-Powell Traverse

Location	Eastern San Gabriel Mountains
Highlights	Subalpine habitat, panoramic views, possible bighorn sheep sightings
Distance & Configuration	8-mile point-to-point
Elevation Gain/Loss	2,400'/3,700'
Hiking Time	5 hours
Optional Map	Tom Harrison *Angeles High Country* or Trails Illustrated *Angeles National Forest*
Best Times	May–November
Agency	Angeles National Forest/San Gabriel Mountains National Monument
Difficulty	Moderately strenuous
Trail Use	Suitable for backpacking, dogs allowed
Permit	National Forest Adventure Pass
Google Maps	Dawson Saddle

Note: This area is near the eastern edge of the Bobcat Fire.

Massive Mount Baden-Powell stands head and shoulders above the foggy or smoggy marine layer that often enshrouds the lowlands of the Los Angeles Basin and the Inland Empire. From Baden-Powell's flattish top, the brown Mojave Desert floor stretches interminably inland toward some hazy vanishing point. The disembodied summit ridges of mountain ranges as far west as Ventura County and as far south as San Diego County seem to float over opaque blankets of haze. Santa Catalina, and sometimes other Channel Islands, are visible on an average early-summer morning.

Named in honor of Lord Baden-Powell, the British Army officer who started the Boy Scouts movement in 1907, Baden-Powell soars higher (9,399') than any other mountain in the San Gabriel mountain range—except for the Mount San Antonio (Old Baldy) complex to the east. Many thousands of hikers troop to Baden-Powell's summit yearly, most of them by way of the trail from Vincent Gap on Angeles Crest Highway. Baden-Powell's summit is the last major milestone on the 52-mile trek from Chantry Flat to Vincent Gap known as the Silver Moccasin Trail. The five-day-long Silver Moccasin backpack is a rite of passage for LA-area Scouts (see Hike 31).

If you want to climb Mount Baden-Powell without having to retrace your steps, you can try a one-way hike, described here, from Dawson Saddle to Vincent Gap. The effort is only a bit more than what's involved in the usual round-trip from Vincent Gap, and you'll visit two other peaks as well. All three peaks offer their own unique and panoramic perspective of the rugged Sheep Mountain Wilderness to the south. As the name suggests, this wilderness protects the habitat of the Nelson bighorn sheep, which number several hundred in the San Gabriel Mountains. Early-morning sightings of the bighorn are not unusual on and near Mount Baden-Powell.

At a moderate pace, including a few short breaks and a stop for lunch, the 9-mile hike should take you about 6 hours. Snow accumulations can blanket the area until June. Thereafter, little or no water can be found on the route, so carry plenty of it. The start and end points of the hike are 5 miles apart by way of Angeles Crest Highway, so you should plan to bring either two cars for a car shuttle, or one car plus a bicycle (to be left near the end point for use in returning to your car at the start point after the hike is over). Those planning a bicycle shuttle may prefer to do this hike in reverse so they can coast down the road on the bike. If you don't want to set up a shuttle or the Bobcat Fire

Mount Baden-Powell Traverse

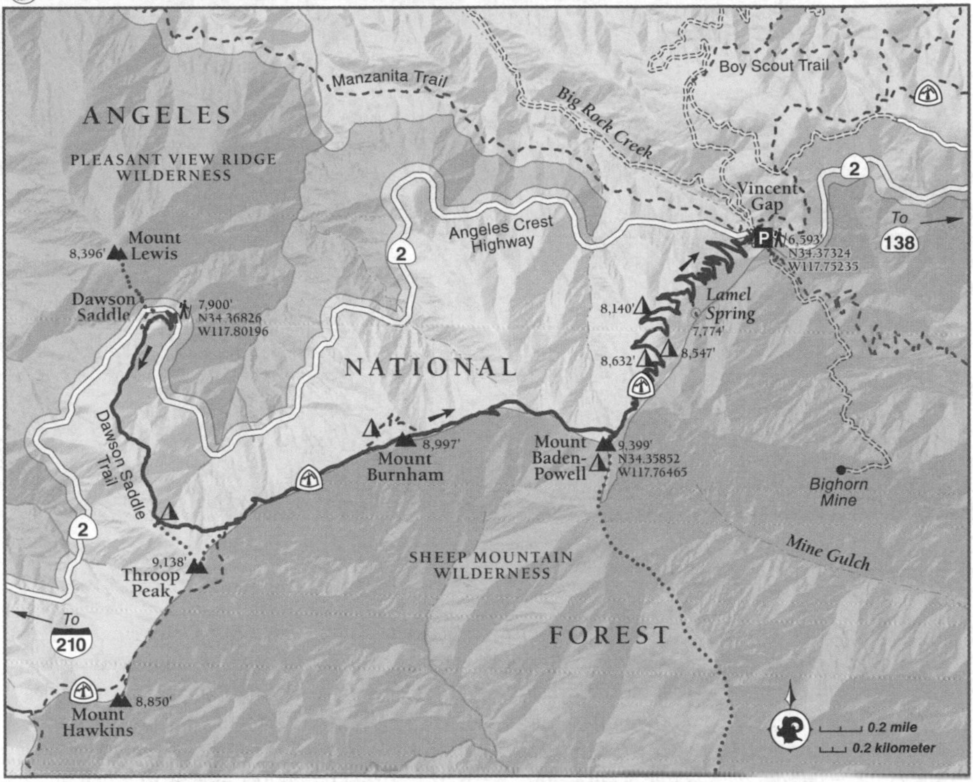

closure is still in effect, you can do this trip as an 8-mile out-and-back from Vincent Gap with 2,800 feet of elevation gain.

Mount Baden-Powell is also a popular winter ascent because Caltrans usually plows the road to Vincent Gap. The icy climb demands crampons, an ice ax, and suitable experience. Most winter climbers return the way they came.

To Reach the Trailhead: From I-15 below the Cajon Pass, take Highway 138 west, and then Highway 2 (the Angeles Crest Highway) west through Wrightwood. Continue 10 miles to the Vincent Gap Trailhead at mile marker 02 LA 74.75. Alternatively, if the Angeles Crest Highway has reopened after the Bobcat Fire, you can reach the trailhead from La Cañada-Flintridge by driving 50 miles east on Highway 2.

Your hike ends at Vincent Gap, but it begins about 5 miles west of Vincent Gap at a point just east of Dawson Saddle at mile marker

02 LA 69.6. There's room for parking along Angeles Crest Highway there, across from where the trail starts. To park at either trailhead, you must display an Adventure Pass. If you prefer to arrange a bicycle shuttle between the trailheads, do the hike in reverse so you can enjoy the downhill ride along the highway.

Description: Beginning at the highway just east of Dawson Saddle, the Dawson Saddle Trail immediately switchbacks uphill (south) through pines and firs to gain the top of a long, gradually ascending ridge that culminates at Throop Peak. Building this trail, which was completed in 1982, required an impressive 3,540 hours of volunteer labor by Boy Scouts. Note that another unsigned, steeper trail starts at Dawson Saddle and joins the main trail in 0.25 mile. About halfway up the trail, lodgepole pines dominate the forest, but keen eyes will spot a few limber pines, which are relatively rare in Southern California. Look closely at the

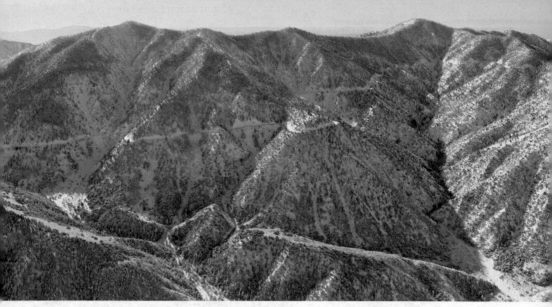

This hike follows the skyline from Dawson Saddle (far right) over Throop (right) to Baden-Powell (left).

needles: lodgepole-pine needles come in bundles of two, while limber pines have bundles of five. Where the trail veers east off the ridge to bypass Throop Peak, step off the trail to find a sheltered campsite on a flat part of the ridge that could accommodate a large Scout troop.

After 1.8 miles you join the Pacific Crest Trail. From this junction, the first side trip takes you southwest on the PCT for 200 yards and then off-trail in the same direction another 300 yards to Throop Peak. This summit and the other two you'll reach later have a hikers' register.

Return to the Dawson Saddle Trail junction, and continue northeast on the PCT, which follows the main, semishaded ridgeline. You will descend to a saddle and then ascend to Mount Burnham's north flank, from which switchbacks take you over to its east shoulder (3 miles). Double back (go west) if you want to take the easy side trip to the summit.

After bagging Mount Burnham, continue east, climbing another breathless 400 feet, to reach the next junction at 4.2 miles. Just above it is Baden-Powell's summit and an impressive monument constructed by the Boy Scouts. Weather-beaten lodgepole and limber pines dot the summit area.

Back at the junction, take the main, heavily traveled trail that descends the northeast ridge

of Baden-Powell. After 40 knee-jarring switchbacks, you reach the end of the descent at the large Vincent Gap parking area on Angeles Crest Highway. About halfway down this trail, from the corner of the 25th switchback, a side trail leads about 200 yards east to a dribbling pipe at Lamel Spring. The spring occasionally dries up in drought years, so you're better off carrying your own water for the full day.

This is a great slope to observe the progression of conifers with altitude. The summit of Mount Baden-Powell is covered in limber and lodgepole pines. Limber pines have 1.5- to 2.5-inch needles in tight bundles of five, medium cones, and famously flexible branches, while lodgepoles have short needles in bundles of two; round, golf ball–size cones; and thin, flaky bark. The ancient limber pine grove is likely a remnant from the last ice age, during which the species was distributed more widely and at lower elevations. One of the most striking specimens is the signed Wally Waldron Tree, named for a longtime Scout leader who led the construction of the Mount Baden-Powell monument. Limber pines disappear below about 9,000 feet on your descent, although they persist down to 8,000 feet on the east ridge, their lowest elevation in Southern California. By 8,650 feet, the beautiful pure stand of lodgepoles gives way to a mixed forest, including white fir and sugar pine. Fir has needles in rows rather than bundles, and the cones grow on the top of the trees and disintegrate in place rather than falling to the ground. Sugar pines have famously long cones, seasonally dripping with sap, and 2.5- to 4-inch needles in bundles of five. The lodgepoles become scarce below 8,100 feet. Jeffrey pines become common below 7,600 feet, with 5- to 10-inch needles in bundles of three and 4- to 8-inch oval cones. Sugar pines are scarce below 7,000 feet. Incense-cedars, with bright-green scales rather than needles, appear around 6,900 feet shortly before you reach the trailhead. Two stands of nonnative giant sequoias were planted at Vincent Gap, recognizable by their awl-shaped leaves.

Backpackers will find room for at least two tents at each saddle on the Angeles Crest. These sites, as well as the north ridge of Baden-Powell, have tremendous views but are exposed to the wind. Larger sheltered sites are located along the trail 0.4 mile before the Throop Peak junction, on the northeast shoulder of Burnham, and about 0.5 mile above Lamel Spring.

HIKE 31 Silver Moccasin Trail

Location	San Gabriel Mountains
Highlight	Backpack across the most beautiful portions of the San Gabriels.
Distance & Configuration	52-mile point-to-point
Elevation Gain/Loss	14,600'/10,200'
Hiking Time	3–7 days
Optional Map	Tom Harrison *Angeles High Country* and *Angeles Front Country*
Best Times	May–November
Agency	Angeles National Forest/San Gabriel Mountains National Monument
Difficulty	Strenuous
Trail Use	Suitable for backpacking, equestrians, dogs; suitable for mountain biking from *Three Points* to *Chantry Flat*
Permit	National Forest Adventure Pass required at both trailheads
Google Maps	Chantry Flat

Note: Portions of this trail were impacted by the 2020 Bobcat Fire.

The Silver Moccasin National Recreation Trail (11W06) runs the length of the San Gabriel Mountains. Starting through chaparral and woods and past a waterfall in Big Santa Anita Canyon, it visits the secluded West Fork San Gabriel River, Chilao's peaceful forest, Cooper Canyon Falls, and the Angeles Crest, culminating on the summit of Mount Baden-Powell. The trail was named by the Boy Scouts and is a rite of passage for thousands of Scouts seeking the coveted 50 Miler or Silver Moccasin badge, but the path had been used for centuries by Native Americans and Anglo settlers for hunting and trade before becoming formalized in the 1930s. The Silver Moccasin Trail coincides with the Gabrielino Trail from Chantry Flats to West Fork Campground, with the Pacific Crest Trail (PCT) from Three Points to Vincent Gap, and with the Angeles Crest 100 ultramarathon route. The trip is long enough for you to adapt to the rhythm of trail life and lose track of time and civilization. You won't find a better trip of this length in Southern California.

There is no good group camping between West Fork and Chilao or between Cooper

Silver Moccasin Trail

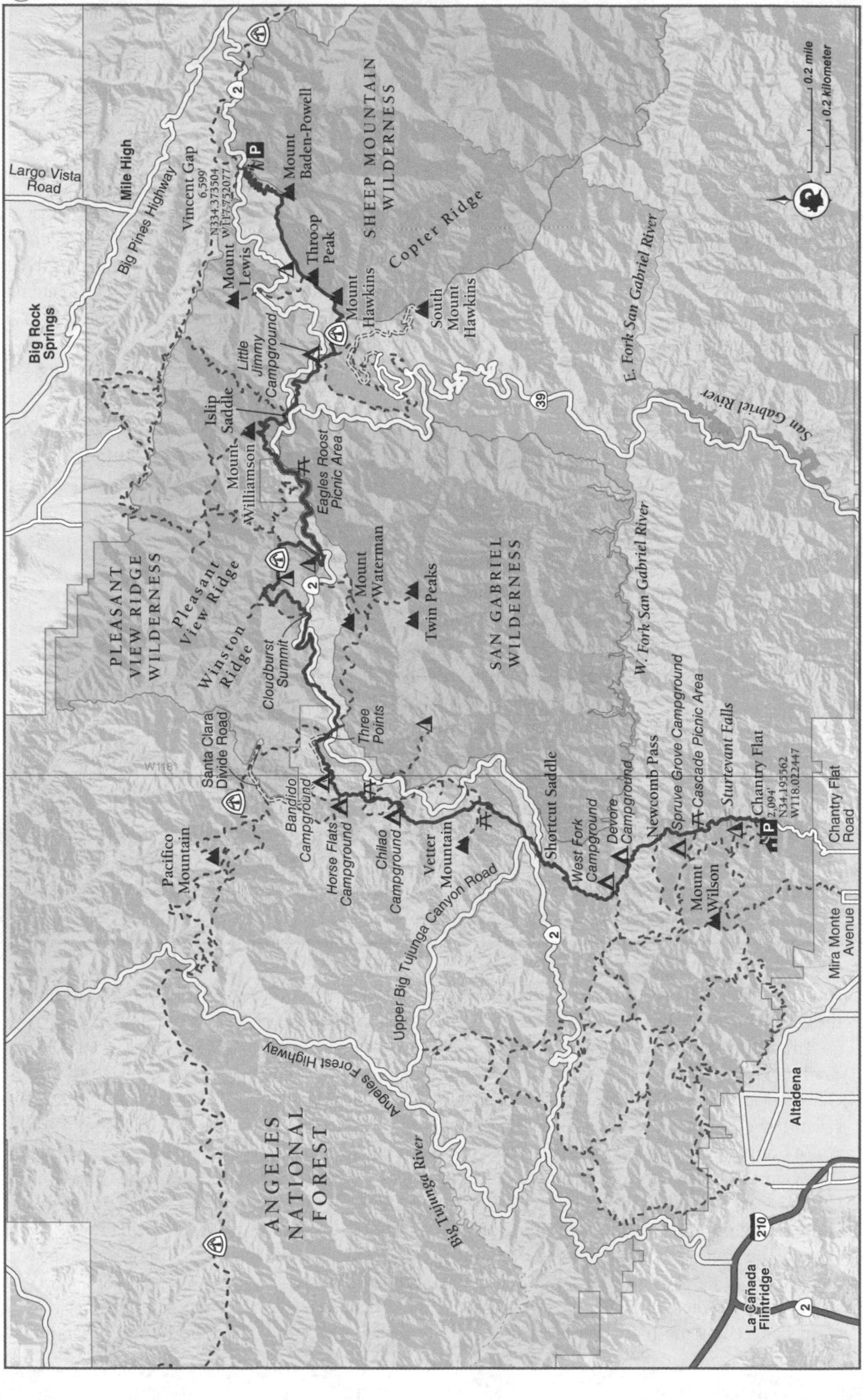

Canyon and Little Jimmy, so you'll have some strenuous hiking days even if you allow a week for the trip. In the winter and spring, the ridge near Mount Baden-Powell is icy and requires an ice ax and crampons and suitable experience; unprepared hikers have died here. By late spring, water can be unreliable for 34 miles between West Fork and Little Jimmy. Check with the U.S. Forest Service before your trip, and cache water jugs near the Angeles Crest Highway crossings if necessary (be sure to carry out the jugs when you collect them). You can find information about water at Cooper Canyon, Buckhorn Campground, and Lamel Spring at the Pacific Crest Trail Water Report (pctwater.com). The PCT is indefinitely closed between the Buckhorn Trail and Eagles Roost to protect the endangered mountain yellow-legged frog, so this trip involves a potentially dangerous walk along the shoulder of the Angeles Crest Highway to bypass the closure. Be careful of poison oak along the trail.

The PCT segment from Vincent Gap to Three Points is closed to mountain bikers, but the Silver Moccasin segment from Three Points to West Fork is considered one of the best rides in the range for advanced cyclists.

To Reach the Trailhead: This hike begins at Chantry Flat and ends at Vincent Gap on the Angeles Crest, so you will need to arrange a car shuttle or have a friend drop you off and pick you up. The 71-mile shuttle between the trailheads takes about 1.5 hours without traffic. To leave a vehicle at Vincent Gap, take I-15 north to Exit 131 (Palmdale/Silverwood Lake). Go left (west) on Highway 138 for 8.5 miles. Turn left (west) on Highway 2 and drive 14.1 miles to the gap at mile marker 2 LA 74.8. To reach Chantry Flat, return to I-15, and take it south 15 miles to the 210 Freeway (Exit 115 B). Go west about 32 miles to Exit 32 for Santa Anita Avenue in Arcadia. Drive north 5 miles to the parking lots at Chantry Flat, passing a vehicle gate that's open 6 a.m.–8 p.m. The lot fills early on weekends, so you may have to backtrack and park along the shoulder.

Description: From the Chantry Flat Trailhead, start down the Gabrielino Trail, which begins as a gated paved road descending into Big Santa

West Fork Campground

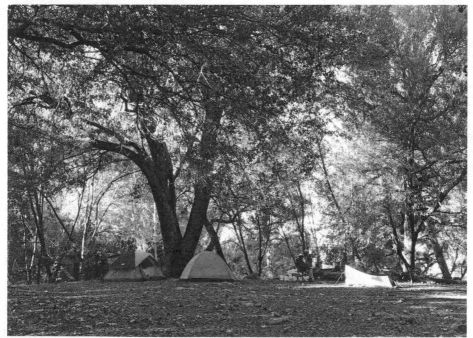

Anita Canyon. The pavement ends at 0.6 mile as you bridge Winter Creek and hike up alder-lined Big Santa Anita Canyon on a roadbed that passes some cabins and soon narrows to a foot trail.

At 1.4 miles come to a four-way junction in a tranquil oak woodland. The right branch goes to Sturtevant Falls, which is a worthy 0.3-mile detour if the creek is flowing well, but generally not impressive in the summer. The left branch is recommended for equestrians or hikers who dislike heights. The middle branch is the most scenic, traversing the face above the waterfall and then following the fern-lined creek past cascades and pools. The left and middle trails reconverge at 2.2 miles.

Continuing up the canyon, reach Cascade Picnic Area at 2.7 miles, where you'll find picnic tables and restrooms near the stream. You'll see many check dams built from concrete blocks resembling Lincoln logs. These dams were installed in the 1960s by the U.S. Forest Service and the Los Angeles County Flood Control District in an effort to reduce the flow of rock and sand into the Big Santa Anita Reservoir. It is hard to imagine that a road once ran through here to bring cement mixers and cranes up the canyon, or that forest managers once believed that pouring cement on a pristine creekbed was a good idea. There's something in nature that doesn't love a dam, and floods and vegetation are gradually restoring the canyon to its original character.

At 3.3 miles reach Spruce Grove Trail Camp, which has water seasonally. (*Spruce* is an older name for the big-cone Douglas-firs that thrive on this side of Mount Wilson.) At 3.5 miles the signed Sturtevant Trail veers left to reach Sturtevant Camp in 0.1 mile. This historic camp was established in 1893 and now has four cabins that you could rent; you must make reservations at sturtevantcamp.com. In a pinch, you could also get water there. However, we stay on the Gabrielino Trail, which steepens as it climbs through chaparral to Newcomb Pass at 5.7 miles.

Switchback down the north side of the pass, crossing the often-closed Rincon–Red Box jeep road, to DeVore Trail Camp on the West Fork of the San Gabriel River at 7.1 miles. Follow the trail west (upstream) to West Fork Trail Camp at 8.2 miles. Both of these fine trail camps have a remote feel as well as reliable water from the

river—this may be the last dependable water for a long time. This canyon was severely impacted by the Bobcat Fire. The Gabrielino Trail continues west, but you'll stay on the Silver Moccasin Trail, which veers north into Shortcut Canyon and then climbs to Shortcut Saddle at mile marker 2 LA 43.30 on the Angeles Crest Highway (Highway 2) at 11.8 miles.

Descend to cross seasonal Big Tujunga Creek at 12.8 miles; then begin a hot climb through chaparral recovering from the 2009 Station Fire. At 14.5 miles pull over a low saddle to cross a service road by a picnic table. At 14.7 miles cross another paved road near the Charlton Flats picnic grounds. The trail curves around the hillside, passing a spur to Vetter Mountain at 15.3 miles; then it meets paved Forest Service Road 3(FS) N16B in the picnic grounds at 15.5 miles. Hike north through a gate; then leave the road at a hairpin turn and continue north along the East Fork of Alder Creek. Eventually, the trail climbs out to meet FS 3N21 near the Chilao Campground Little Pines Loop, just north of the Angeles Crest Highway at mile marker 2 LA 49.69 (17.6 miles). The first-come, first-served campground sometimes has piped water.

Continue on the Silver Moccasin Trail through a pine forest, over a low ridge, and down to the edge of the Upper Chilao Picnic Area at 18.2 miles, where you might again find a faucet. At 18.6 miles recross FS 3N21 at the Chilao Trailhead. Pass Horse Flats Campground (no water) at 19.7 miles and then the Bandido Group Camp (also no water) at 20.1 miles. The trail now turns east and parallels the paved Santa Clara Divide Road to its junction with the Angeles Crest Highway at Three Points (mile marker 2 LA 52.85), where you'll find trailhead parking and an outhouse, 22.2 miles.

Your route now coincides with the PCT and exits the Station Fire burn area but continues to pass patchy scars from the Bobcat Fire. Climb near the Angeles Crest Highway, crossing it three times to reach Cloudburst Summit at 27.0 miles by mile marker 2 LA 57.04. Follow the circuitous trail down (or shortcut down the dirt service road) into Cooper Canyon to find a spacious and scenic trail camp shaded by pines at 29.7 miles. Seasonal water flows in the nearby

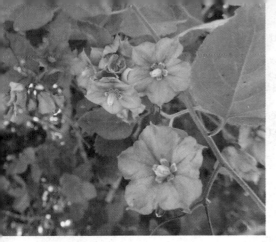

Purple nightshade

creek. At 31.0 miles reach a junction with the Buckhorn Trail. Cooper Canyon Falls is just to the east and is well worth a visit if the creek is flowing. The PCT is closed ahead indefinitely to protect the habitat of the endangered mountain yellow-legged frog. Unless the closure has been lifted, our route turns right and climbs the Burkhart Trail, passing two waterfalls, to reach Buckhorn Campground at 32.6 miles. You may find working water spigots at the campground.

Walk up through the campground and find the paved exit road leading east to meet the Angeles Crest Highway at mile 2 LA 59.05 (33.4 miles). You now face a dull and dangerous walk along the shoulder of the highway to Eagles Roost picnic area at 2 LA 61.65 (36.1 miles). The PCT resumes along Kratka Ridge, a low ridge with stunning views, then crosses back to the north side of the highway at 2 LA 62.50 (37 miles). It then climbs high onto the shoulder of Mount Williamson, passes a spur leading to Williamson's summit, and drops back to cross the highway once more at Islip Saddle, 2 LA 64.0 (39.9 miles).

Beyond the saddle, begin a long, gradual climb toward Mount Baden-Powell. Watch for red currants, which ripen by late summer. At 42.2 miles reach the spacious Little Jimmy Trail Camp, named for cartoonist Jimmy Swinnerton, who drew the *Little Jimmy* comic strip and spent his summers here from 1890 to 1910. The camp has picnic benches and stone ovens. If the sites near the trail are full or noisy, look farther back for more-private spots. Less than a quarter mile beyond the camp, you'll find reliable Little Jimmy Spring beside two huge incense-cedars and many wildflowers.

Continuing on the PCT, reach aptly named Windy Gap at 42.5 miles. Pressure differences between the desert and valley air masses funnel air through this low point in the Angeles Crest. A web of trails radiates from the gap; be sure to continue east on the PCT. At 42.9 miles pass an undeveloped, large campsite at the edge of the burn zone from the 2002 Curve Fire. Continue past climbers' trails leading to Middle Hawkins, Mount Hawkins, and Throop Peak to reach a signed junction with the Dawson Saddle Trail at 45.5 miles.

The next section of the trail, along the Angeles Crest, is perhaps the best part of the whole trip. You'll find a small exposed tent site with amazing views here and at each saddle between Throop and Baden-Powell. At 46.6 miles bypass Mount Burnham on the north side. You'll find another campsite large enough for a troop of Scouts on the northwest slope of the mountain. Major Fredrick Burnham was a cofounder of the Boy Scouts movement. At 47.9 miles reach a short trail on the right leading to the 9,399-foot summit of Mount Baden-Powell. A monument here celebrates Lord Robert Baden-Powell (1857–1941), who founded the Boy Scouts in 1907. You can find more exposed camping on the ridge south of the peak. The only trees growing this high are lodgepole and limber pines, which favor the tallest mountains in Southern California. Lodgepole pines have needles in bundles of two and round, golf ball–size cones, while limber pines have needles in bundles of five and longer, 4- to 6-inch cones on their flexible branches. The Wally Waldron Tree at the junction below the summit is a twisted limber pine believed to be 1,500 years old.

The trip ends with 40 knee-jarring switchbacks that descend to Vincent Gap. Halfway down, you'll pass three undeveloped campsites and then a signed spur at a switchback that leads 100 yards to seasonal Lamel Spring, in a ravine.

POSSIBLE ITINERARY			
DAY	CAMP	MILES	ELEVATION GAIN
1	West Fork	8.2	2,700'
2	Chilao	9.4	3,400'
3	Cooper Canyon	12.1	2,600'
4	Little Jimmy	12.5	3,600'
5	(exit)	9.5	2,300'

HIKE 32   Mount Islip

Location	Crystal Lake Recreation Area
Highlight	Ocean-to-desert views
Distance & Configuration	8-mile loop
Elevation Gain	2,400'
Hiking Time	4 hours
Optional Map	Tom Harrison *Angeles High Country*
Best Times	May–November
Agency	Angeles National Forest/San Gabriel Mountains National Monument
Difficulty	Moderately strenuous
Trail Use	Suitable for backpacking, dogs allowed
Permit	None required
Google Maps	Crystal Lake Recreation Area

Note: This area was at the edge of the 2020 Bobcat Fire burn zone.

Mount Islip is named for George Islip, a mountain man who lived in San Gabriel Canyon before 1880. The south approach of the peak, one of the significant high points in the San Gabriel Mountains, feels a bit like real mountain climbing, despite its rather straightforward ascent by way of marked trails. You begin amid spreading oaks and tall conifers in Crystal Lake Basin, rise through progressively smaller and sparser timber, and finally reach the nearly bald and often windblown summit. On clear days it offers a comprehensive view, both north over the Mojave Desert and south over the metropolis.

For the slight effort of an extra half mile on the way up or down, you can spend the night at Little Jimmy Campground, one of the nicest trail camps in the San Gabriels. In the spring, ice may linger on the steep north-facing slopes and you may prefer to take the Big Cienega Trail in both directions.

To Reach the Trailhead: From I-210 in Azusa, drive north on Azusa Avenue, which becomes San Gabriel Canyon Road (Highway 39) as it passes flood-control basins at the mouth of San Gabriel Canyon. Continue 24 miles north through the canyon to the Crystal Lake Recreation Area turnoff. Drive a half mile past the Crystal Lake Visitor Center to the main hikers' parking lot.

Description: Start hiking on the marked Windy Gap Trail. On the way to Windy Gap, you cross the Mount Hawkins Truck Trail twice (at the first crossing the road is paved, and at the second it's dirt), pass the Big Cienega Trail, and then tackle the steep, upper slopes of the cirque-like rim overlooking Crystal Lake basin. Windy Gap is the lowest spot on the north side of that rim and earns its name when high-pressure air masses over the Mojave Desert push their way into the Los Angeles Basin. Ghostly stands of dead trees testify to the inferno of the 2002 Curve Fire that swept through the basin.

At Windy Gap (2.5 miles), you meet the Pacific Crest Trail, which joins from the right (east). Continue north 0.7 mile on the PCT

Crystal Lake Basin is a good place to look for blazing stars in the summer.

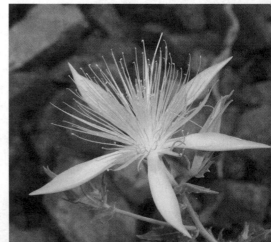

Mount Islip

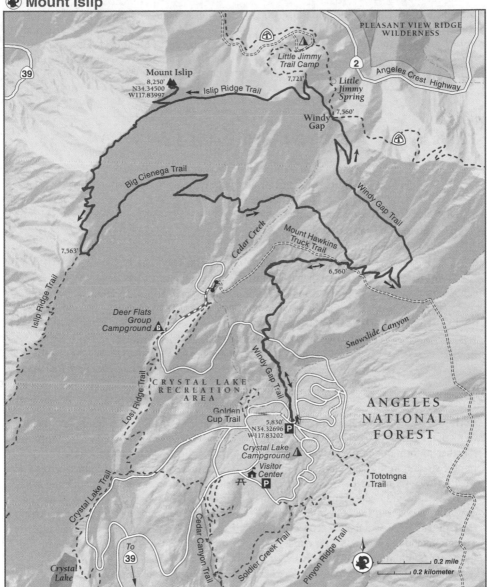

to the next junction. Going right takes you to Little Jimmy Campground, but this trip goes left up the sunny east ridge of Mount Islip to its summit. (*Note:* Hard snow or ice can linger on the steep, north-facing slopes north of Windy Gap until sometime in May. You can avoid that stretch if need be by going straight up the east shoulder of Mount Islip from Windy Gap; that route becomes snow-free earlier in the season.)

On the summit (3.5 miles), you'll discover the shell of an old stone cabin and footings of a fire lookout tower that stood on Islip from 1927 until 1937, when the lookout was moved southeast to a better site, South Mount Hawkins. That structure was completely destroyed in the 2002 Curve Fire.

On your return, for the sake of variety, you can follow the Islip Ridge and Big Cienega Trails. Two switchbacks below the summit of

Mount Islip, turn right on the Islip Ridge Trail, which goes down Islip's south ridge all the way to Crystal Lake. You, however, travel partway down Islip Ridge Trail and then veer east on Big Cienega Trail (4.7 miles). After gradually descending along wooded south-facing slopes, you join the Windy Gap Trail just north of the upper crossing of Mount Hawkins Truck Trail (6.7 miles). Turn right and return to the hikers' parking lot.

HIKE 33   Down the East Fork

Location	San Gabriel River, San Gabriel Mountains
Highlights	An epic trek along a cascading stream, with nearly a vertical mile of descent
Distance & Configuration	16-mile point-to-point
Elevation Gain/Loss	200'/4,800'
Hiking Time	11 hours
Recommended Map	Tom Harrison *Angeles High Country*
Best Times	May–November
Agency	Angeles National Forest/San Gabriel Mountains National Monument
Difficulty	Strenuous
Trail Use	Suitable for backpacking, dogs allowed
Permit	National Forest Adventure Pass required at Vincent Gap; self-issued permit required if starting from the East Fork Trailhead
Google Maps	Vincent Gap

Born from snow-fed rivulets, the many tributaries of the East Fork San Gabriel River gather together to form one of the liveliest and most remote streams in the San Gabriel Mountains. At The Narrows of the East Fork, the water squeezes through the deepest gorge in Southern California. From the bottom of The Narrows, the east wall soars about 5,200 feet to Iron Mountain, and the west wall rises about 4,000 feet to the South Mount Hawkins divide.

On this grand journey down the upper East Fork, you'll descend nearly a mile in elevation, travel from high-country pines and firs to sun-scorched chaparral, and cross three important geologic faults: the Punchbowl, Vincent Thrust, and San Gabriel Faults. During the course of a single day, you could experience a temperature increase of as much as 60°F.

You can do this hike in one incredibly long day with an early start, or you can camp overnight on one of the shaded streamside terraces near the midpoint of the trek. You'll find sites every mile or so; the best camping sites include former trail camps at Fish and Iron Forks and the lower part of The Narrows.

The upper part of the canyon receives few visitors and remains pristine, while the lower portion is heavily traveled by day hikers and "prospectors" panning for gold in the creek. If everyone hauls out a bit of the detritus left behind by thoughtless users, the canyon will become more attractive.

This route passes through the Sheep Mountain Wilderness. Currently, a wilderness permit is required only if you start the trip from the south at the East Fork Trailhead; they're available at a self-service trailhead kiosk at the parking area.

Navigation on the trip is easy throughout—you simply head downcanyon the whole way. Consult a detailed map often if you want to confirm exactly where you are. Heavy runoff after a storm or major snowmelt can create hazardous stream crossings, which is one of the reasons why this trip is recommended

Down the East Fork

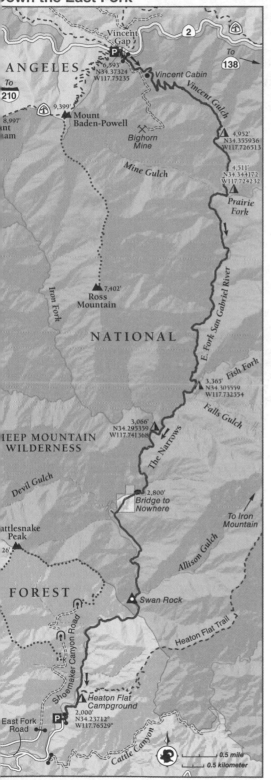

only from late spring through fall. Contact the Angeles National Forest rangers for current conditions. The other reason is that snow may block access to the upper trailhead at Vincent Gap, although Highway 2 is usually plowed to Vincent Gap. Check dot.ca.gov for road conditions; if the highway is listed as "closed 5 miles west of Big Pines," it is open to Vincent Gap.

It's practical to have someone drop you off at the starting point, Vincent Gap, and later pick you up at the hike's end, East Fork Station. That being said, it is important to note that the amount of time required to complete the trip can vary greatly due to problems with adverse weather or swift-flowing water, a stretch of excessive bushwhacking along the banks of the upper river, how heavy a pack you are carrying, and the hiking ability of your party's slowest member. This is not a trip for hikers without plenty of successful experience in off-trail wilderness travel. Allow some flexibility in your planned arrival time at the end.

Cars parked at either the start or the end point will need to display an Adventure Pass.

If you don't want to arrange a car shuttle, you can join the throngs hiking to the Bridge to Nowhere from the East Fork Trailhead. This out-and-back trip is 9.5 miles with 1,000 feet of elevation gain.

To Reach the Trailhead: This trip requires a 1.5-hour, 81-mile car shuttle. Leave a getaway vehicle at the East Fork Trailhead: From the 210 Freeway in Azusa, take Exit 40 for northbound San Gabriel Canyon Road (Highway 39), and drive 12 miles to East Fork Road, on the right. Continue up East Fork Road 6 miles to a parking lot at the end. You can get a self-issued wilderness permit at a box by the outhouse. To reach the Vincent Gap Trailhead, return to the 210 Freeway and take it east about 23 miles to I-15 (Exit 64A), then north about 16 miles to Highway 138 (Exit 131). Drive west on Highway 138 for 8.6 miles; then turn left onto Angeles Crest Highway (Highway 2) and go 14 miles to the Vincent Gap Trailhead parking lot, at mile marker 74.88. Better yet, have somebody drop you off and then pick you up later.

Description: From the parking area on the south side of Vincent Gap, walk down the gated road to the southeast. At a signed junction in 0.2 mile, the Mine Gulch Trail veers left, into Sheep Mountain Wilderness. Take it; the road itself continues toward the Bighorn Mine, an abandoned stamp mill from the gold rush era.

Intermittently shaded by big-cone Douglas-firs, white firs, Jeffrey pines, and live oaks, the path descends along the south slope of Vincent Gulch. The gulch itself follows the Punchbowl Fault, a splinter of the San Andreas. At 0.7 mile, on a flat ridge spur, look for an indistinct path on the right that leads about 100 yards, passing a tangle of downed trees, to an old cabin believed to have been the home of Charles Vincent. Vincent led the life of a hermit, prospector, and big-game hunter in the Baden-Powell and Old Baldy area from 1870 until his death in 1926.

After a few switchbacks, the primitive trail crosses Vincent Gulch (usually dry at this point, but wet a short distance below) at 1.6 miles. Thereafter it stays on or above the east bank. Pass a tributary on the left at 2.0 miles, and then a second one at 2.5 miles. An unsigned trail leads to a fine campsite in the second tributary, but you should be careful to stay right and drop onto the floor of the main drainage.

The trail soon becomes indistinct, and you must pick your own path down the rocky floor of Vincent Gulch. At 3.1 miles, watch for the wreck of a Schweizer sailplane. In February 1974, the plane was caught in a severe downdraft on the flank of Mount Baden-Powell and became trapped in the canyon. The occupants walked away with minor injuries, but the plane was unsalvageable.

A large sign marks the confluence of Prairie Fork, a wide drainage coming in from the east at 4.2 miles from the start. A trail once led up this canyon to Cabin Flat, but it was obliterated by the 1997 Beiderbach Fire and is now heavily overgrown with poison oak and stinging nettles. You veer right (west) down a gravelly wash, good for setting up a camp.

Shortly after, at the Mine Gulch confluence, you bend left (south) into the wide bed of the upper East Fork. For several miles to come, there is essentially no trail. It may take several hours to traverse this stretch, depending on your group's energy and motivation. To help you gauge your progress, you can often see Iron Mountain, the major summit to the south.

Proceed down the rock-strewn floodplain, crossing the creek (and battling alder thickets) several times over the next mile. The canyon becomes narrow for a while, and you must wade or hop from one slippery rock to another. Fish Fork, on the left at 7.9 miles from the start, is the first large stream south of Prairie Fork. One of the best campsites along the canyon can be found here.

If you have time for an intriguing side trip, Fish Fork canyon is well worth exploring. Chock-full of alder and bay, narrow with soaring walls, and with its clear stream tumbling over boulders, the canyon boasts one of the wildest and most beautiful settings in the San Gabriels. About 1.6 miles upstream lies a formidable impasse: there, the waters of Fish Fork drop 12 feet into an emerald-green pool set amid sheer rock walls. A bigger waterfall, inaccessible by means of this approach, lies farther upstream.

At 8.2 miles, you may observe a thin column of water dropping over the cliff at the mouth of Falls Gulch on the left. In another mile, you enter The Narrows. A rough trail, worn in by hikers, traverses this 1-mile-plus section of fast-moving water. You'll pass swimmable (if chilly) pools cupped in the granite and schist bedrock and cross the stream when necessary. Listen and watch for water ouzels (dippers) by the edges of the pools. Old mining trails once threaded the canyon walls here and to the north, but they are all virtually obliterated now.

At the lower portals of The Narrows at 10.7 miles, you come upon the enigmatically named Bridge to Nowhere. During the 1930s, road builders managed to push a highway up along the East Fork stream to just this far. The arched, concrete bridge, similar in style to those built along Angeles Crest Highway, was to be a key link in a route that would carry traffic between the San Gabriel Valley and the desert near Wrightwood. Fate intervened. A great flood in 1938 thoroughly demolished most of the road, leaving the bridge stranded. A later attempt to construct a road through the East Fork gorge also resulted in failure. High on the canyon's west rim lies Shoemaker Canyon Road, a "road to nowhere."

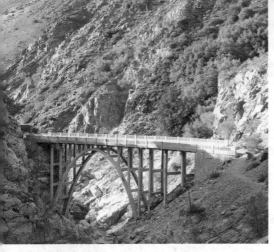

Bridge to Nowhere

Below the bridge, on remnants of the old road washed out in 1938, you'll run into more and more hikers, anglers, and other travelers out for the day. The east side of the canyon generally has a decent trail, but that occasionally becomes harder to find when you are forced over to the west side. At 12.7 miles, Swan Rock, an outcrop of metamorphic rock branded with the light-colored imprint of a swan, comes into view on the right. At 15.0 miles you come upon Heaton Flat Campground. From there a final, easy 0.5-mile stroll takes you to the East Fork Station and trailhead at the end of East Fork Road.

HIKE 34   Old Baldy Loop

Location	Eastern San Gabriel Mountains
Highlights	Panoramic views along the Devils Backbone and atop LA County's highest point
Distance & Configuration	10.5-mile loop
Elevation Gain	3,900'
Hiking Time	6 hours
Optional Map	Tom Harrison *Angeles High Country*
Best Times	June–October
Agency	Angeles National Forest/San Gabriel Mountains National Monument
Difficulty	Strenuous
Trail Use	Suitable for backpacking, dogs allowed
Permit	None required
Google Maps	Manker Flat

Mount Baldy is one of the most popular hikes in Southern California. Its summit, the highest in the San Gabriel Mountains and Los Angeles County, offers breathtaking views, yet the route is straightforward for a hiker of average ability. There are many routes on the mountain, but this one is especially enjoyable because it makes a loop up past the Baldy Bowl and down along the stunning Devils Backbone to the ski area at the Baldy Notch. From here, one can follow a dirt service road back to Manker Flats. This is a deceptively dangerous route when icy, and only experienced mountaineers with ice ax, crampons, and sufficient knowledge should attempt it under winter or spring conditions.

If you are looking for the easiest way to the summit, take the ski lift to Baldy Notch and hike the Devils Backbone, 6 miles out-and-back with 2,300 feet of elevation gain.

To Reach the Trailhead: From the 210 Freeway in Claremont, take Exit 52 for Base Line Road. Go west on Base Line for 0.2 mile; then turn right (north) on Padua Avenue. In 1.8 miles turn right onto Mount Baldy Road. Follow it 11.7 miles to Manker Flats, where you can park along the road.

Description: From Manker Flats, walk west through a gate and up a service road. In 0.5 mile the road makes a hairpin turn, and you

⊕ Old Baldy Loop

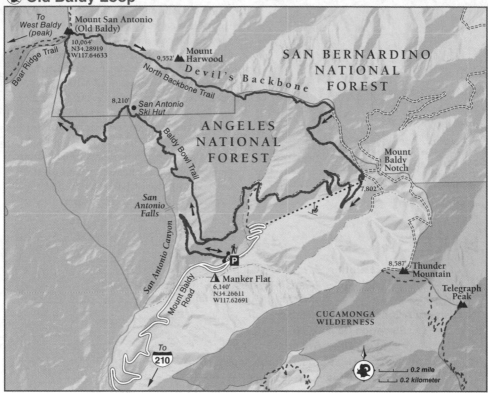

have an excellent view of San Antonio Falls. At 0.9 mile look for the Baldy Bowl Trail switchbacking up the slope to the left. It is easy to miss; if you get to a point directly overlooking Manker Flats, you have gone too far.

Follow the trail through an open forest up to a Sierra Club ski hut, built by volunteers in 1937, on the right at 2.4 miles. Use of the hut is by reservation only, through the Angeles Chapter of the Sierra Club. Trail campers without reservations are invited to camp in the so-called Rock Garden about 200 yards southwest of the hut.

The ski hut marks the halfway point of the ascent in distance and elevation gain. Just beyond, cross the head of San Antonio Creek beneath the scree-filled Baldy Bowl. This area is a backcountry skier's paradise in the winter and early spring. On a rare quiet day, it is also a good place to look for bighorn sheep.

The trail continues around the southwest edge of Baldy Bowl, crossing a field of talus and switchbacking up to the ridge (3.1 miles). *Note:*

Shady spots along this part of the trail remain icy long after most of the mountain has melted out. Expert mountaineers have had serious and fatal slips on this seemingly innocuous stretch of trail.

Now follow the ridge north. At 3.5 miles, at a sign labeled BALDY BOWL TRAIL, look for a use trail dropping into the canyon. On October 5, 1945, a Curtiss C-46 Commando grazed the cloud-covered ridge of Mount Baldy and tumbled down the canyon. You can find wreckage strewn down the gully, with the largest wing section 0.1 mile below the trail. Our trip, however, climbs on to the windswept summit above treeline (4.1 miles). Rock rings provide partial shelter while you picnic. Camping can be magnificent on a calm night, or an ordeal in adverse weather. Most days you can easily make out the other two members of the triad of Southern California giants—San Gorgonio Mountain and San Jacinto Peak—about 50 miles east and southeast, respectively. On days of crystalline clarity, the Old Baldy panorama includes 90

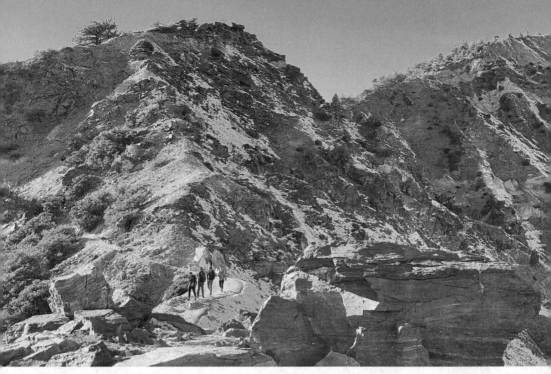
The Devil's Backbone is the most dramatic portion of Mount Baldy.

degrees of ocean horizon, a 120-degree slice of the tawny desert floor, and the far-off ramparts of the southern Sierra Nevada and the Panamint Range, as much as 160 miles away.

After taking in the magnificent scenery, descend east along the Devils Backbone Trail. Beware that five trails depart the summit ridge and that many hikers have headed the wrong way, especially when visibility is poor. This spectacular trail passes along the south side of Mount Harwood and then follows a knife-edge ridge down to the ski area at Baldy Notch. The Devil's Backbone, once a hair-raiser, lost most of

its terror when the Civilian Conservation Corps constructed a wider and safer trail, complete with guardrails, in 1935–36. The guardrails are gone now, but there's plenty of room to maneuver, unless there are strong winds or ice on the trail. Devil's Backbone offers grand vistas of both the Lytle Creek drainage on the north and east and San Antonio Canyon on the south.

From the lodge at Baldy Notch (7.2 miles, 7,800'), follow the service road descending to the southwest. Pass the original junction with the Baldy Bowl Trail before reaching Manker Flats.

HIKE 35   Baldy via Bear Ridge

Location	Eastern San Gabriel Mountains
Highlights	Strenuous and spectacular climb via Mount Baldy's original trail
Distance & Configuration	13-mile out-and-back
Elevation Gain	5,800'
Hiking Time	7 hours
Optional Map	Tom Harrison *Angeles High Country*
Best Times	June–October

Agency	Angeles National Forest/San Gabriel Mountains National Monument
Difficulty	Strenuous
Trail Use	Dogs allowed, suitable for backpacking
Permit	None required
Google Maps	Mount Baldy Trout Pool

The great south ridge of Mount Baldy rises directly from Mount Baldy Village to the summit and climbs nearly 6,000 feet in 3.5 horizontal miles. The trail offers the greatest sustained elevation gain of any in the San Gabriel Mountains. According to the Winter 1934 issue of *Trails Magazine,* "This is a hard one-day trip, but is often done." Nowadays you will avoid the usual Baldy crowds until reaching the summit. Most hikers will appreciate trekking poles. Start early in summer because the switchbacks above Bear Flat are long and shadeless. The ridge is icy in the winter and can be deadly.

This trail was built in the summer of 1889 by Fred Dell and his crew. Dell was the owner of Dell's Camp, a resort in San Antonio Canyon. The trail, passable by horses, cut about 4 miles off the previous approach of taking a miner's trail to Baldy Notch and then hiking the backbone. The work was financed by Dr. B. H. Fairchild of Claremont, who hoped to persuade Harvard to place an observatory on the summit. A November blizzard discouraged the Harvard astronomers, and the observatory stayed on Mount Wilson, but hikers still enjoy the trail. From 1910 to 1913, William Dewey used the trail to operate the Baldy Summit Inn, six tent cabins on the mountaintop. The venture ended when the tents burned in a cooking fire.

Baldy via Bear Ridge

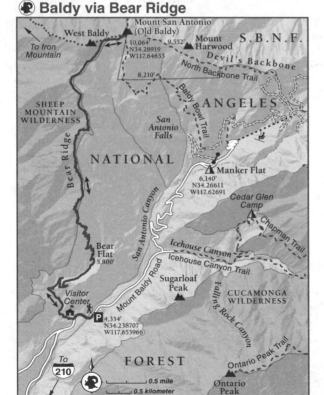

To Reach the Trailhead: From the 210 Freeway in Claremont, take Exit 52 for Base Line Road. Go west on Base Line Road 0.2 mile; then turn right (north) on Padua Avenue. In 1.8 miles turn right on Mount Baldy Road. Follow it 7.6 miles to the Mount Baldy Trout Pools, where you will find plenty of parking across the road above Mount Baldy Village.

Description: Walk 0.3 mile back down Mount Baldy Road and take a right on Bear Canyon Road just below the visitor center. Hiker parking is not permitted along this road. Walk up Bear Canyon Road past numerous cabins.

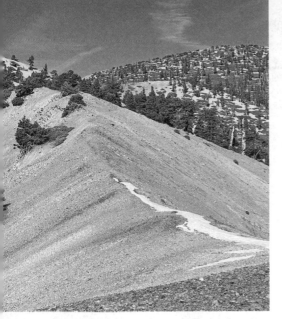

Upper Bear Ridge

When the road ends at 0.7 mile, turn right onto the Bear Canyon Trail (7W12, here signed MT. BALDY TRAIL). Switchback up through the canyon live oaks and big-cone Douglas-firs, then across a sunbaked slope and back into the canyon to reach Bear Flat (2 miles, 5,400').

The 2008 Bighorn Fire burned from Bear Flat up to the ridge, and the slopes are now smothered in dense ceanothus, scrub oak, and manzanita. The trail makes 16 switchbacks through the burn zone before reaching the first intact Jeffrey pines. Enjoy views of Icehouse Canyon and the surrounding peaks. Another rack of less-distinct switchbacks brings you to

Bear Ridge, the halfway point on the trip (3.4 miles, 7,200'). Sugar pines and white firs join the forest, and the thick chaparral gives way to an open understory of manzanita. You could pitch a tent here at a small clearing.

Hike up the ridge, enjoying more great views. At 4.4 miles, near the 8,400-foot contour, the ridge merges with a second ridge to the east, rising from Lookout Mountain, and dramatic views open into Cattle Canyon. At 4.9 miles (9,000'), cross a section known as The Narrows, where the ridge drops steeply on both sides. For the remainder of the trip, you are in a beautiful open forest of lodgepole pines, often sculpted by weather into unusual shapes until they vanish entirely on the bald summit.

The final stretch is gentler, climbing the upper ridge and traversing across the southeast side of West Baldy to reach the high point of the San Gabriel Mountains (6.5 miles). This is a good place to watch for elusive desert bighorn sheep. The trail passes close by West Baldy before reaching the true summit. You could spend a memorable night on the summit, but the winds can be ferocious. Return the way you came.

VARIATION

If you left a bike or car at Manker Flats, descend the Devils Backbone or Baldy Bowl Trail (see Hike 34). These options are highly recommended because they are spectacular, you avoid retracing your steps, and you save your knees from the brutal descent.

HIKE 36   Cucamonga Peak

Location	Eastern San Gabriel Mountains
Highlights	Alder-shaded stream, stupendous valley views
Distance & Configuration	12-mile out-and-back
Elevation Gain	4,300'
Hiking Time	7 hours
Optional Map	Tom Harrison *Angeles High Country*
Best Times	May–November
Agency	San Bernardino National Forest/Front Country Ranger District
Difficulty	Strenuous
Trail Use	Dogs allowed, suitable for backpacking

Permit National Forest Adventure Pass and
Cucamonga Wilderness permit required
Google Maps Icehouse Canyon Trailhead

Cucamonga Peak's south and east slopes feature some of the most dramatic relief in the San Gabriel range. At 8,859 feet, the peak stands sentinel only 4 miles from the edge of the broad inland valley region known as the Inland Empire. Go all the way to the top for the view, but don't be too disappointed if you see only haze and smog. So much beautiful high country can be seen along the way that reaching the top is just icing on the cake.

Most of the hike lies within Cucamonga Wilderness, which requires a permit for both day and overnight use east of Icehouse Saddle. You can obtain your permit by calling the San Bernardino National Forest Front Country Ranger District Office at 909-382-2851 or applying online from the Forest Service website (fs.usda.gov/sbnf).

Near Cucamonga's summit you'll tackle a steep, north-facing gully that can retain snow into May. Be sure to discuss with a ranger the possible hazards of snow and ice if it's early or late in the year.

To Reach the Trailhead: Exit I-210 at Mills Avenue in Claremont, and follow Mills north toward the mountains. After 1.8 miles Mills veers right and becomes Mount Baldy Road. An 8-mile climb up through San Antonio Canyon on Mount Baldy Road takes you to the small village of Mount Baldy and a national-forest ranger station on the left where you can pick up the needed wilderness permit.

Continue 1.5 miles past the village to a short spur road on the right signed NO OUTLET. Park at the end of that spur, which is the trailhead for

Cucamonga Peak

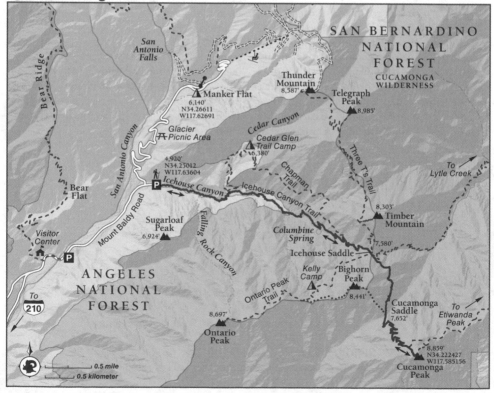

the Icehouse Canyon Trail, and don't forget to post an Adventure Pass on your car. This popular trailhead sometimes fills up by midmorning on busy weekends.

Description: Walk up the Icehouse Canyon Trail following the alder-shaded, boulder-filled streambed, which may be dry at its lowermost end. The first couple of miles along the canyon are a fitting introduction to a phase of Southern California scenery unfamiliar to many visitors and newcomers. Huge big-cone Douglas-fir, incense-cedar, and live oak trees cluster on the banks of the flowing stream, which dances over boulders and fallen logs. Moisture-loving flowering plants like columbine sway in the breeze. Some of the old cabins along the lower canyon survive, while others, destroyed by flood or fire, have left evidence of their existence in the form of foundations or rock walls.

Old newspaper reports suggest that an ice-packing operation existed in or near Icehouse Canyon during the late 1850s. The ice was packed down San Antonio Canyon on mules to a point accessible to wagons, whereupon it was carted, as quickly as possible, to Los Angeles for use in making ice cream and for chilling beverages. Whether ice was quarried in this canyon or in another, Icehouse Canyon's name is apt enough: cold air flowing downcanyon produces refrigerator-like temperatures on many a summer morning and deep-freeze temperatures in winter.

Chapman Trail (a longer, alternate route) intersects on the left (north) at 1.0 mile. At Columbine Spring (2.4 miles, the last water during the warmer months), the trail starts switchbacking up the north wall. After passing the upper intersection of the Chapman Trail at 2.9 miles, you continue to pine-shaded Icehouse Saddle at 3.5 miles, where trails converge from many directions. The trail to Cucamonga's summit contours southeast, descends moderately, and climbs to a 7,654-foot saddle at 4.4 miles, between Bighorn and Cucamonga Peaks. Thereafter, it switchbacks up a steep slope dotted with lodgepole pines and white firs.

At 5.8 miles, the trail crosses a shady draw 200 feet below and northwest of the Cucamonga Peak summit. An indistinct path goes straight up to the top, 6.0 miles from your starting point at the Icehouse Canyon trailhead. Return the same way, or take the alternate route, the Chapman Trail, if you'd like to explore a longer but scenic descent from Icehouse Saddle.

The Diving Board on Cucamonga Peak

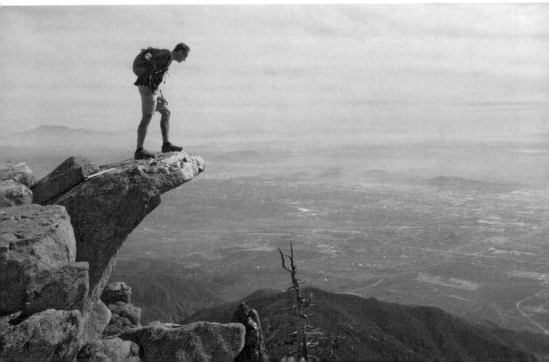

HIKE 37   The Three T's

Location	Eastern San Gabriel Mountains
Highlights	Great views, ridgeline traverse
Distance & Configuration	13-mile point-to-point with a short shuttle
Elevation Gain/Loss	5,000'/4,000'
Hiking Time	8 hours
Optional Map	Tom Harrison *Angeles High Country*
Best Times	May–November
Agency	Angeles National Forest/San Gabriel Mountains National Monument
Difficulty	Strenuous
Trail Use	Dogs allowed, suitable for backpacking
Permit	National Forest Adventure Pass
Google Maps	Icehouse Canyon Trailhead

Timber, Telegraph, and Thunder Mountains form the undulating northeast wall of San Antonio Canyon. This superb romp over the three T's begins up Icehouse Canyon and descends through the ski resort at Baldy Notch. For an easier hike that shaves off 3 miles and more than half the elevation gain, take the ski lift from the top of Mount Baldy Road up to the notch, and do the trip in reverse.

Although this trip enters the Cucamonga Wilderness, no wilderness permit is currently required unless you visit Cucamonga Peak or other trails east of Icehouse Saddle.

To Reach the Trailhead: This trip requires a short car or bicycle shuttle; a walk between trailheads on the curvy road would be unpleasant. Exit I-210 at Mills Avenue in Claremont, and

The Three T's

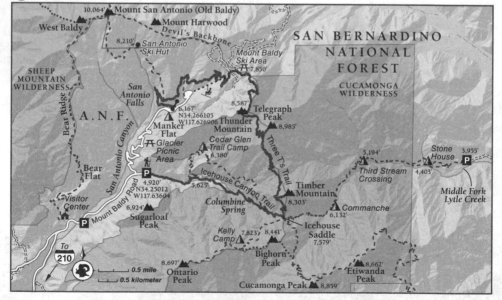

follow Mills north toward the mountains. After 1.8 miles Mills veers right and becomes Mount Baldy Road. An 8-mile climb up through San Antonio Canyon on Mount Baldy Road takes you to the small village of Mount Baldy. Continue 4.2 miles up the road to Manker Flats, where you will leave one vehicle. Drive or pedal 2.7 miles down the hairpin turns, and turn left into Icehouse Canyon, where you park at the trailhead on the left.

Description: Follow the Icehouse Canyon Trail 3.8 miles to the signed five-way junction at Icehouse Saddle (see Hike 36). Turn left and climb north toward Timber Mountain (4.7 miles). The trail curves around the west side, so you will have to make a 0.2-mile detour to reach the true summit. Follow the trail down to a saddle and up to Telegraph Peak (7.1 miles). Again, make a short detour on a use trail to the northeast to reach the summit, which is the highest point of the trip.

Return to the trail and drop steeply to a third saddle, then climb back up to the final summit, reaching Thunder Mountain at 8.7 miles. From here, the Gold Ridge ski road leads down to Mount Baldy Notch (10.1 miles).

From the notch, hike down the service road to Manker Flats. Alternatively, the ski lift runs on weekends and is a tempting way to save your knees from wear and tear.

HIKE 38 Deep Creek Hot Springs

Location	Near Hesperia, the north slope of the San Bernardino Mountains
Highlights	Natural hot-spring pools alongside a mountain stream
Distance & Configuration	3.8-mile out-and-back
Elevation Gain	950'
Hiking Time	2.5 hours
Optional Map	USGS 7.5-minute *Lake Arrowhead*
Best Times	March–November
Agency	San Bernardino National Forest/Mountaintop Ranger District
Difficulty	Moderate
Trail Use	Dogs allowed
Permit	Parking fee
Google Maps	Deep Creek Hot Springs Trailhead

Deep Creek Hot Springs in the San Bernardino National Forest has been a minor magnet for hikers and nature lovers—eccentric and otherwise—for decades. Volunteers have spent years fashioning rock-bound basins that impound water that ranges from about 96°F to about 102°F. Water flowing out of those basins quickly reaches chilly Deep Creek, which has carved a deep cleft in the north slope of the San Bernardino Mountains.

Note: U.S. Forest Service regulations do not allow camping at Deep Creek Hot Springs, and Bowen Ranch is now closed to camping as well. When planning your trip, note that Bowen Ranch does not have a phone, a website, or an e-mail address. Typically, the Forest Service has no definitive information about either Bowen Ranch or about stream or weather conditions at Deep Creek.

To Reach the Trailhead: To get to the most convenient portal for the hot-springs hike, which lies outside the national-forest boundary, go north on I-15 over Cajon Pass. Six miles north of the pass, exit east onto Main Street, and follow it 7.2 miles through Hesperia. Where Main Street curves south, veer left (east) onto Rock Springs Road. Cross the dry bed of the Mojave River, and follow the road 2.8 miles to a junction where its name changes to Roundup Way. Continue east

Deep Creek Hot Springs

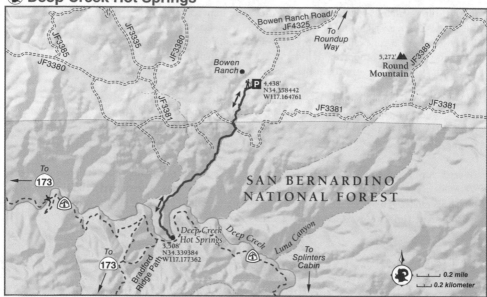

4.4 miles, and then turn right (south) onto the Bowen Ranch Road, a good dirt road.

Proceed 5.4 miles, passing various junctions, to a toll gate and 1920s cabin at the rustic, private Bowen Ranch. Pay the day-use fee at the gate, and be sure to pick up a copy of the hand-drawn "treasure" map that may help you navigate to the hot springs. Park your car at the trailhead, a short distance past the toll gate. Since the ranch lies outside the San Bernardino National Forest boundary, you do not need to display a National Forest Adventure Pass.

Description: Now you're ready to head out on foot toward the springs, almost 2 miles away and nearly 1,000 feet lower in elevation. After an initial 0.5 mile of downhill hiking, briefly

jog left on a dirt road, then veer right on a signed trail entering San Bernardino National Forest land. You lose about 700 feet of elevation as you descend to Deep Creek's canyon floor (1.8 miles).

About halfway down this stretch, where the trail splits, take the right fork to ensure an easier, more gradual descent. Once you reach the canyon bottom, you must decide how to cross the creek to reach the hot pools on the far side. In winter, the water is often swift and bone-chillingly cold. Forest Service regulations allow nude bathing in the Deep Creek Hot Springs drainage area, and typically about half of the visitors do so. For many health reasons, avoid submerging your face in a hot-spring pool! Camping, campfires, and glass containers are strictly prohibited.

Deep Creek Hot Springs

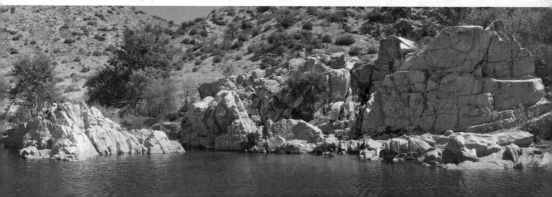

Remember that the uphill, post-soak hike back to the car can be enervating and possibly exhausting in the summer heat. Bring plenty of drinking water (not alcohol, which dehydrates the body) if the weather is warm! Inexperienced hikers have also gotten into deep trouble here when cold rain or snow is falling. The pools may be plenty warm, but inadequately equipped persons who can't get dry after a visit to the pools are at risk for hypothermia.

HIKE 39   Heart Rock

Location	Lake Gregory, San Bernardino Mountains
Highlights	Waterfall by unusual rock formation
Distance & Configuration	1.8-mile out-and-back
Elevation Gain	200'
Hiking Time	1 hour
Optional Map	USGS 7.5-minute *Silverwood Lake*
Best Times	All year; waterfall is best March–June
Agency	San Bernardino National Forest/Mountaintop Ranger District
Difficulty	Easy
Trail Use	Dogs allowed, good for kids
Permit	None required
Google Maps	Heart Rock

The cool waters of Seely Creek flow down the north slope of the San Bernardino Mountains beneath incense-cedars and oaks. Through a fortuitous quirk of geology, they've carved a remarkable heart-shaped basin in the rock alongside a waterfall. Beyond, they rush down the granite slabs into an alluring pool. This short hike follows the bank of Seely Creek to the Heart Rock overlook and the pool. Wear footwear with good tread because the trail is uneven, steep, and rocky at times, although children will probably enjoy the obstacles. The best times for this trip are in the spring when the waterfall is most dramatic and in the early summer when the water is tempting for a dip.

The creek and camp are named for David and Wellington Seely, brothers who established a sawmill here in the 1850s to provide for the Mormon outpost in San Bernardino. Their name has been misspelled "Seeley" on many official documents, including the USGS topographic map.

To Reach the Trailhead: From the I-10 or I-210/CA 210 in San Bernardino, take Exit 73B or 76, respectively, onto Waterman Avenue, which becomes Rim of the World Scenic Byway (Highway 18). At the top of the ridge (11.5 miles from the I-210 exit, 16.8 miles from the I-10 exit), exit onto Highway 138 (Crestline). Proceed north 1.2 miles to the stop sign in the middle of Crestline, and then continue 1.5 miles down to the Camp Seely entrance road at mile marker 138 SBD 35.00. If the gate is locked, park on the shoulder of the highway outside the gate and walk the narrow, paved road across Seely Creek to a second gate, 0.4 mile from the highway, by a post marking trail 4W07. (If the gate is open, you can drive the 0.4 mile to the second gate.)

Follow shady trail 4W07 through incense-cedars and black oaks as it leads north from the parking area. Soon you'll enjoy views of the creek as the trail follows above it.

At 0.9 mile, look for an unmarked three-way fork in the trail. From here, the route devolves into a maze of footpaths. To the right, descend a rocky path to a boulder overlooking Heart Rock and the waterfall. Keep a close eye on young children because the overlook is perched above a sheer cliff.

🎯 Heart Rock

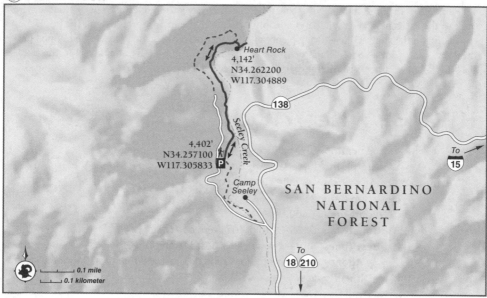

The path straight from the fork joins another path descending from the overlook to reach the base of the falls and a pleasant pool slightly farther downstream. This is a good place for a picnic. Unfortunately, thoughtless visitors leave their trash here; if you bring a garbage bag and pack out some of the litter, the site will be better for everyone.

The left fork leads back up to the paved road, which parallels the trail; however, the trail you took is more scenic, so return the way you came.

Waterfall beside Heart Rock

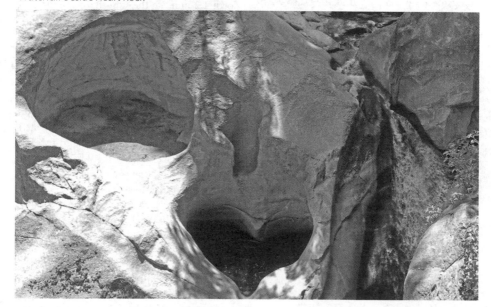

HIKE 40   Cougar Crest Trail

Location	Big Bear Lake, San Bernardino Mountains
Highlights	Pinyon–juniper forest, lake and mountain views
Distance & Configuration	5 miles to PCT or 7 miles to Bertha Peak (out-and-back)
Total Elevation Gain	800' or 1,450'
Hiking Time	2.5 hours or 3.5 hours
Optional Map	USGS 7.5-minute *Fawnskin*
Best Times	April–November
Agency	San Bernardino National Forest/Mountaintop Ranger District
Difficulty	Moderate
Trail Use	Dogs allowed, good for kids (to Cougar Crest)
Permit	National Forest Adventure Pass
Google Maps	Cougar Crest Trailhead

Big Bear Lake, with the sloping mountain rim that rises above the serene and mostly undeveloped north shore, offers excellent hiking through a splendid juniper forest. Here, the Cougar Crest Trail ascends to a junction with the 2,600-mile-long Pacific Crest Trail (PCT)—the world's longest maintained footpath.

To Reach the Trailhead: From the 210 freeway in northeast San Bernardino, take Exit 81 for Highway 330, which becomes Highway 18 in Running Springs. As soon as you reach Big Bear Lake, about 27.5 miles from the 210 freeway, turn left on Highway 38. Drive along the north shore for 5 miles to the large Cougar Crest Trailhead on the left (north) side of the road near mile marker 038 SBD 53.50. Be sure to display your Adventure Pass in your car, or park on the shoulder of the highway, where no pass is required.

Description: From the trailhead kiosk, head up the paved Cougar Crest Trail. In 0.1 mile, the paved path veers right to the Big Bear Discovery Center, but you stay straight on the broad Cougar Crest Trail. Traces of mining activity are evident as you climb along a shallow draw filled with a delightful mix of outsize pinyon pines and western junipers and occasional straight and tall Jeffrey pines. The sweet and pungent scents exuded by the wood and needles of these trees mingle intoxicatingly on a warm day.

After a long mile, the old road becomes a narrow trail and begins to curl and switchback along higher and sunnier slopes. Big Bear Lake comes into view occasionally, its surface azure in the slanting illumination of a spring or summer morning or dotted with silvery pinpoints of light on a late-fall day.

The trail reaches a divide, bends right, and for a short distance traverses a cool (or

San Gorgonio peers over the ridge beyond Big Bear Lake.

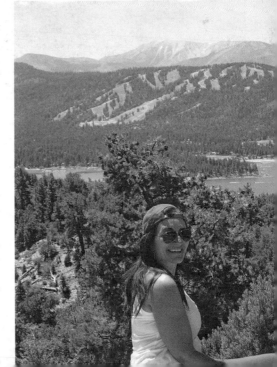

Cougar Crest Trail

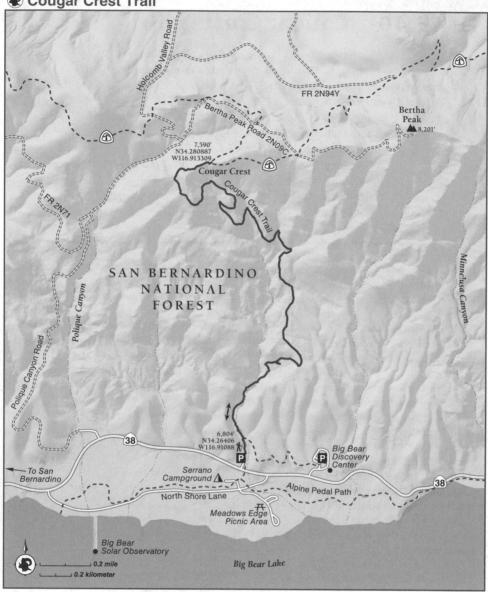

sometimes cold and icy) north-facing slope. At 2.5 miles and 800 feet of climbing, the Cougar Crest Trail joins the Pacific Crest Trail, the latter reserved for hikers and horses (mountain bikes and other mechanical conveyances are prohibited on the entire PCT between the Mexican and Canadian borders). Most hikers enjoy a snack on a bench beneath a magnificent western juniper and then turn around here.

VARIATION

If you want a longer hike, bear right and start contouring east, high on the sunny, south-facing slope. Spread before you now is the lake (technically a shallow reservoir), which half-fills a 10-mile-long trough in the mountains, and various resort and residential communities spread along the shore and beyond. Behind the lake and about 12 miles distant, the rounded, often-snow-mantled ramparts of San Gorgonio Wilderness gleam.

The southern view does not significantly improve as you press on, though the high point ahead—Bertha Peak—will furnish a better view in other directions. When the PCT crosses a rock-strewn service road (2.9 miles from the start), leave the nicely graded trail and start climbing east on the road. A sweaty, 0.7-mile ascent takes you to a small microwave relay station atop Bertha Peak. Outside the relay station's perimeter fence, you'll find a peak baggers' register, plus fine views over the treetops into Holcomb Valley and the Mojave Desert to the north.

HIKE 41 Grand View Point

Location	Big Bear Lake, San Bernardino Mountains
Highlights	Forested trail with lake and mountain views
Distance & Configuration	7-mile out-and-back
Total Elevation Gain	1,100'
Hiking Time	4 hours
Optional Map	USGS 7.5-minute *Big Bear Lake*
Best Times	April–November
Agency	San Bernardino National Forest/Mountaintop Ranger District
Difficulty	Moderate
Trail Use	Dogs allowed, good for kids, suitable for mountain biking
Permit	National Forest Adventure Pass
Google Maps	Aspen Glen Picnic Area

Grand View Point, high on the ridge above Big Bear Lake, offers a memorable view across the Santa Ana River Canyon to the tall summits of the San Gorgonio Wilderness. A network of trails leads up from the Aspen Glen Picnic Area to the point. Take this popular hike on a clear day when you can fully appreciate the vistas. This whole ridge south of Big Bear is laced with fire roads and singletrack trails that draw mountain bikers from across Southern California. This trail is also enjoyable in the snow, and you are likely to have good tracks to follow.

To Reach the Trailhead: From the 210 Freeway in San Bernardino, take Exit 81 for Highway 330, which becomes Highway 18 in Running Springs. About 31 miles from the 210, in Big Bear Lake Village at mile marker 018 SBD 47.43, where a sign points to Mill Creek Road and picnic grounds, turn right (south) onto Tulip Lane. Proceed 0.5 mile to the Aspen Glen Picnic Area, on your right.

Description: Follow the Pineknot Trail (1E01) from the trailhead sign at the south end of the picnic area. The trail climbs through a forest of black oak, white fir, and Jeffrey pine, with an understory of boulders, buckthorn, and wildflowers. This area is particularly appealing in the late spring when the flowers are in bloom and in October when the oak leaves turn golden.

In a quarter mile, come to a junction with the Cabin Trail (1E24). Both trails rejoin ahead, but the Pineknot Trail has better views and is more popular, while the Cabin Trail draws mountain bikers seeking a loop ride.

The Pineknot Trail climbs, crosses a ridge, and then drops to cross the creek in Red Ant

Grand View Point

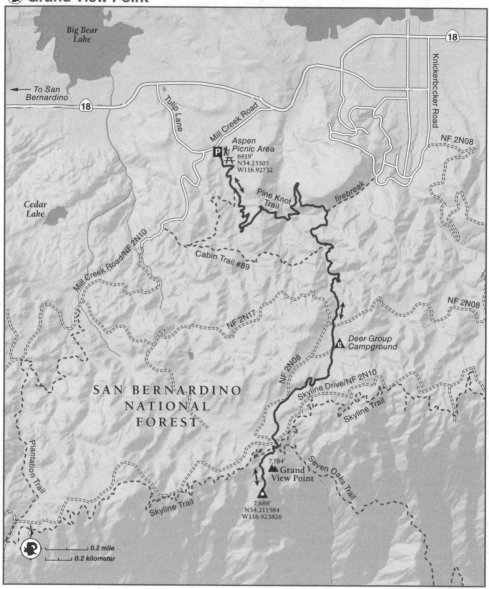

Canyon. Climb back up to a ridge and turn south. When the trail comes close to the creek again, watch for an unsigned junction with the Cabin Trail on the right (1.7 miles).

The main trail continues straight (south) and crosses Forest Road 2N08 (2.4 miles). It then levels out, passes Deer Group Campground, and parallels 2N08 to reach Forest Road 2N10 at the top of the ridge (3.3 miles). Cross the road to meet the Skyline Trail, then follow the signed Grand View Point Trail 0.3 mile southeast to the clearing on Grand View Point.

HIKE 42   Forsee Creek Trail

Location	San Gorgonio Wilderness, San Bernardino Mountains
Highlight	Peak bagging amid Southern California's highest mountains
Distance & Configuration	13-mile out-and-back (to Trail Fork Camp)
Elevation Gain	3,700'
Hiking Time	8 hours
Recommended Map	Tom Harrison *San Gorgonio Wilderness*
Best Times	May–November
Agency	San Bernardino National Forest/Mill Creek Visitor Center
Difficulty	Strenuous
Trail Use	Dogs allowed, suitable for backpacking
Permit	San Gorgonio Wilderness permit required
Google Maps	Forsee Creek Trail 1E06

Note: The Forsee Creek and San Bernardino Peak Trails are temporarily closed due to damage caused by the 2020 El Dorado Fire. Check the San Gorgonio Wilderness Association website (sgwa.org) to see if the trails have reopened.

Tucked amid the tall, straight trunks of lodgepole pines at nearly 2 miles above sea level, the wind-sheltered and mostly bug-free Trail Fork Camp is a peak bagger's delight. Just above the trail camp lies the lightning-tortured roof of Southern California—San Bernardino Mountain—containing four named high points

reached by an easy, half-day stroll. Farther east lies the big daddy of Southern California summits—San Gorgonio Mountain—reached by an all-day (13-mile round-trip) hike involving only moderate elevation change.

The trek to Trail Fork Camp and the crest beyond is itself a challenging day hike. It's somewhat easier if you take one full day to hike in and a partial day to return. The high peaks of San Gorgonio Wilderness tend to create their own local storms in summertime, so be aware of thunderstorm forecasts before embarking on

Sunset over the San Bernardino Divide

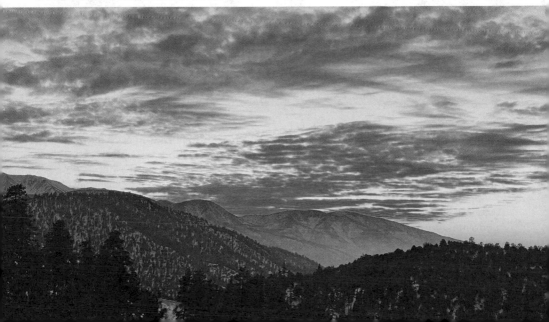

Forsee Creek Trail

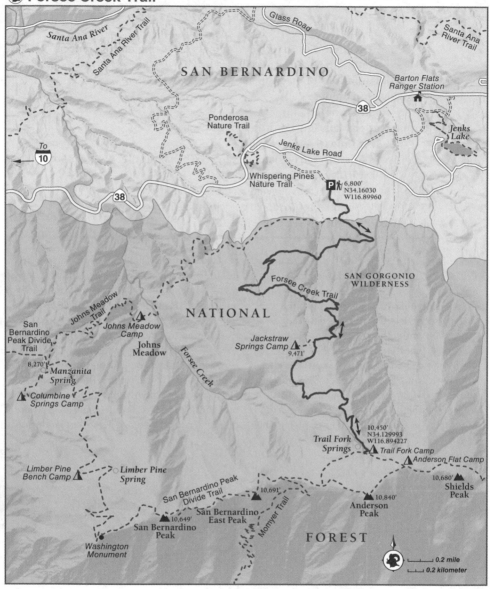

your journey. Rain gear and a tent with a water-proof fly are musts during such conditions; better yet, consider canceling or postponing your trip if there is tropical moisture in the area.

A free wilderness permit is required to enter the San Gorgonio Wilderness, and quotas fill well in advance during summer weekends. Obtain your permit at sgwa.org/wilderness-permits.

To Reach the Trailhead: To reach the trailhead from I-10 at Redlands, take Highway 38 east through Mentone (and past the Mill Creek Visitor Center), up onto the forested highlands of the San Bernardino Mountains (almost 44 miles). Just before mile marker 038 SBD 25.51, 18 miles beyond Mill Creek Visitor Center, turn right on Jenks Lake Road. After 0.3 mile turn right on a rough dirt road signed FORSEE CREEK TRAIL, and proceed cautiously another 0.6 mile to a large clearing used for parking.

Description: From the trailhead, make your way steadily uphill under shade-giving Jeffrey pines, incense-cedars, white firs, black oaks, and a few sugar pines, quickly passing a side trail to Johns Meadow. Most summers, thin streams of water cascade down two or three gullies traversed by the first 2 miles of trail. After an hour or two of unrelenting labor, you leave the yellow-pine vegetation behind and enter a zone dominated by lodgepole pines. Much higher up, the lodgepoles (with two needles per cluster) are joined by limber pines (with five needles per cluster and rubbery branch tips).

At 4.2 miles Jackstraw Springs Trail Camp (which is prone to mosquitoes in the summer) lies down a side path to the right. At 6.2 miles the trail bends sharply right and arrives at a junction. Just below, hidden in a clump of bushes, lies Trail Fork Springs—oftentimes the first trickle in the headwaters of Forsee Creek. Retrace your steps about 100 yards on the Forsee Creek Trail to find the steep, narrow side path leading east up to Trail Fork Camp. Several flat sites for camping can be found hereabouts amid the lodgepoles and weathered outcrops of banded metamorphic rock. A bald area on a flat ridge just northeast is the perfect spot to admire a view stretching north toward Big Bear Lake and to toast the last rays of the setting sun.

VARIATIONS

If time and energy permit, pay a visit to nearby Shields and Anderson Peaks, 0.7 mile and 0.4 mile away, respectively. On the crest between these peaks lie scraggly pines, many battered and stripped of their bark by lightning strikes. North of the crest, in protected pockets, uniformly spaced lodgepole pines grow tall and straight with dark "bathtub rings" around their waists indicating snow accumulations several feet deep.

An optional peak-bagging foray to the west might include both of the San Bernardino peaks, plus the historic Colonel Henry Washington Monument, which commemorates the original San Bernardino baseline and meridian

survey point, established in 1852. (The monument lies off-trail; you'll find it by walking 160 yards straight up the ridge from the southwesternmost switchback in the San Bernardino Peak Divide Trail.) For more than 150 years, all land surveys of Southern California have referred to Colonel Washington's initial baseline. Due west of the monument, starting from the foot of the mountain, today's Base Line Road stretches radially outward many miles across the flat, alluvial plain occupied by San Bernardino and several of its satellite cities. As viewed from the monument on clear days, Base Line Road seems to point toward a vanishing point in or beyond the San Gabriel Valley.

It's possible to return to the trailhead via a longer (17 miles total) route that loops around via Johns Meadow. Descend the San Bernardino Peak Divide Trail west and north to an 8,270-foot trail junction near Manzanita Springs, then head northeast on the often-steep, unmaintained trail toward Johns Meadow. East of Johns Meadow, the trail is maintained.

On the Forsee Creek Trail with a little guy
Alfred Kwok

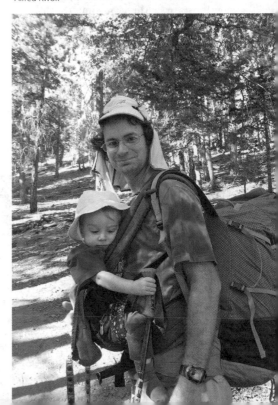

HIKE 43   Dollar Lake

Location	San Gorgonio Wilderness, San Bernardino Mountains
Highlight	Sparkling glacial tarn
Distance & Configuration	12-mile out-and-back
Elevation Gain	2,700'
Hiking Time	7 hours
Optional Map	Tom Harrison *San Gorgonio Wilderness*
Best Times	May–November
Agency	San Bernardino National Forest/Mill Creek Visitor Center
Difficulty	Strenuous
Trail Use	Dogs allowed
Permit	National Forest Adventure Pass and San Gorgonio Wilderness permit required
Google Maps	South Fork Trail 1E04

Sparkling and silvery like a freshly minted silver dollar, Dollar Lake lies cupped amid a talus-frosted natural bowl, not far below the great divide of San Bernardino Mountain. Snow lingers late—sometimes into August—on the steep slopes overlooking the lake. It's hard to believe that this splendid landscape, reminiscent of the High Sierra, exists here in Southern California, only 20 air miles from the suburban housing tracts of San Bernardino.

A day hike to Dollar Lake (via the South Fork Trail) in the San Gorgonio Wilderness is not only possible but rather straightforwardly easy for any well-conditioned hiker willing to rise early and get to the trailhead by 8 or 9 a.m. A free wilderness permit is required to enter the San Gorgonio Wilderness, and quotas fill well in advance during summer weekends. Obtain your permit from sgwa.org /wilderness-permits.

To Reach the Trailhead: To reach the trailhead from I-10 at Redlands, take Highway 38 east through Mentone (and past the Mill Creek Visitor Center), up onto the forested highlands of the San Bernardino Mountains (about 44 miles). Just before mile marker 038 SBD 25.51, 18 miles beyond Mill Creek Visitor Center, turn right on Jenks Lake Road. Proceed 3 miles to the large South Fork Trailhead parking lot on the left. You'll need to display an Adventure Pass on your parked car.

Poopout Hill burned but still has magnificent views.

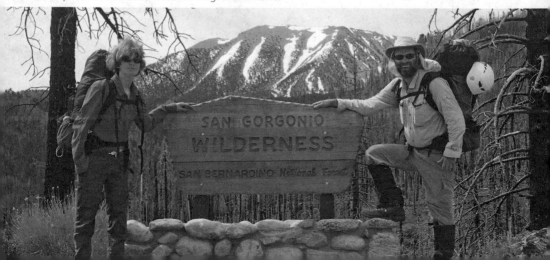

🐾 Dollar Lake

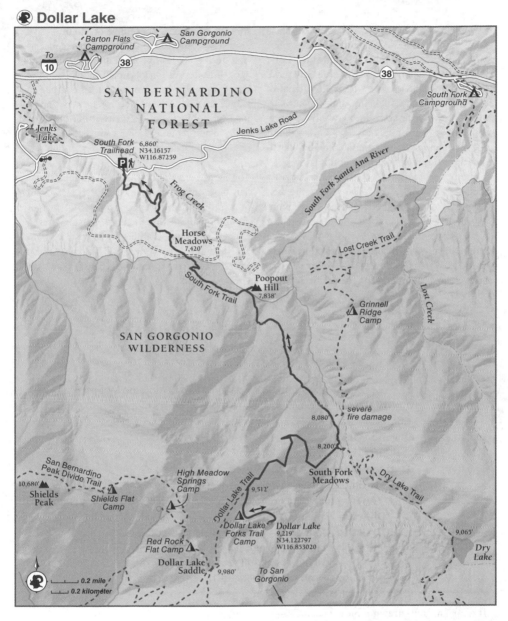

Description: The South Fork Trail crosses Jenks Lake Road, heading south, and commences a moderate ascent up a shady canyon. Much of the forest from here to South Fork Meadows tragically burned in the 2015 Lake Fire, which was started by an arsonist near Big Bear. Soon, the trail switches back, climbs out of the canyon, and climbs southeast toward a cabin and picnic area at Horse Meadows (1.0 mile). Near the meadow's upper edge, you cross a dirt road now closed to public use. At 2.0 miles, reach a short spur on the left leading to Poopout Hill, a worthy viewpoint where San Gorgonio Mountain is framed between the trees.

Continue your ascent through a skeletal forest. The trail draws close to the South Fork Santa Ana River. Remain on the right bank of the creek, staying right at the signed junction with the Dry Lake Trail (3.7 miles). To the left is South Fork Meadows, where many small tributaries combine and funnel into the South Fork. Days or weeks later, some of this water will travel down the wide Santa Ana River flood-control channel through Anaheim and Santa Ana. Much of the water seeps into gravelly or sandy soils downstream and recharges underground aquifers, never reaching the ocean. You stay to the right and do not cross the South Fork.

Your ascent continues on the crooked, mostly shaded Dollar Lake Trail. The yellow-pine belt fades, while stout and straight lodgepole pines appear in greater numbers. At 5.3 miles, just past a large, manzanita-covered patch on the mountainside, you'll come to a junction where a side trail starts slanting down toward Dollar Lake, a short half mile away. The San Bernardino

Mountains are the only range of mountains in Southern California to show evidence of glaciation during the last Ice Age (about 10,000 years ago). The depression occupied by Dollar Lake was dammed by a terminal moraine, a pile of rubble left when the last glacier retreated. Camping is prohibited within a quarter mile of Dollar Lake, including on the ridges above the lake.

VARIATIONS

The loop from the South Fork Trailhead over San Gorgonio via Dollar and Dry Lakes is an outstanding 21-mile hike with 4,700 feet of elevation gain. Along the way, you could camp at Dry Lake View, Trail Flat, or Dry Lake, or on the summit of San Gorgonio. The easiest and fastest way up the mountain is by way of Vivian Creek (see Hike 44).

HIKE 44 San Gorgonio Mountain via Vivian Creek

Location	San Gorgonio Wilderness, San Bernardino Mountains
Highlight	Standing atop Southern California's highest spot
Distance & Configuration	18-mile out-and-back
Elevation Gain	5,700'
Hiking Time	10 hours
Optional Map	Tom Harrison *San Gorgonio Wilderness*
Best Times	April–November
Agency	San Bernardino National Forest/Mill Creek Visitor Center
Difficulty	Strenuous
Trail Use	Dogs allowed, suitable for backpacking
Permit	National Forest Adventure Pass and San Gorgonio Wilderness permit required
Google Maps	Vivian Creek Trailhead 1E08

The barren, talus-strewn summit of San Gorgonio Mountain (or Greyback, after its steely-gray appearance from the valleys below) receives dozens of hikers on most fine-weather weekends. No hiker, however, has an easy time of it. Either variation of the popular northern approach (via Dollar Lake or Dry Lake) requires more than 20 miles of round-trip hiking. On

the southern approach by way of the Vivian Creek Trail, described here, you begin hiking at a point several hundred feet lower than the northern (South Fork) trailhead, but you save some miles of distance on the round-trip.

The Vivian Creek Trail, the original path to the top of San Gorgonio, was built around the turn of the 20th century. Today, about eight

San Gorgonio Mountain via Vivian Creek

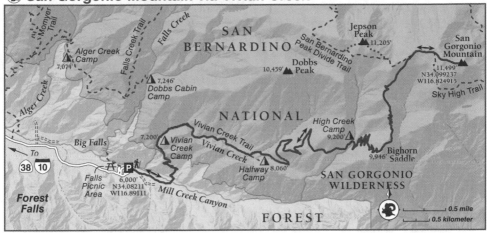

routes (or variations on routes) culminate at the summit. After 1988, when the north-side Poopout Hill trailhead closed, the Vivian Creek Trail once again became the fastest and easiest way up the mountain. This south-facing route also has the advantage of a longer season; most of the snow on the upper parts of the trail is gone by May or June—a month or more before the north-facing routes are similarly clear.

Of those who approach the summit by way of Vivian Creek, perhaps half do so over a two- or three-day period, hauling their overnight gear to camps such as Halfway or High Creeks and day hiking from there. Others, in excellent condition and traveling lightly, have taken as little as 7 hours total, with a half hour spent at the top and some jogging on the way down. At a leisurely pace with plenty of breaks, a daylong summit hike could take a mind- and

San Gorgonio Mountain from the south after a winter storm

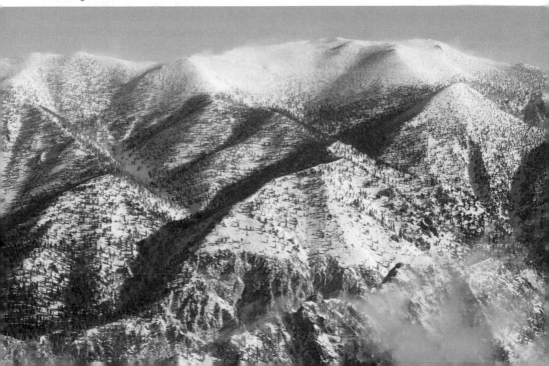

leg-numbing 14 hours. That approach is OK in June or July (assuming you start hiking at dawn), but you probably wouldn't want to try it during November, when daylight lasts 11 hours or less.

A free wilderness permit is required to enter the San Gorgonio Wilderness, and quotas fill well in advance during the summer weekends. Obtain a permit at sgwa.org/wilderness-permits.

To Reach the Trailhead: To reach the trailhead from I-10 at Redlands, take Highway 38 east for 8.5 miles, past Mentone to Mill Creek Visitor Center; then continue up Mill Creek Canyon another 6.2 miles to a hairpin turn where you veer right onto Valley of the Falls Drive. Proceed 4.5 miles through the cabin community of Forest Falls, all the way to the end of the road and a spacious trailhead parking lot. Be sure to display your Adventure Pass on your car.

Description: From the trailhead, walk east (uphill) past a vehicle gate and follow a dirt road 0.6 mile to its end. Go left across the wide, bouldery wash of Mill Creek, and find Vivian Creek Trail going sharply up the oak-clothed canyon wall on the far side. The next half mile is excruciatingly steep, and this pitch is worse on the return, when your weary quads must absorb the punishment of each lurching downhill step.

Mercifully, at the top of the steep section, the trail levels momentarily and then assumes a moderate grade up alongside Vivian Creek. A sylvan Shangri-la unfolds ahead. Pines, firs, and cedars reach for the sky. Bracken fern smothers the banks of the melodious creek, which dances over boulders and fallen trees. After the first October frost, the bracken turns a flaming yellow, made all the more vivid by warm sunlight pouring out of a fierce blue sky. You can camp here, 1.4 miles from the start.

Near Halfway Camp (3.0 miles), the trail begins climbing timber-dotted slopes covered intermittently by thickets of manzanita. Dobbs Peak, just below timberline, comes into view to the north, though the nearly treeless San Bernardino Mountain divide remains hidden. After several zigs and zags on north-facing slopes, you swing onto a brightly illuminated south-facing slope. Serrated Yucaipa Ridge looms to the south, rising sheer from the depths of Mill Creek Canyon. Soon thereafter, the sound of bubbling water heralds your arrival at High Creek at 5.4 miles and the trail camp of the same name. Be ready for a chilly night if you stay here; cold, nocturnal air often flows down along the bottom of this canyon from the 10,000-plus-foot peaks above.

Past High Creek Camp, the trail ascends gently on several gratuitously long switchbacks through lodgepole pines and, at length, attains Bighorn saddle on a rocky ridge (6.9 miles). The pines thin out and appear more decrepit as you climb crookedly up along this ridge toward timberline; a patch burned at the edge of the Apple Fire. This fire ignited in Cherry Valley in July 2020, when a vehicle malfunctioned, and swept across 33,424 acres, including the southeastern portion of the San Gorgonio Wilderness. At 8.4 miles the San Bernardino Peak Divide Trail intersects from the left. Stay right and keep climbing on a moderate grade across stony slopes dotted with cowering krummholz pines. Soon, nearly all vegetation disappears.

On the right you pass Sky High Trail, which bends around the mountain and descends toward Dry Lake and South Fork Meadows in the north. Keep straight and keep going. A final burst of effort puts you on a boulder pile marking the highest elevation in Southern California (9 miles from your starting point). From this vantage, even the soaring north face of Mount San Jacinto to the south appears diminished in stature.

Several campsites surrounded by enclosures of piled-up stones are scattered around the summit plateau. These comprise Summit Trail Camp, a fine place to stay overnight if the weather is calm and clear (most typically in September and October). At night, planets and stars gleam overhead, but they must compete for attention with the glow of millions of lights below.

HIKE 45   Whitewater Canyon

Location	Whitewater Preserve, San Bernardino Mountains
Highlights	Desert river, possible bighorn sheep sightings
Distance & Configuration	4.0-mile out-and-back (to Red Dome)
Elevation Gain	400'
Hiking Time	2 hours
Optional Map	wildlandsconservancy.org/preserves/whitewater
Best Times	October–April, 8 a.m.–5 p.m.
Agency	The Wildlands Conservancy
Difficulty	Moderate
Trail Use	Dogs allowed, suitable for backpacking, good for kids
Permit	Notify a ranger before you leave a vehicle overnight.
Google Maps	Whitewater Preserve

The Whitewater River is the largest waterway between the Mojave and Colorado Rivers. The Wildlands Conservancy has established an outstanding nature preserve in the river canyon at the site of the former Whitewater Trout Farm. This trip explores the desert and river along a short segment of the Pacific Crest Trail (PCT), part of the Sand to Snow National Monument.

Whitewater Canyon

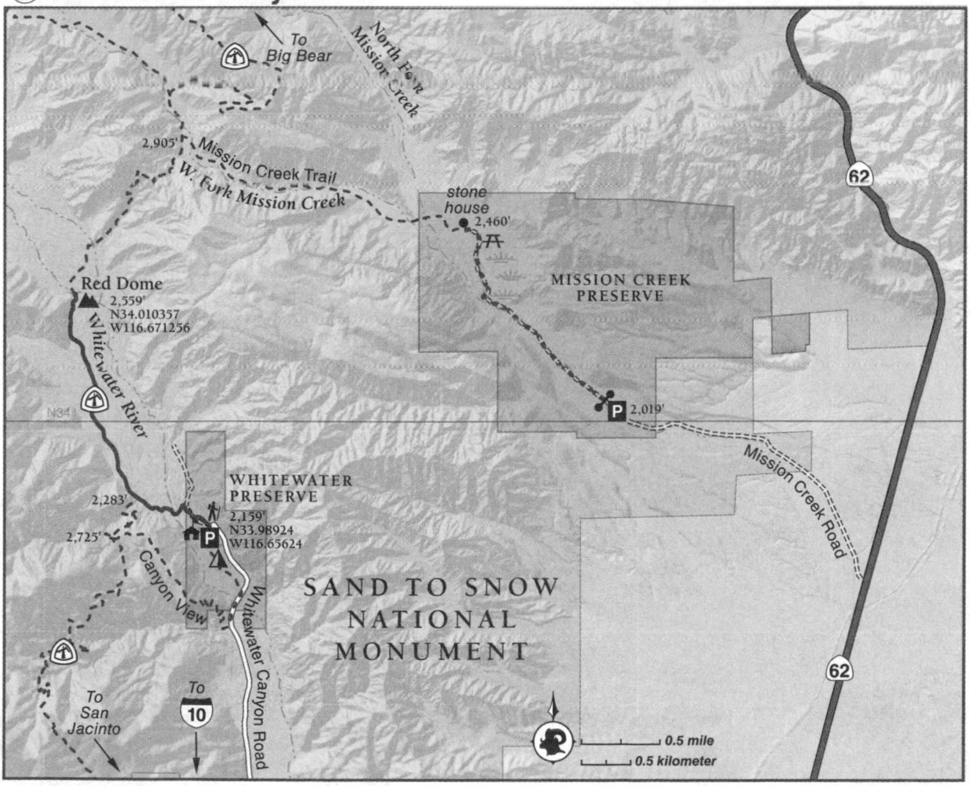

The best time to visit is in the spring, when wild-flowers are in bloom and the river earns its name. Animals large and small visit the canyon for water and food; watch for prints and scat. Scan the cliffs above the preserve headquarters for bighorn sheep. This trip is a short out-and-back walk, but those desiring a longer trip can make many variations. If you're not staying overnight, be sure to be out by 5 p.m. when the gate closes.

To Reach the Trailhead: From I-10 west of Palm Springs, take Exit 114, and turn right at the end of the exit ramp onto Tipton Road. Follow this frontage road east less than a quarter mile, and turn left onto Whitewater Canyon Road. Proceed 4.9 miles to the end of the road at the parking area for Whitewater Preserve.

Description: Sign in at the ranger station, then walk north along a rock-lined path from the trailhead kiosk. After passing a pair of palm trees, veer west and cross the Whitewater River wash. The trail varies from year to year as floodwaters reshape the canyon floor, but the path is usually marked. Even if it is hard to follow, watch for and eventually pick up the well-defined trail on the west side. Follow it through a grove of desert willows to a junction with the PCT at the mouth of a tributary canyon, 0.5 mile from the start.

Stay straight and follow the PCT north to a bend where the Whitewater River veers west (1.9 miles). On the right side of the trail is a small volcanic lump called Red Dome. The PCT makes a poorly defined crossing of the wash here before heading over a ridge into the Mission Creek drainage. If you are out for a short hike, this is a good place to savor the river and then return the way you came.

VARIATION

If you arrange for a vehicle at Mission Creek Preserve, 15 miles away via I-10 and Highway 62, you can turn this trip into an enjoyable 8-mile one-way trip between the two Wildlands Conservancy preserves.

Crossing Whitewater River

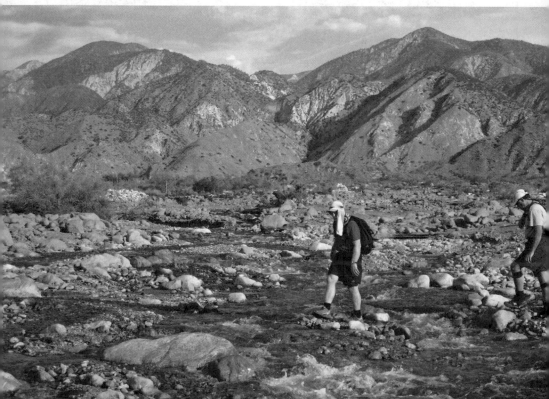

HIKE 46   Big Morongo Canyon

Location	Big Morongo Canyon Preserve, north of Palm Springs
Highlights	Riparian splendor amid the desert, excellent birding
Distance & Configuration	1- to 3-mile loop
Total Elevation Gain/Loss	50'–300', depending on route
Hiking Time	30 minutes–2 hours
Optional Map	Big Morongo Canyon Preserve Trail System (bigmorongo.org/trails)
Best Times	October–May
Agency	Big Morongo Canyon Preserve
Difficulty	Easy
Trail Use	Good for kids
Permit	None required
Google Maps	Big Morongo Canyon Preserve

Nearly 300 species of birds have been spotted along a 6-mile stretch of Big Morongo Canyon, just outside the town of Morongo Valley. Animals frequenting the canyon—which is now protected as a wildlife corridor between the desert and mountains as part of the Sand to Snow National Monument—include bighorn sheep, bobcats, mountain lions, and mule deer. The 31,000-acre Big Morongo Canyon Preserve, administered by the federal Bureau of Land Management, encompasses the wettest parts of the canyon. The preserve sits astride a melding of coastal chaparral and desert habitats and is regarded as one of the most important wildlife oases in the California desert. The exotic freshwater marsh found here owes its existence to seepage of water up along a geologic fault associated with a great rift between tectonic plates—the San Andreas Fault Zone—not far to the south.

The uppermost (wet) part of Big Morongo Canyon Preserve lies about 2,000 feet above low-lying Palm Springs and the Coachella Valley, so the summer heat is intense but rarely intolerable here. Still, it's best to stick with the cooler months, or visit in the early-morning or late-afternoon hours. The preserve is open daily from 7:30 a.m. to sunset.

To Reach the Trailhead: From I-10 near Palm Springs, drive 11.3 miles north on Highway 62 to Morongo Valley. Just past the business district, turn right on East Drive, and look for the preserve entrance on the left.

Description: For a rewarding 1.2-mile stroll through contrasting habitats, walk past the visitor information display and pick up the Desert Willow Trail on the left. It guides you between a sun-blasted terrace covered in alkali goldenbush and a huge thicket of honey mesquite. You dip to cross the Big Morongo Wash and pass a spur trail, the Yucca Ridge Trail, 0.4 mile from the start.

Continue on the Desert Willow Trail into the heart of Big Morongo's riparian oasis. You meander on boardwalks amidst a junglelike assemblage of willows, cottonwoods, alders,

Mesquite beans, a favorite of the Cahuilla people

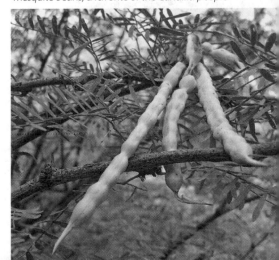

🏞 Big Morongo Canyon

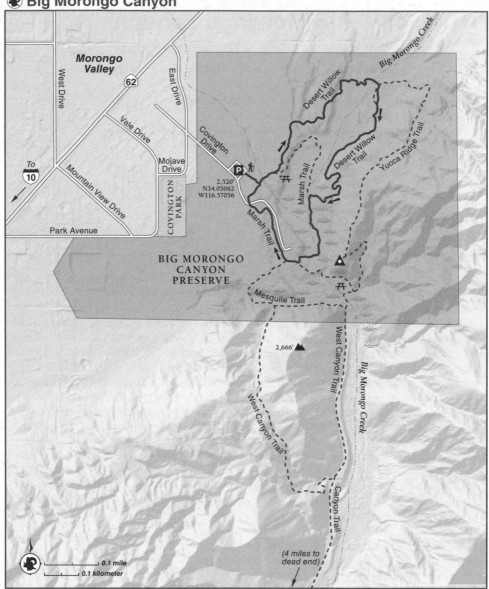

and fan palms (the latter two apparently introduced, though they lie not far from the edge of their normal range). Watercress and water parsnip have overrun the surface of the shallow waters below your feet.

At 0.8 mile, you come to a T-intersection with the Marsh Trail. Off to the right a quarter mile is your parked car. To the left, you pass the Mesquite Trail before looping back to the trailhead.

HIKE 47   Pushawalla Palms

Location	Coachella Valley Preserve, east of Palm Springs
Highlights	Palm oases, ridge walk
Distance & Configuration	6.5-mile loop
Elevation Gain	1,000'
Hiking Time	4 hours
Best Times	October–March
Agency	Center for Natural Lands Management
Difficulty	Moderate
Permit	None required
Google Maps	Pushawalla Palms Trailhead

The 17,000-acre Coachella Valley Preserve, located on the San Andreas Fault between Palm Springs and Joshua Tree National Park, was established in 1986 to protect the sand dune habitat of the endangered Coachella Valley fringe-toed lizard. The crushed rock and clay in the fault zone are nearly impermeable to groundwater, forcing the water to the surface and creating a series of springs that support spectacular palm oases in the midst of the parched desert.

Pushawalla Palms

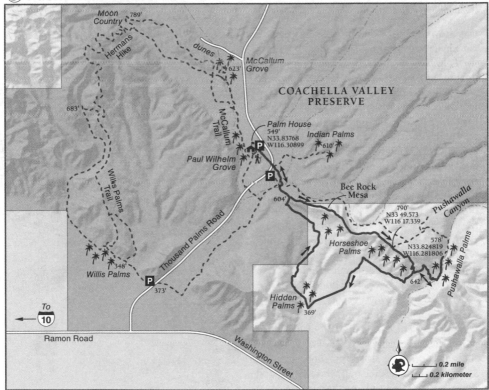

This loop tour of the southeastern part of the preserve features three separate palm groves and expansive views from a narrow ridge.

The Coachella Valley Preserve System is managed by multiple agencies. The Thousand Palms Oasis, on the west side of Thousand Palms, has the main parking lot and Palm House visitor center. That portion is closed on Mondays and Tuesdays. This hike visits the Pushawalla, Horseshoe, and Hidden Palms Oases on the east side of the road and is open daily. Check cnlm .org/portfolio_page/coachella-valley for current conditions.

To Reach the Trailhead: From I-10, take Exit 131, heading north on Monterey Avenue; then immediately turn right onto Ramon Road. Drive east for 4.5 miles. Turn left on Thousand Palms Road, and proceed 2.0 miles to the visitor center parking area on the left. If the lot is closed or you don't plan to stop at the visitor center, you can park 0.3 mile back down Thousand Palms Canyon Road at a turnout on the east side.

Description: If you haven't already been to Coachella Valley Preserve, consider stopping at the Palm House in the Thousand Palms Oasis next to the parking area (if it is open). Docents can tell you about current conditions and wildlife. A sign on the south side of the visitor center parking lot indicates the start of the trail to the Pushawalla, Horseshoe, and Hidden Palms Oases. The trail leads across the desert and crosses Thousand Palms Road at the alternative parking turnout (0.2 mile). At a signed junction just beyond, turn right and follow frequent signposts to steps leading onto Bee Rock Mesa (0.5 mile). At the crest of the ridge, a sign points east along the ridgetop toward Pushawalla Palms and south down to Hidden Palms. This trip heads to Pushawalla and will loop back to this point by way of Hidden Palms.

Follow the narrow, exposed ridge for a mile, enjoying the panoramic views. Pass above Horseshoe Palms. Near the end of Bee Rock Mesa, the Pushawalla Palms trail descends off the north side to a signed junction on a flat. Stay right and follow the trail across the flat and down a narrow ridge to another junction (2.0

miles). Stay left for Pushawalla Palms; you will return to this junction later to take the other fork to Horseshoe and Hidden Palms. Descend a narrow gully and arrive at the oasis in Pushawalla Canyon. During the wet months, the canyon bottom will often have a trickle of water, though it is unsuitable for drinking. Turn left and explore up the canyon to find the two main palm groves (2.6 miles).

Return through the narrow gully to the junction from which you just came, and head west toward Horseshoe Palms, nestled at the foot of the ridge. The maze of trails through the valley can be confusing; follow the trail markers that eventually lead you onto an old jeep track down the middle of the valley. After passing Horseshoe Palms, come to a fork in the road at a hitching post. Take the trail on the right into Hidden Palms Oasis.

When the road ends, continue north on a trail that eventually rejoins jeep tracks. The maze of paths in this area can be confusing. At another fork beneath power lines near the toe of the main ridge, veer right and return to the signed junction on Bee Rock Mesa (5.6 miles). Descend the stairs and retrace your steps to your vehicle.

Pushawalla Palms Oasis

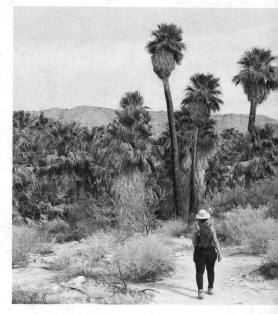

HIKE 48   Black Rock Panorama Loop

Location	Joshua Tree National Park
Highlights	Desert vegetation and views
Distance & Configuration	6.5-mile loop
Elevation Gain	1,200'
Hiking Time	4 hours
Recommended Map	Tom Harrison *Joshua Tree National Park* or Trails Illustrated *Joshua Tree*
Best Times	October–April
Agency	Joshua Tree National Park
Difficulty	Moderate
Permit	None required
Google Maps	Black Rock Canyon Trail

Black Rock Canyon is near the western edge of Joshua Tree National Park and connects to the main park only by the remote California Riding and Hiking Trail. While it lacks the outlandish rock formations characteristic of the main park, it does have an exceptionally lush and beautiful assortment of prickly desert vegetation. An extensive trail network fans out from the Black Rock Campground. The best moderate hike in this area, the Panorama Loop explores a series of washes, climbs up to a ridgeline with splendid views, and then returns via another wash system.

To Reach the Trailhead: From the 210 Freeway in Yucca Valley, take Exit 117 for Highway 62. In 21.3 miles, turn south on Joshua Lane at the sign for the Black Rock Campground (opposite Highway 247, 0.4 mile east of mile marker 062 SBD 12.00). Follow Joshua Lane as it curves east, then back south, and ends at a T-junction in 4.4 miles. Turn right, and then immediately turn left on Black Rock Canyon Road, which leads into the campground. Park by the Black Rock backcountry board on the east side of the road shortly past the entrance. The road is divided, and the trailhead is easy to miss.

Description: From the backcountry board, follow the trail east for 0.1 mile to a sandy wash. Follow the trail south in the wash, passing the California Riding and Hiking Trail, Short Loop

Trail, Burnt Hill Trail, and West Side Loop. At 1.6 miles, the canyon narrows and you pass Black Rock Spring. Its tiny trickle is mostly of interest to bees and other critters.

At 1.8 miles, the loop splits at a signed junction. Navigation is easiest if you take the right fork and make a counterclockwise loop. At 2.2 miles, pass a sign on the right pointing to Warren Point. The trail follows a shallow wash through a forest of Joshua trees before joining the ridgeline. At 3.5 miles, reach the

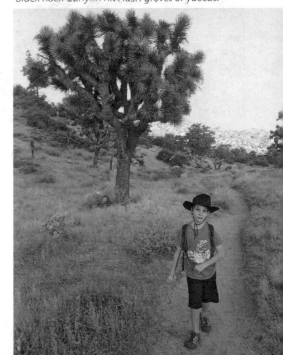

Black Rock Canyon has lush groves of yuccas.

Black Rock Panorama Loop

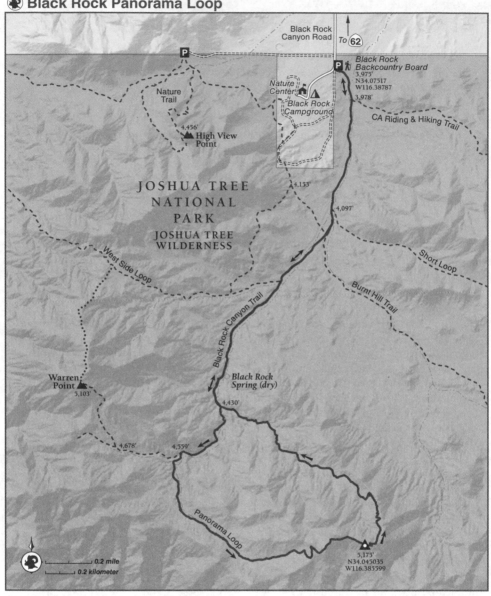

highest point on the ridge, with excellent views of San Gorgonio and of the intricate canyons in the Little San Bernardino Mountains. The steep, sandy trail veers left (north) down the ridge and then northwest down the canyon. At 4.8 miles arrive back at the split in the loop. Hike north down the wash back to the trailhead.

HIKE 49 Wonderland of Rocks Traverse

Location	Joshua Tree National Park
Highlight	Scrambling amid gigantic boulders
Distance & Configuration	6-mile point-to-point
Elevation Gain/Loss	200'/1,200'
Hiking Time	6 hours
Recommended Map	Tom Harrison *Joshua Tree National Park* or Trails Illustrated *Joshua Tree*
Best Times	October–April
Agency	Joshua Tree National Park
Difficulty	Strenuous
Permit	National park entry fee
Google Maps	Keys West Backcountry Registration Board (start); Rattlesnake Canyon Picnic Area (end)

More than 100 million years ago, a molten mass of rock lay several miles underground, cooling and crystallizing by agonizingly slow degrees. As the mass solidified, it contracted slightly, and fractures developed within it. Over geologic time, this mass moved upward, while

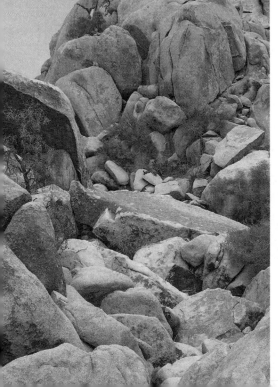

Wonderland Ravine is full of enormous boulders.

older, overlying layers of rock were eroded away. As the younger rock neared the surface, groundwater seeping into the fractures chemically transformed some of the rock crystals into clay. Large, more-or-less rectangular blocks of rock with rounded corners became isolated from each other in a matrix of loose clay. Once exposed above the surface, the clay quickly washed away, leaving open crevices between the blocks. Various mechanical forces and chemical weathering further chipped away at the boulders and rounded them even more.

The products of all this uplift and shaping are the monzogranite boulders we see today spectacularly exhibited in the Wonderland of Rocks section of Joshua Tree National Park. Everywhere you look, your mind is dazzled by huge, pancake- or loaflike stacks of rocks (where horizontal fractures predominate), by rocks in columns or spires (where vertical fractures predominate), and by huge domes. Each unique structure has been fashioned by a particular set of events occurring over millions of years.

The one-way traverse across the Wonderland of Rocks described here is known by some as the Wonderland Connection. Make no mistake: this is no easy stroll. Its "strenuous" rating is solely because of the fiercely jumbled landscape you must cross during the latter part of the trip; you should be adept at both boulder-hopping and scrambling across tilted rock surfaces. Much of the travel involves meticulously lowering

⊕ Wonderland of Rocks Traverse

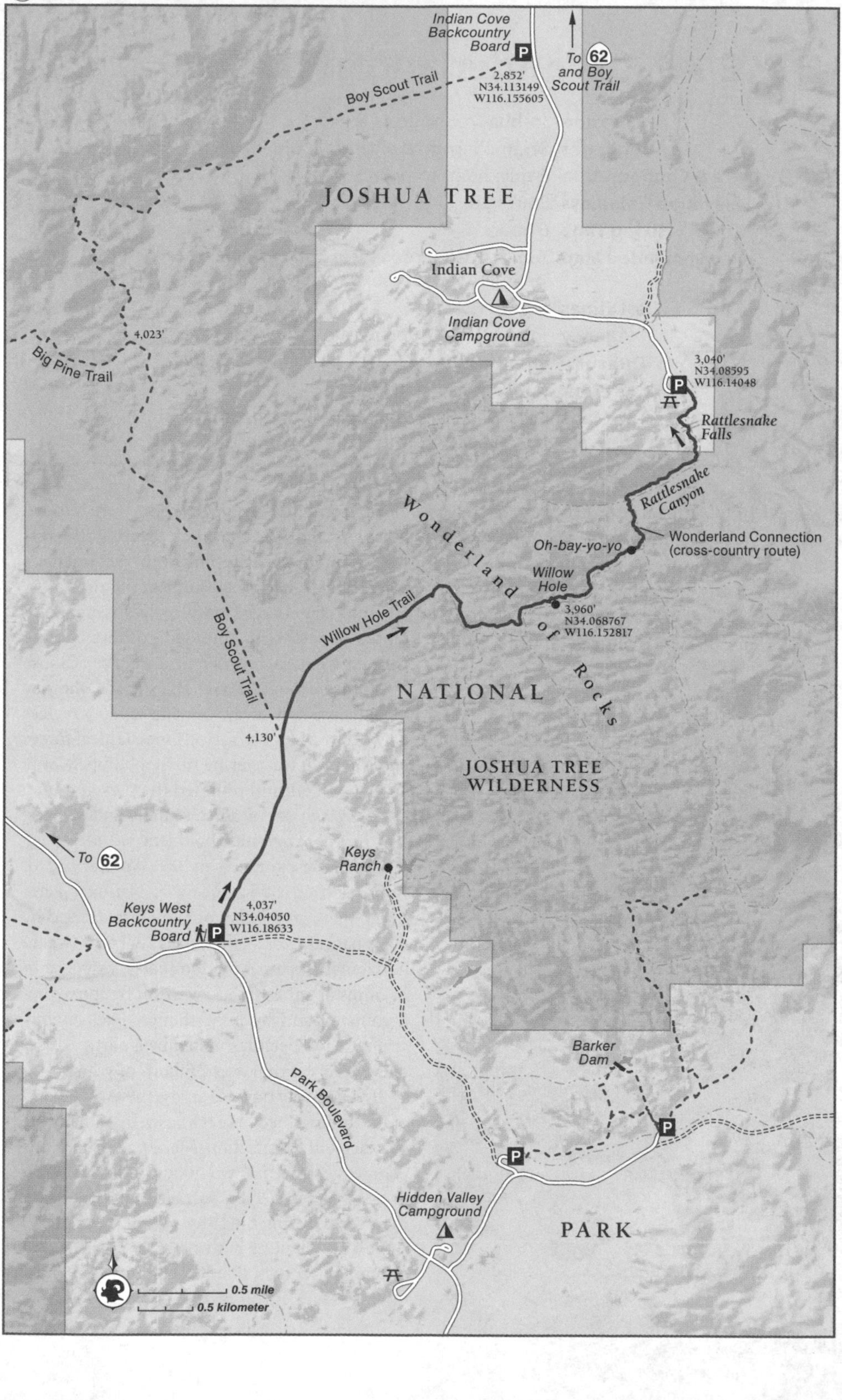

Indian Cove
Backcountry
Board **P**

2,852'
N34.113149
W116.155605

↑ To **62**
and Boy
Scout Trail

Boy Scout Trail

JOSHUA TREE

Indian Cove

△ Indian Cove
Campground

3,040'
N34.08595
W116.14048

P
🏕

*Rattlesnake
Falls*

↑

4,023'

Big Pine Trail

*Rattlesnake
Canyon*

Oh-bay-yo-yo

*Willow
Hole*

Wonderland Connection
(cross-country route)

W o n d e r l a n d

Willow Hole Trail

3,960'
N34.068767
W116.152817

N A T I O N A L

o f   R o c k s

Boy Scout Trail

4,130'

**JOSHUA TREE
WILDERNESS**

To **62**

Keys
Ranch ●

Keys West
Backcountry
Board 🚶 **P**

4,037'
N34.04050
W116.18633

Park Boulevard

Barker
Dam

P

P

P

Hidden Valley
Campground
△
🏕

P A R K

⊕

⊢——————⊣ 0.5 mile
⊢——————⊣ 0.5 kilometer

yourself downward over angular boulders—not recommended for the faint of heart. Camping is prohibited in the Wonderland area; you must plan your visit as a day trip.

To Reach the Trailheads: Arrange one vehicle at the Rattlesnake Canyon Picnic Area in Indian Cove and a second one at the Keys West backcountry board (Boy Scout Trailhead) in the main park. The shuttle involves a half-hour drive, even though the two trailheads are only a few miles apart as the crow flies over the Wonderland of Rocks. To reach Indian Cove from Highway 62, drive 8.8 miles east from Park Boulevard in the town of Joshua Tree; then turn south onto Indian Cove Road, 0.4 mile east of mile marker 062 SBD 27.00. Pass the entrance station in 1.1 miles and the backcountry board in another 0.5 mile; then continue 1.4 miles to the campground. Turn left (east) and pass through the campsites to reach the picnic area at Rattlesnake Canyon in another 1.3 miles. To reach the Boy Scout Trailhead, return to Park Boulevard in Joshua Tree and turn left (south). Pass the West Entrance Station and reset your odometer. In 6.4 miles, reach the large paved parking area for the Keys West backcountry board on the north side of the road, 0.8 mile east of mile marker 20.

Description: From the Keys West backcountry board, follow the Boy Scout Trail (formerly a dirt road) 1.2 miles north across sandy flats dotted with Joshua trees to the Willow Hole Trail, intersecting it on the right. Follow the Willow Hole Trail northeast to where it enters a dry wash, and then continue downhill in the wash. The wash soon becomes a canyon bottom flanked by stacks of boulders. At 3.5 miles you arrive at Willow Hole—large pools flanked by a screen of willows.

Following a beaten-down path, you then work your way through the willows on the right, over a low ridge and across a hard-to-identify gap between two rock piles. If you find yourself scrambling on difficult boulders, you're on the wrong path. Follow the narrow canyon bottom below, which carries water draining from the pools at Willow Hole during the wetter parts of the year. Your remaining route is entirely downhill, but negotiating a canyon section clogged with boulders impedes your progress.

At 0.7 mile beyond Willow Hole, the wash opens up in a broad clearing. Just north of this clearing, accessed by an obscure trail, is Oh-Bay-Yo-Yo, a cavelike shelter beneath a huge boulder. Take care of this special spot and leave no trace. This trip continues along the wash to a confluence with a second wash on the right.

Stay in the main canyon as it veers north and descends sharply for 0.3 mile to join Rattlesnake Canyon. Exercise care while descending this hazardous stretch. You can find fascinating caves under the gigantic talus blocks. (It was here, during a prearranged rendezvous and car-key exchange between original author Jerry Schad's party and a party traveling in the opposite direction, that one set of keys was dropped into the boulder maze and almost irretrievably lost. The lesson: always have an extra key in a magnetic box on the car frame or hidden nearby.)

Once you reach Rattlesnake Canyon, only a bit more than a mile of hiking remains. The going is easy for a while as you follow the sandy wash downhill (northeast). Some cottonwood trees brighten the otherwise desolate scene of sand and soaring stone walls. As the canyon bends left for a final descent to the flats of Indian Cove below, you face more episodes of serious scrambling. Keeping to the left canyon wall past some interior live oak trees, work your way around a slotlike canyon worn in the granitic rock. Down in the bottom of the slot are potholes worn by the abrasive action of flash flooding. A little more scrambling and a short walk down the canyon's sandy wash takes you to the end of the hike, the picnic area at Indian Cove.

VARIATION

If you can't arrange a vehicle shuttle, you can also return by way of the Boy Scout Trail that starts near the north end of Indian Cove. This option is 14 miles and takes about 10 hours of walking.

HIKE 50   Ryan Mountain

Location	Joshua Tree National Park
Highlights	Panoramic mountain and desert views
Distance & Configuration	2.8-mile out-and-back
Elevation Gain	1,000'
Hiking Time	2 hours
Optional Map	Tom Harrison *Joshua Tree National Park* or Trails Illustrated *Joshua Tree*
Best Times	September–May
Agency	Joshua Tree National Park
Difficulty	Moderate
Trail Use	Good for kids
Permit	National park entry fee
Google Maps	Ryan Mountain Trail, Park Boulevard

Elongated Ryan Mountain rises above the boulder-studded plains of Lost Horse and Queen Valleys in Joshua Tree National Park. The view from the top is arguably the best in the park, encompassing the blocky summits of San Jacinto and San Gorgonio, the intricately dissected Wonderland of Rocks, and a succession of shimmering basins and skeletal mountain ranges stretching east toward the Colorado River and south toward Baja California. The popular trail from the mountain's base to its top is well worn, yet steep and rocky, with more than 600 painstakingly built stone stairs.

To Reach the Trailhead: From the national park's headquarters and main visitor center on Highway 62 outside Twentynine Palms, drive 16 miles southwest on Utah Trail/Park Boulevard. Alternatively, starting from the town of Joshua Tree, drive 17 miles southeast on Park Boulevard. Your hike begins at the Ryan Mountain parking area, at mile marker 13.

Ryan Mountain

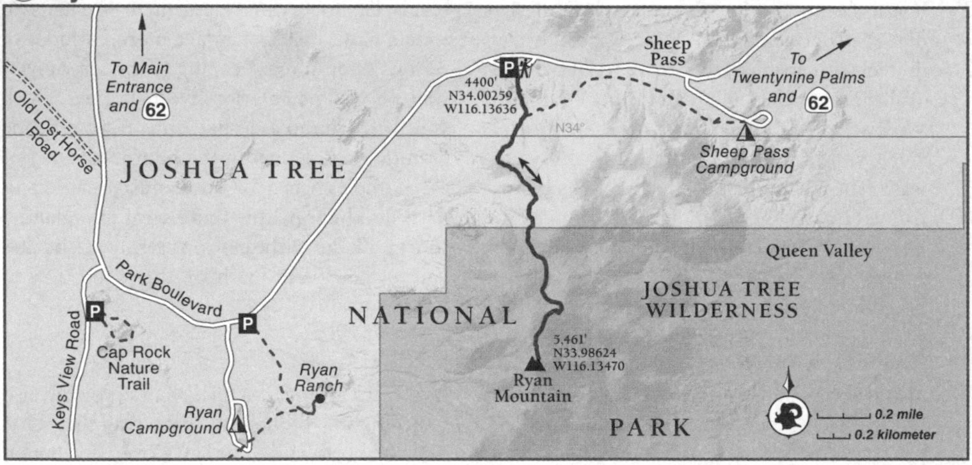

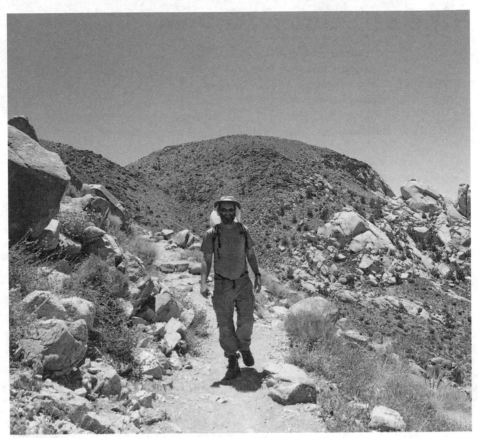

Ryan Mountain Trail   Kiby McDaniel

Description: From the parking area, head straight, uphill along the north and west flanks of the mountain, amid scattered juniper and pinyon pine. Look at the rocks to the west; you may note one that looks like the head and trunk of an elephant, while the other resembles the open mouth of a panther. Soon the geologic character of the rock underfoot changes. You cross the boundary between the White Tank monzogranite, the same rock you see exposed in boulder piles in the valleys below, and the Pinto gneiss, a much older rock into which the monzogranite rock was intruded (many miles underground) some 130 million years ago. The Pinto gneiss, which is foliated with layers of dark minerals, was metamorphosed (changed in form by intense heat and pressure) around 1.5 billion years ago, during an era when life on Earth consisted of nothing more than single-celled organisms. Watch for climbers on the monzogranitic Saddle Rocks, the largest rock formations in the park.

If you can, try a morning-twilight ascent of Ryan Mountain in the late fall or early winter. As the sun rises, look down and watch the interplay of light and shadow across the Joshua tree–dotted plains and on the monzogranite boulder piles, which rise like battlements out of the alluvium. From the top, you can see San Gorgonio and San Jacinto and are centrally located to pick out the high summits of Joshua Tree, including Queen, Quail, Eagle, and Keys View.

HIKE 51   Lost Horse Mine

Location	Joshua Tree National Park
Highlights	Mining history
Distance & Configuration	4.2-mile out-and-back
Elevation Gain	500'
Hiking Time	2 hours
Optional Map	Tom Harrison *Joshua Tree National Park* or Trails Illustrated *Joshua Tree*
Best Times	October–April
Agency	Joshua Tree National Park
Difficulty	Moderate
Trail use	Good for kids
Permit	National park entry fee
Google Maps	Lost Horse Mine Trailhead

The Lost Horse Mine, one of the few highly profitable gold mines in Southern California, yielded 10,000 ounces of gold between 1894 and 1931. The story of the mine was related by William Keys, a longtime resident of the area: Johnny Lang, a rancher, had his horses taken by a gang of cattle rustlers. Lang learned of the mine from a prospector and, to protect himself from further threats from the gang, went in with three partners to buy the rights to it. They purchased the mine for $1,000, naming it Lost Horse.

Five years later, J. D. Ryan, a wealthy rancher from Montana, joined the partnership and hauled in a massive steam-powered 10-stamp mill. The mill crushed the ore from the mine. The resulting powder was mixed with water to form a slurry, which was treated with mercury to separate the gold from the debris. The amalgam was then smelted to extract the gold, which was shipped in 200-pound bricks to Banning. To power the steam mill, Ryan ran a pipeline 3.5 miles from the well at his ranch to the mine. The hills around the mine are still sparsely vegetated because the junipers and yuccas were felled as fuel for the steam mill.

According to Keys, Ryan caught Lang stealing gold from the night shift and forced Lang to sell out. Lang later retrieved some of the bullion

that he had secreted away near the mine, but he died of exposure along Keys View Road in the winter of 1925. Keys buried him near the Lost

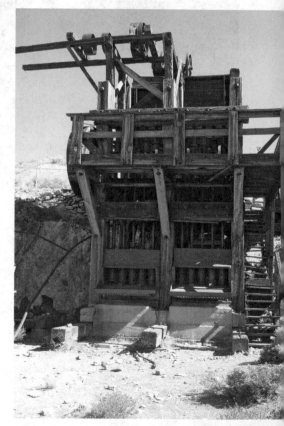

Lost Horse Mill

🔊 Lost Horse Mine

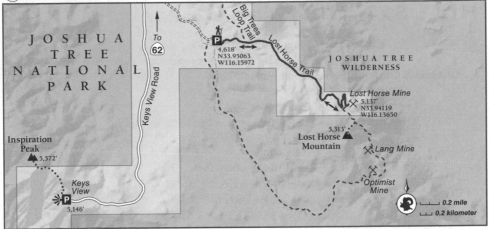

Horse Mine turnoff. As you hike this popular trail to the mine, imagine this Wild West drama unfolding, keep an eye out for hidden treasure, and take care that your hiking partner doesn't double-cross you.

To Reach the Trailhead: From the main Park Boulevard through Joshua Tree National Park, 0.8 mile east of mile marker 16, turn south on Keys View Road. In 2.4 miles, turn left at a good signed dirt road to Lost Horse Mine. The road, which is open for day use only, ends in 1 mile at a parking area with an outhouse.

Description: The wide trail, formerly a wagon road, begins at the east end of the parking area. It starts up the wash and then promptly veers left at a sign. This is a good place to learn to identify Mojave yucca (with hairlike threads on the edge of the blades) and nolinas (similar in stature, but with no hairs). At 0.3 mile, pass the signed Big Tree Trail to Ryan Campground on the left. Our trail tends east beneath a volcanic hill.

The trail gradually climbs to the southeast. Enter the burn zone of the 2009 Lost Horse Fire. In 1 mile, cross a low ridge. Views open up to the east; soon after, the Lost Horse Mine comes into view. Look for the remains of a stone cabin on the right. At 2.0 miles, reach a trail and old roadbed forking left toward the mine.

Lost Horse Mine is fenced off. The shaft formerly reached a depth of 500 feet, with lateral tunnels every 100 feet. As the wooden frame decayed and the tunnels began to collapse, a sinkhole started to form. The park service has plugged the shaft and shored up the mill, but stay clear of the fence for your safety. You can also explore the foundations of the old cabins and the cyanide-settling tanks.

VARIATION

Those looking for a longer hike can make this into a 6-mile loop. Continue southeast up the right fork of the main trail to a saddle at 2.2 miles, where you could make a short detour to the top of Lost Horse Mountain. Descend the steep and rugged remains of an old mining road into a beautiful system of ridges and gullies. Pass the remains of Lang Mine at 2.7 miles.

The trail climbs onto a ridge, then turns west along the south flank of Lost Horse Mountain to a chimney at Optimist Mine (3.2 miles). At 4.5 miles, the trail crosses and joins a dry wash leading through a secluded valley of Joshua trees. Finally, curve right to return to the trailhead where you started.

HIKE 52   Lost Palms Oasis

Location Joshua Tree National Park
Highlights A palm oasis and desert vegetation
Distance & Configuration 7.5-mile out-and-back
Elevation Gain 700'
Hiking Time 4 hours
Optional Map Tom Harrison *Joshua Tree National Park* or
Trails Illustrated *Joshua Tree*
Best Times October–March
Agency Joshua Tree National Park
Difficulty Moderately strenuous
Permit National park entry fee
Google Maps Cottonwood Spring

Lost Palms Oasis showcases Joshua Tree National Park at its best. The trail leads you across cactus-clad hills before plunging into a deep canyon studded with the park's trademark granite boulders that conceal the largest stand of California fan palms in the park. Lost Palms is in a day-use area; camping is prohibited.

Lost Palms Oasis

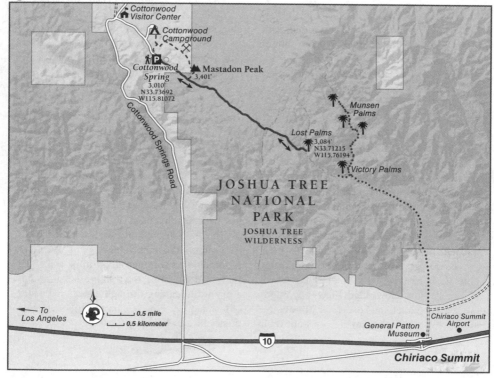

To Reach the Trailhead: Drive east on I-10 for 32 miles past Indio, then exit north on Cottonwood Springs Road to Joshua Tree National Park. Proceed 7.2 miles to Cottonwood Visitor Center, where you pay your park admission fee. Turn right (east), and proceed 1.1 miles to the Cottonwood Spring Trailhead parking area at the end of the road.

Description: A trail descends southeast from the trailhead into the small Cottonwood Spring Oasis, once home to Cahuilla Indians. The protein-rich bean pods from the thorny mesquite tree were one of their major food sources. Look for the deep mortars in the granite boulders where women ground the beans into flour.

Continue southeast to a signed junction at 0.6 mile. The left fork leads to Mastodon Peak, but this trail goes right. Walk across the flat desert past countless cholla cacti, yuccas, and ocotillos. Continue in and out of dry washes in the badlands before reaching the end of the official trail on the canyon rim, 3.5 miles from the start.

You may take a short detour to the right for an overlook of Lost Palms Oasis. An unmaintained but popular trail to the left makes a steep and rocky descent into the oasis on the canyon floor. Your efforts are rewarded at the bottom of the canyon, where you can enjoy the splendid palm oasis.

HIKE 53 Ladder Canyon

Location	Mecca Hills, north of the Salton Sea
Highlights	Slot canyon and fault-churned landscape
Distance & Configuration	4.3-mile loop
Elevation Gain	750'
Hiking Time	3.5 hours
Optional Maps	USGS 7.5-minute *Mecca, Mortmar* and *Cottonwood Basin*
Best Times	October–April
Agency	Bureau of Land Management/Palm Springs–South Coast Field Office
Difficulty	Moderately strenuous
Trail use	Good for kids
Permit	None required
Google Maps	Painted Canyon Trailhead

Ladder Canyon is the informal name given to a slotlike ravine incised into the sedimentary strata of the Mecca Hills on the eastern fringe of the Coachella Valley. Several ladders at strategic spots within the canyon assist or make feasible passages over abrupt dry falls (drop-offs) along the bottom. On rare occasions—mostly during summer thundershowers—these drop-offs briefly come alive with cascading, muddy water.

Ladder Canyon is a tributary of the superbly scenic Painted Canyon, which worms its way into the Mecca Hills Wilderness, which is administered by the Bureau of Land Management. The famed San Andreas Fault Zone passes through here, giving you a glimpse of what hundreds of miles of horizontal displacement and tens of miles of stretching (over many millions of years) can do to a landscape consisting of little else but stark rock formations.

Ladder Canyon was once a hidden treasure but has now become extremely popular; go early or expect crowds. Unfortunately, the popularity comes with other trappings of civilization, including graffiti and car break-ins. Don't leave anything of value in your vehicle.

Ladder Canyon

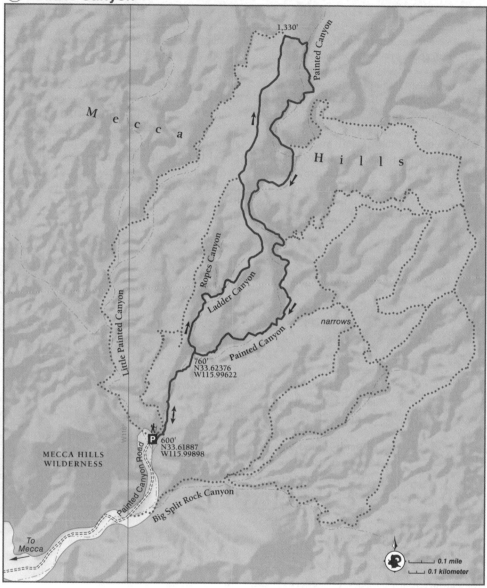

To Reach the Trailhead: The Mecca Hills lie about 120 miles east of Los Angeles. From I-10 east of Indio, turn south onto Highway 86S. Drive 10 miles to 62nd Avenue near the town of Mecca. Drive east 2 miles on this road to its end at Johnson Street, then turn right. Proceed another 2 miles, then turn left on 66th Avenue, which becomes Box Canyon Road. In 4.1 miles, turn left onto Painted Canyon Road at a sign. This dirt road is usually passable by low-clearance cars unless it has washed out. Proceed 4.7 miles to the parking area in Painted Canyon. There are many options for dispersed camping along Painted Canyon Road before the parking area.

Description: Start hiking into the narrow canyon with sheer sandstone walls on the right (northeast), which is upper Painted Canyon.

All around you are fantastic formations of sandstone and shale (former sea bottom) that have been tilted upward at steep angles due to tensional forces along the San Andreas Fault. During the cooler part of the year, low-angle sunlight partially illuminates the canyon bottom, spotlighting scattered smoke trees growing in the sandy wash, making them appear like gray puffs of smoke when seen from a distance.

At 0.4 mile, a slotlike ravine nearly blocked by fallen sandstone boulders (and possibly marked by a LADDER CANYON sign) can be seen along the canyon wall to the left. Some mild scrambling and clambering up several near-vertical ladders allow you to gain elevation quickly. Volunteers maintain the ladders, but it's always wise to inspect them yourself before trusting them.

At 0.8 mile from the start, there's a fork where the now-wider ravine divides into two nearly equal tributaries. Take the left fork for the easier route. (Using the right-fork tributary, you would quickly climb to the west rim of Painted Canyon and later rejoin the main route.) By 1.5 miles you reach the head of the left-fork ravine and find yourself just below and west of a rounded ridge (a large rock cairn lies on a knoll to the left). An informal trail swings up that ridge and follows its course steadily uphill in the direction of some radio towers about 2 miles north.

In the direction opposite the radio towers, a gorgeous view of the Coachella Valley and Salton Sea unfolds as you climb. The below-sea-level Salton Sea is the largest inland body of water in California—blue and inviting from a distance, but not especially picturesque or sweet-smelling up close. The sea has been the recipient of nearly a century's worth of irrigation runoff from the Coachella and Imperial Valleys (and more recently wastewater from the Mexicali region of northern Baja California), which has created a noxiously polluted body of water plagued by ever-increasing salinity levels. The vast, sunken landscape before you, flanked by mountains on both the east and west sides, resulted from tensional forces that continue to pull apart the Pacific and North American tectonic plates in this part of California.

At 2.0 miles, in a saddle on the ridge, the trail turns abruptly right and darts down a rocky slope into the wide, sandy wash of upper Painted Canyon. Make a right and start to enjoy the entirely downhill remainder of the hike. Painted Canyon deepens as you descend, exposing a geological wonderland of primarily dark metamorphic rocks. At 2.7 miles, a deep tributary canyon comes in from the left, offering a good side trip of a half mile or more if you are curious and energetic. At 3.3 miles, a ladder facilitates easy passage over an otherwise frightening descent over a dry fall in the main canyon. The rest is easy going on a wide bed of coarse sand past the Ladder Canyon turnoff and back to your car.

Ladder Canyon slot

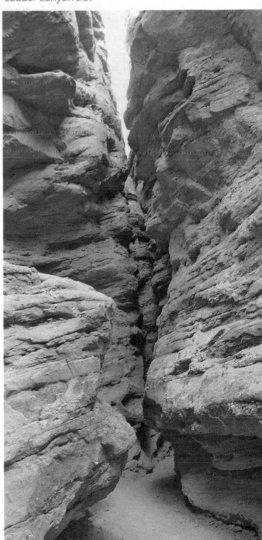

HIKE 54   Murray Hill

Location	Santa Rosa Mountains
Highlights	Views, a peak, and some desert vegetation
Distance & Configuration	7-mile out-and-back
Elevation Gain	1,900'
Hiking Time	5 hours
Optional Map	N/A
Best Times	October–March
Agency	Santa Rosa and San Jacinto Mountains National Monument
Difficulty	Moderately strenuous
Trail use	Suitable for equestrians, bikers
Permit	None required
Google Maps	Garstin Trailhead

Prominent from many directions, pyramid-shaped Murray Hill offers panoramic views over the Palm Springs area and the Santa Rosa Mountains. It is best climbed on a clear, cool day. Its diminutive name belies the fact that Murray Hill is a steep and strenuous hike that challenges and rewards the intrepid explorer. The summit is named for Scottish rancher Welwood Murray, who founded the Palm Springs Hotel in 1887 and drew attention to the area as a spa and resort. Murray Hill can be approached from the west, north, or south. This trip describes the western approach via the Garstin and Wild Horse Trails, but you can enjoy a longer loop or a one-way trip in combination with other trails. Many of the trails in this area were built by and named for members of the Desert Riders, an active equestrian group in the Coachella Valley. Peninsular desert bighorn sheep frequent the area; watch for their raisin-size scat, and scan the slopes in hopes that you might see the elusive animals.

To Reach the Trailhead: From I-10, take Highway 111 south into Palm Springs. The road becomes North Palm Canyon Drive and then South Palm Canyon Drive. Most lanes turn left to become East Palm Canyon, but stay right (straight) and continue on South Palm Canyon Drive for 1.9 miles. Turn left onto East Bogart Trail, and follow it 0.9 mile over a bridge across Palm Canyon Wash. Immediately turn left on Barona Road, and park at the end.

Description: The trail starts at a post at the end of Barona Road and leads east. In 150 yards, it reaches a signed fork. The Henderson Trail veers left and heads northeast along the toe of the ridge, but turn right and follow Garstin Trail up steep switchbacks hewn from the hillside. Your efforts are rewarded by steadily widening views to the west.

Shortly before reaching the top of the hill, the trail forks. The right fork is recommended; it follows the ridgeline for 0.1 mile before

Murray Hill

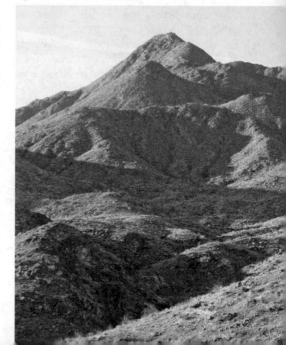

🐾 Murray Hill

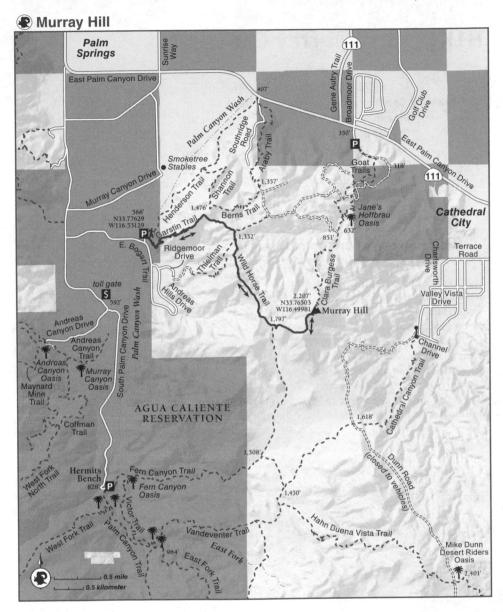

rejoining its sister. Soon after, 1.2 miles from the start, come to a junction with Berns Trail on top of the ridge.

From here, Murray Hill stands prominently to the southeast. Your goal is to head there via the Wild Horse Trail without getting lost on the maze of poorly marked paths crisscrossing the mountains. Turn right and head toward Murray Hill. At 1.5 miles, stay right at a fork. Just beyond, at a four-way junction with the Thielman Trail, go straight onto the Wild Horse Trail. Continue up the ridge to a junction, 2.7 miles. The right fork drops to Fern Canyon, but this trip stays left onto the Clara Burgess Trail, which climbs the fine ridgeline to the summit of Murray Hill.

HIKE 55   Murray Canyon

Location	Palm Springs
Highlights	Palm oases, waterfalls
Distance & Configuration	4-mile out-and-back
Elevation Gain	500'
Hiking Time	3 hours
Optional Map	Indian Canyons *Murray Canyon*
Best Times	January–April
Agency	Agua Caliente Band of Cahuilla Indians
Difficulty	Moderate
Trail Use	Good for kids, suitable for equestrians
Permit	Indian Canyons entry fee
Google Maps	Murray Canyon Trail

Murray Canyon is named for Scottish rancher Welwood Murray, who founded the Palm Springs Hotel in 1887 and brought attention to the area as a spa and resort. The canyon cuts a groove down the rugged eastern slope of the Desert Divide. The trail visits several palm oases before ending at the Seven Sisters, a series of stone pools with a 12-foot waterfall. Murray Creek runs through the winter and spring. The trail crosses the creek more than a dozen times,

Seven Sisters Waterfall

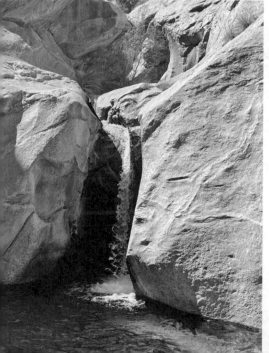

and the rocks can be slippery, so a trekking pole is helpful; this trip isn't recommended for those unsure of their balance. It is usually possible to cross on logs and keep your feet dry, but you might have to wade in high water, and the creek is impassable during rare floods. The falls are a great destination for a picnic, but don't expect to find solitude on this popular trail. The Indian Canyons are open 8 a.m.–5 p.m.

To Reach the Trailhead: From I-10, take Highway 111 south into Palm Springs, where the road name changes to North Palm Canyon Drive then South Palm Canyon Drive. About 12.4 miles from the freeway, most lanes turn left to become East Palm Canyon Drive, but stay straight (south) to continue on South Palm Canyon Drive. Follow South Palm Canyon Drive 2.8 miles to the Indian Canyons tollgate. Beyond the gate, immediately turn right and follow Andreas Canyon Road 0.8 mile to the Andreas Canyon parking area. Turn left, cross a bridge, pass the Bent Palm Picnic Area, and park at the Murray Canyon Trailhead in 0.2 mile.

Description: Follow the trail south across the desert at the base of a ridge, past brittlebushes and creosote. In 0.2 mile, pass the Andreas Canyon South Trail on your left. At 0.7 mile, make a switchback down to cross Murray Creek at a palm oasis. On the far side, pass another junction on the left with the Coffman Trail.

At 1.0 mile, reach the mouth of Murray Canyon. The trail follows the winding canyon,

Murray Canyon

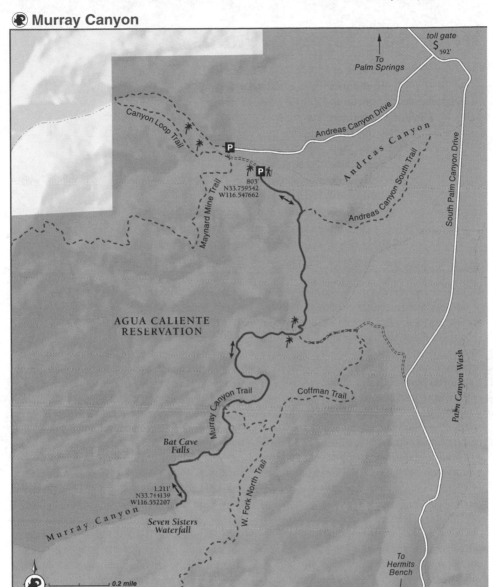

crossing the creek repeatedly. The California fan palms and honey mesquite bushes growing along the creek were important sources of food for the Cahuilla Indians.

At 1.4 miles, reach a second junction on the left with the Coffman Trail, which leads over the ridge out of the canyon. Just beyond, find a hitching line. Equestrians should leave their horses here because the last 0.5 mile of the canyon is unsuitable for riding. When you come

to the only steep climb on the trail, look right at a huge overhanging rock known as the Bat Cave. A modest waterfall flows from the ceiling of the cave.

Continue the brief steep climb and go over some slick rocks to reach a pool and small waterfall at trail's end. Do not try to explore farther; it is prohibited by the tribal rangers and would require potentially hazardous rock climbing.

HIKE 56   Pines to Palms

Location	Santa Rosa Mountains
Highlights	Palm oasis and desert
Distance & Configuration	15-mile point-to-point
Elevation Gain/Loss	100'/3,500'
Hiking Time	7 hours
Optional Map	Indian Canyons overview map
Best Times	October–March
Agency	Agua Caliente Band of Cahuilla Indians
Difficulty	Strenuous
Trail Use	Suitable for backpacking
Permit	Indian Canyons entry fee
Google Maps	Palm Canyon Trail 4E01 (southern trailhead); Hermits Bench (northern trailhead)

Palm Canyon should be on every serious Southern California hiker's to-do list. The canyon separates the San Jacinto Mountains and Desert Divide on the west from the Santa Rosa Mountains on the east and offers magnificent scenery in all directions. As it descends from the pinyon pines of the mountains to the cacti of the desert, it takes you past most of the Seussian plant life of the Upper and Lower Sonoran zones. The enormous palm oasis at the north end (bottom) of the trail is a fitting conclusion to a long but rewarding day. Those looking for a more casual hike suitable for children will enjoy roaming the oasis from the trailhead at Hermits Bench.

This hike presents a couple of logistical challenges. The northern trailhead at Hermits Bench is only open 8 a.m.–5 p.m. If you are not out before the gates close, the rangers will initiate a search. The drive between trailheads takes about 45 minutes, so if you leave a vehicle at Hermits Bench when it opens, drive to the upper trailhead, and begin walking at 9 a.m., you will have at most 8 hours to complete the 15-mile trek. Some prefer to do the trip as an overnight backpack, with a trusted friend handling the drop-off and pickup. Note that camping is prohibited on the reservation land comprising the northern half of the canyon (beginning about 2 miles north of Agua Bonita Spring).

To Reach Hermits Bench (the northern trailhead): Leave a car where the trip ends at Hermits Bench. From I-10, take Highway 111 south into Palm Springs. The road becomes North Palm Canyon Drive, then South Palm Canyon Drive. Most lanes turn left to become East Palm Canyon, but stay right (straight) to continue on South Palm Canyon Drive 2.8 miles to the tollgate at the entrance to Indian Canyons. Notify the ranger of your plans. Continue 2.5 miles to the trailhead parking at Hermits Bench.

To Reach Palm Canyon (the southern trailhead): Head back north and turn right on East Palm Canyon Drive, which becomes Highway 111. Go east and southeast 11 miles, then turn right on Highway 74 and follow it 18 miles. Just past mile marker 074 RIV 77.85, turn right onto Pine View Drive, and proceed 0.2 mile to the end of the paved road.

Description: Walk north from the Palm Canyon Trailhead up a dirt road. In 0.1 mile, veer right at a blank steel trail marker. Hike north through ribbonwood and chaparral, enjoying the sweeping views of Palm Canyon's upper reaches. At 1.3 miles, come to a signed four-way junction, and continue straight on jeep tracks leading north on the ridge. (The trail to the left also reaches Palm Canyon, but it may be overgrown and more difficult to follow.)

🄡 Pines to Palms

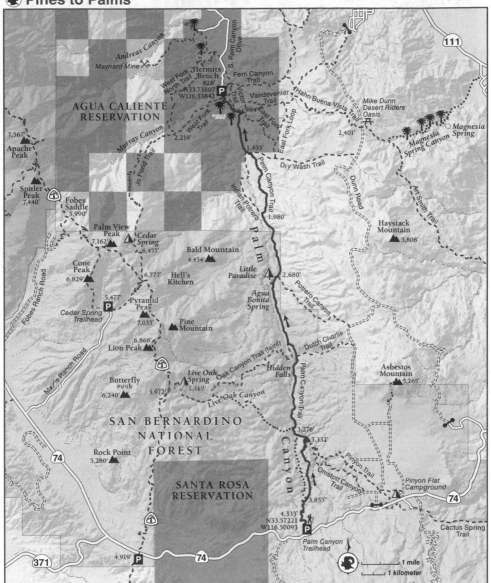

Your route hugs the rolling ridgeline and then switchbacks northeast down into Omstott Canyon. Turn left and follow the trail down the canyon. Go around a bend and meet the Palm Canyon Trail at a post (3.9 miles).

The trail along upper Palm Canyon is narrow, lightly traveled, and faint in places. This land is used for cattle ranching, and several gates control the cattle; close them behind you. Stay on Palm Canyon Trail. Within 0.2 mile, pass a fork where the unmaintained Live Oak Canyon Trail leads west. Then pass Dutch Charlie Trail to the east, 6.3 miles, and the faint Oak Canyon Trail veering southwest through the mesquite. (If you have time, you might try following it around a bend to Hidden Falls.)

The next section of trail is notable for its abundance of yuccas. At 8.3 miles, reach a

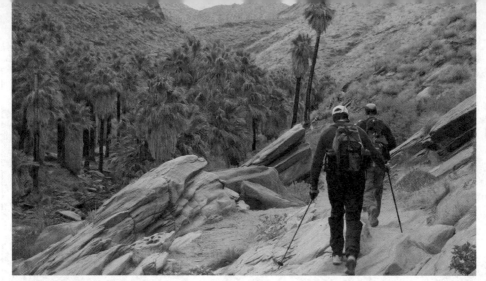
Palm Canyon Oasis

signed junction. Agua Bonita Spring is on the canyon bottom to the west, and water can be found here much of the year. Look for bedrock mortars where the Cahuilla once ground their food. At 8.6 miles, the Potrero Canyon Trail veers off to the right. Palm Canyon becomes deeper and more rugged. The rocky badlands to the west are called Hells Kitchen. At 10.4 miles, reach a junction with the Indian Potrero Trail. Either fork is enjoyable, and they rejoin in at 12.4 miles at a junction with the aptly named Dry Wash Trail.

Continue north to an enormous palm oasis at the junction with the Victor, Vandeventer, and East Fork Trails (13.5 miles). Stay left on the Palm Canyon Trail for another mile, passing many more palms before climbing up to Hermits Bench.

HIKE 57 San Jacinto Peak: The Easy Way

Location	San Jacinto Mountains
Highlight	Broad view of Southern California from summit
Distance & Configuration	11-mile out-and-back
Elevation Gain	2,600'
Hiking Time	6 hours
Optional Map	Tom Harrison *San Jacinto Wilderness*
Best Times	May–November
Agency	Mount San Jacinto State Park
Difficulty	Moderately strenuous
Trail use	Suitable for backpacking
Permit	San Jacinto Wilderness permit required
Google Maps	Palm Springs Aerial Tramway

San Jacinto Peak is a close second, after San Gorgonio Mountain, on the roster of Southern California high points, but its more sharply defined and imposing bulk makes it instantly identifiable from almost anywhere. According to legend, upon witnessing the sunrise from the summit one morning, the famed naturalist John Muir exclaimed, "The view from San Jacinto is the most sublime spectacle to be found anywhere on this earth!"

Despite his propensity for superlatives and the lack of historical evidence that he actually

San Jacinto Peak: The Easy Way

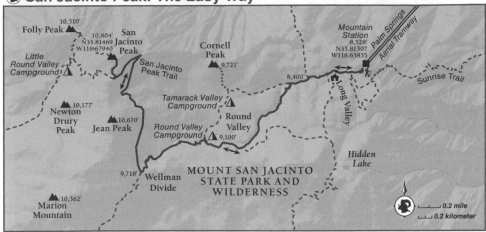

Folly Peak ▲ 10,510'
10,804'
N33.81469 San
W116.67940 Jacinto
Peak

Little
Round Valley
Campground △

San Jacinto
Peak Trail

Cornell
Peak
▲ 9,721'

8,400'

Mountain
Station
8,528'
N33.81307
W116.63855

Palm Springs
Aerial Tramway

Sunrise Trail

▲ 10,177'
Newton
Drury
Peak

▲ 10,670'
Jean Peak

Tamarack Valley
Campground △

Round Valley
Campground △

Round
Valley
9,100'

Long Valley

Hidden
Lake

9,718'
Wellman
Divide

MOUNT SAN JACINTO
STATE PARK AND
WILDERNESS

▲ 10,362'
Marion
Mountain

0.2 mile
0.2 kilometer

climbed San Jacinto, Muir may have been right. We may never know. Since his visit more than a century ago, more than 20 million people have come to settle within a 150-mile radius around the mountain. Air pollution dims today's view, even on the clearest days. Still, 100-mile visibility is not uncommon—out to the Channel Islands in the west, down to the northern Sierra of Baja California to the south, and east into Arizona. San Gorgonio and the San Bernardino Mountains rear up in the north, 15–20 miles away, blocking vistas of the Mojave Desert.

The north face of San Jacinto, which at one point soars 9,000 feet up in 4 horizontal miles, is one of the most imposing escarpments in the United States. Expert climbers have made the grueling ascent from the north in as little as 9 hours. Fortunately, several easier, well-graded trails let you bag the summit from other directions with a lot less effort. Every summer, thousands of people take advantage of the easiest route of all, the 5.5-mile trail between the mountain station of the Palm Springs Aerial Tramway (8,516') and the top of San Jacinto (10,804'). Well-conditioned hikers accustomed to high altitudes will find this a moderate trip. Others can still get plenty of pleasure out of shorter trips that don't stray very far from the mountain station. The slopes hereabouts feature some of the most inviting high-country forests and meadows south of the Sierra Nevada.

To prepare for your trip, call the Palm Springs Aerial Tramway at 760-325-1391 or visit pstramway.com for information and operating hours. The tramway usually closes in late September for maintenance; otherwise, it operates daily year-round. If you intend to camp overnight, reserve a campsite at Round Valley or Tamarack Valley in advance (parks.ca.gov /pages/636/files/DPR409.pdf).

Palm Springs Aerial Tramway

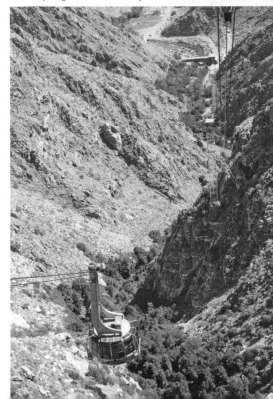

To Reach the Trailhead: From eastbound I-10, take the Palm Springs exit (Highway 111), and drive 8.5 miles to Tramway Road, on the right. Drive 4 miles up Tramway Road to where it ends in the parking lot for the lower terminus (Valley Station) of the Palm Springs Aerial Tramway. Purchase a round-trip ticket, and ride the tramway up to the Mountain Station, where you can find visitor amenities, such as a restaurant and gift shop.

Description: A paved pathway leads 0.2 mile down from the Mountain Station to the San Jacinto State Wilderness ranger hut in Long Valley, where you must obtain a wilderness permit for travel beyond Long Valley. From the ranger hut, follow the wide trail leading steadily uphill for 2 miles to Round Valley, mostly through a coniferous forest of Jeffrey pine, sugar pine, and white fir. Backpacking campsites are located in the Round Valley area and at Tamarack Valley, 0.5 mile north of Round Valley via a side trail. Continue your ascent, somewhat steeper now, through thinning lodgepole pines to a trail junction at Wellman Divide, 3.2 miles from the start. This is where you get your first impressive view—south over tree-covered summits, foothills, and distant desert and coastal valleys.

After an almost obligatory (common, anyway) water or snack break at Wellman Divide, continue your leisurely uphill grind toward San Jacinto Peak. You traverse north for more than a mile across a boulder-strewn slope covered by scattered lodgepole pines and a carpet of low-growing alpine shrubs. Abruptly, you change direction at a switchback corner, climb southwest for a while, and arrive on a saddle just south of the peak itself (5.2 miles). Veer right, follow the path up along the right (east) side of the summit, pass a stone hut, and then scramble from boulder to boulder for a couple of minutes to reach the top.

Hopefully the weather will allow you to rest a spell in the warm sun, cupped amid the jumbo-size rocks, and savor the lightheaded sensation of being on top of the world. Make sure you leave the summit of San Jacinto Peak in time to catch the last downhill tram ride. The steep, paved climb back to the Mountain Station may feel like the hardest part of the entire hike.

HIKE 58 San Jacinto Peak: The Hard Way

Location	San Jacinto Mountains
Highlight	Greatest elevation gain of any day hike in the Lower 48
Distance & Configuration	21-mile point-to-point
Elevation Gain/Loss	10,600'/2,600'
Hiking Time	13 hours or more
Optional Map	Tom Harrison *San Jacinto Wilderness*
Best Times	May–early June; October–early November
Agency	Santa Rosa and San Jacinto Mountains National Monument
Difficulty	Very strenuous
Trail Use	Suitable for backpacking
Permit	Free San Jacinto Wilderness permit at Long Valley Ranger Station
Google Maps	North Lykken Trailhead

This hike, known as the Cactus-to-Clouds Hike by Palm Springs hiking enthusiasts, is an absolute hoot—if you survive. For three decades now, ever-increasing numbers of adventurers have set foot in Palm Springs on a former Cahuilla footpath scaling the east slope of San Jacinto. For some, the goal has been San Jacinto Peak, 14 trail-miles away and 10,400 feet higher. Other hikers have settled for Long Valley, where the Mountain Station of the Palm

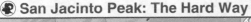

San Jacinto Peak: The Hard Way

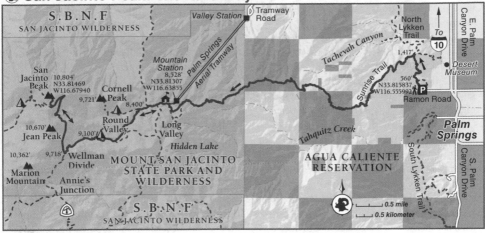

Springs Aerial Tramway sits—a "mere" 9 miles and 8,000 feet higher.

You must prepare for this hike with plenty of vigorous physical conditioning. Fortunately the San Jacinto and nearby San Bernardino and San Gabriel Mountains have many great routes for you to train. Conditioning hikes should include at least 5,000 feet of elevation gain, plus exposure to elevations of 9,000 feet or more.

Because the climate encountered on the full climb ranges from low desert to Arctic/alpine, you should try this hike only during the most moderate seasons—either late spring or early fall. If you go too early in the spring season, you might encounter treacherous patches of icy snow below Long Valley. In fall, you must wait until typical morning temperatures on the lower trail sink to less than lethally hot levels. The first snows usually arrive in November or December. For stable weather, it's hard to beat late October.

On a cool day during these moderate-season periods, you'll probably consume the better part of a gallon of water before your first dependable fill-up at Long Valley. In warm weather, a typical hiker will need a gallon or more. If you go all the way to San Jacinto Peak, remember that you must return to Long Valley and the tram station for a ride back down the mountain. The mileage quoted above in the capsulized summary includes the round-trip from Long Valley to the peak and back. When you arrive at the Mountain Station, you may need to purchase a one-way ticket for the tram ride down. Once you arrive

at the bottom, you can call a taxi to get back to the starting point. Call the Palm Springs Aerial Tramway at 760-325-1391, or visit pstramway .com, for information about the tramway and its operating schedule.

A predawn start on the trail—preferably 2 hours before sunrise—is mandatory to beat the worst of the heat and ensure you have enough daylight on your return trip. The ridge-running Skyline Trail is only lightly maintained but gets enough use to be well defined. If you are considering hiking downhill, remember that for much of the year, the desert is dangerously hot after sunrise.

To Reach the Trailhead: Ramon Road, a major east–west thoroughfare through the south side of Palm Springs, intersects that city's main north–south drag, Palm Canyon Drive, just south of the main business district. From that intersection, go 0.4 mile west on Ramon Road to where it dead-ends at the foot of Mount San Jacinto. Park off the street near the North Lykken Trailhead.

Description: Follow a dirt road north from the end of Ramon Road, and almost immediately you'll see the Carl Lykken Trail on the left. Climb about 1 mile and 1,000 feet up this maintained riding and hiking trail to reach a rocky saddle. A rougher trail, originating at the Palm Springs Desert Museum, comes up from the east and joins the saddle as well. Our Skyline Trail, also rough, takes off up the ridge to the west, past inscriptions that warn of the arduous ascent ahead.

Vistas of Coachella Valley and the vast sweep of the Colorado Desert expand as you trudge uphill, step after step, curling up along one side of the sinuous ridge, then the other. In a few hours, you will ascend through low-desert, high-desert, and chaparral plant associations into a boreal zone of pines and firs.

At about 5 miles (from Ramon Road), the trail might be more difficult to follow amid the manzanita chaparral. If you lose the trail, back up immediately and try to find it. You must stay on the route in order to negotiate the steep, rocky, brushy terrain ahead. At about 6.5 miles (5,800'), the trail crosses a shallow ravine, veers left, traverses through some oaks just above the creek, crosses the ravine again, and then climbs out of the ravine toward a ridge. It wanders up this ridge, sparsely dotted with timber, to about 7,600 feet, where it veers right (northwest) and traverses several steep gullies on a deeply shaded (in the fall, at least), northeast-facing slope. The section ahead is very dangerous if it is covered by hard-packed snow or ice and you don't have an ice ax and crampons. As you near a sheer rock outcropping, the trail abruptly bends left (southwest) and climbs almost straight up a steep slope to the lip of terracelike Long Valley, at an elevation of 8,400 feet.

You've come 10 miles from Ramon Road and gained 8,000 feet. If you choose to bail out at this point, simply head north through Long Valley a few hundred yards to the tramway station. Otherwise, pick up a wilderness permit at the Long Valley ranger hut below the tramway station.

From the ranger hut, follow the wide trail leading steadily uphill to Round Valley (12 miles), mostly through a coniferous forest of Jeffrey pine, sugar pine, and white fir. Continue the somewhat steeper ascent beyond Round Valley through thinning lodgepole pines to a trail junction at Wellman Divide (13 miles).

Beyond Wellman Divide, a more leisurely uphill grind takes you inexorably up toward San Jacinto Peak. You traverse north for more than a mile across a boulder-strewn slope covered by scattered lodgepole pines and a carpet of low-growing alpine shrubs. Abruptly, you change direction at a switchback corner, climb southwest for a while, and arrive on a saddle (15 miles) just south of the peak itself. Veer right, follow the path up along the right (east) side of the summit, pass a stone hut, and then scramble from boulder to boulder for a couple of minutes to reach the top. The view is dizzying, not only because of the sheer height, but also because you have ascended into thin air to a level where about one-third of Earth's atmosphere lies below you.

Your journey is not over yet! Make sure you leave the summit of San Jacinto Peak in time to catch the last downhill tram ride.

HIKE 59   San Jacinto Peak: The Middle Way

Location	San Jacinto Mountains
Highlights	Broad vistas and an atmosphere reminiscent of the Sierra Nevada
Distance & Configuration	15-mile out-and-back
Elevation Gain	4,400'
Hiking Time	9 hours
Optional Map	Tom Harrison *San Jacinto Wilderness*
Best Times	April–November
Agency	San Bernardino National Forest/San Jacinto Ranger District
Difficulty	Strenuous
Trail Use	Suitable for backpacking

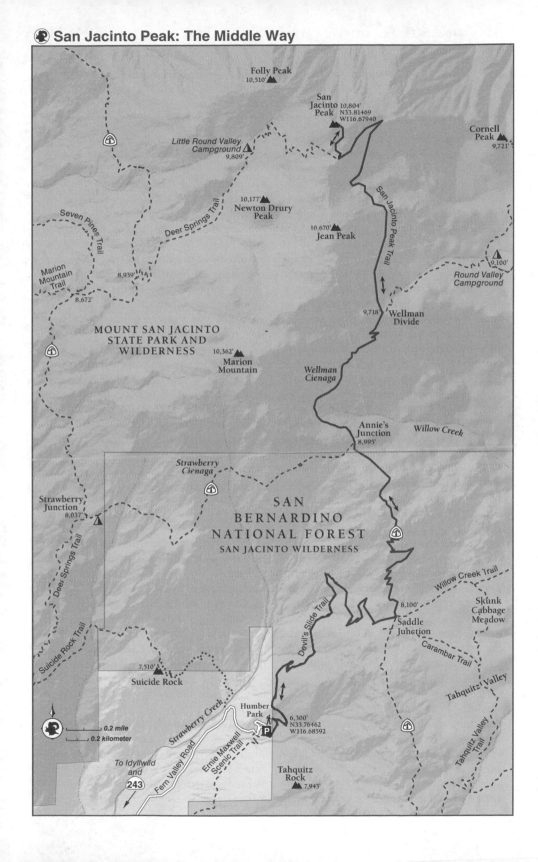

Folly Peak
10,510' ▲

San
Jacinto 10,804'
Peak N33.81469
W116.67940
▲

Cornell
Peak ▲
9,721'

Little Round Valley
Campground △
9,809'

Newton Drury 10,177' ▲
Peak

San Jacinto Peak Trail

Jean Peak 10,670' ▲

Seven Pines Trail

Deer Springs Trail

△ 9,100'

Round Valley
Campground

Marion
Mountain
Trail

8,939'

8,672'

9,718' Wellman
Divide

MOUNT SAN JACINTO
STATE PARK AND
WILDERNESS

10,362' ▲
Marion
Mountain

Wellman
Cienaga

Annie's
Junction
8,995'

Willow Creek

Strawberry
Cienaga

SAN
BERNARDINO
NATIONAL FOREST
SAN JACINTO WILDERNESS

Strawberry
Junction ▲
8,037'

Deer Springs Trail

Willow Creek Trail

Skunk
Cabbage
Meadow

8,100'

Suicide Rock Trail

Devil's Slide Trail

Saddle
Junction

Carambar Trail

7,510' ▲
Suicide Rock

Tahquitz Valley

0.2 mile
0.2 kilometer

Strawberry Creek

Humber
Park

6,300'
N33.76462
W116.68592

Tahquitz Valley
Trail

Ernie Maxwell Scenic Trail

To Idyllwild
and
243

Fern Valley Road

Tahquitz
Rock
▲ 7,943'

Permits San Jacinto Wilderness permit and National Forest
Adventure Pass required
Google Maps Humber Park, Fern Valley Road

The San Jacinto Mountains, like many other units of the Peninsular Ranges (and much of the Sierra Nevada to the north), have gradually sloping west faces and more steeply plunging east faces. Hike 58 tackled the desert-facing east slope of San Jacinto range. This route meanders in a far more leisurely fashion up the forested west slope. The comparison to the Sierra Nevada is an apt one: the climb from the yellow-pine botanical zone in Idyllwild toward the Arctic/alpine zone atop San Jacinto Peak is similar to many trips in the western Sierra Nevada that take hikers up through various forest belts to timberline.

This hike to San Jacinto Peak (midway in difficulty compared to the previous two in this book), follows the popular Devil's Slide Trail out of the resort community of Idyllwild. To control overuse, the U.S. Forest Service has established quotas for this trail on summer weekends and holidays. Apply by mail; the quota fills up well in advance on popular weekends, although early birds may be able to get first-come, first-served permits on the day of the trip. Call the San Jacinto Ranger Station for current information. Quotas or not, all hikers must obtain a wilderness permit (for either hiking or backpacking the route) at the Forest Service ranger station in the center of Idyllwild. The station is located on the east side of Highway 243, one block north of North Circle Drive. You will be driving past or very near this station on your way to the trailhead at Humber Park.

To Reach the Trailhead: Exit I-10 at Banning, and follow Highway 243 south for 25 miles to reach Idyllwild's town center and, on the left (east), North Circle Drive. Drive 0.75 mile northeast on North Circle Drive, veer right on South Circle Drive (crossing over Strawberry Creek), and take the first left, Fern Valley Road. Continue nearly 2 miles to the end of the road, where you will find a parking space (perhaps not on weekends, unless it's early!) in the large lot at Humber Park. A National Forest Adventure Pass is required.

Description: Two trails diverge from the parking lot: the Ernie Maxwell Scenic Trail descends to the right (south), and the Devil's Slide Trail ascends to the left (east and north). You waste no time on that ascent as you switch back and forth along a zigzagging course, intermittently enjoying the shade cast by oak, pine, fir, and cedar foliage. Two rock-climbing destinations are in view as you climb: Suicide Rock generally on the left (west) and the more imposing Lily Rock (or Tahquitz) on the right. During spring and early summer, rivulets of ice-cold water flow down several of the small ravines you cross on your way up.

At the top of the ridge, at Saddle Junction (2.5 miles), you can take a breather on a nearby rock or fallen log. Five trails converge in this flat space. Opportunities for wilderness camping are east of here in the Skunk Cabbage Meadow and Tahquitz Valley areas. These wilderness camping sites could make a suitable base camp for a two- or three-day expedition to the peak and back.

For the next leg, follow the Pacific Crest Trail (PCT) left (north) from Saddle Junction toward Wellman Divide. You ascend along a bouldery ridge, through statuesque Jeffrey pines and white firs, enjoying intermittent vistas east, south, and west. At Annie's Junction (4.4 miles), the PCT swings left (west), contouring more or less across the south flank of Marion Mountain. Strawberry Cienaga, a permanently soggy area in the upper Strawberry Creek drainage and a possible side trip, lies 1 mile down that trail. Our way, however, continues north through scattered lodgepole pines and white firs, past a boggy spot called Wellman Cienaga, and reaches Wellman Divide at 5.4 miles.

At Wellman Divide, the trail to the right descends to Round Valley and Long Valley, while our way stays left (north), climbing moderately but inexorably toward San Jacinto Peak. You traverse north for more than a mile across a boulder-strewn slope covered by scattered

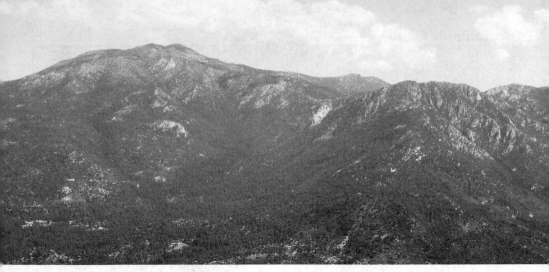

San Jacinto rises high above Idyllwild.

lodgepole pines and a carpet of low-growing alpine shrubs. Abruptly, you change direction at a switchback corner, climb southwest for a while, and arrive in a saddle just south of the peak itself (7.4 miles). Veer right, follow the path up along the right (east) side of the summit, pass a stone hut, then scramble from boulder to boulder for a couple of minutes to reach the top. When it's time to go, retrace your route to the trailhead.

VARIATION

Alternatively, you can loop around the west side of the mountain to make a terrific 20-mile tour of San Jacinto by way of Little Round Valley and Strawberry Junction.

HIKE 60   Tahquitz Peak

Location	San Jacinto Mountains
Highlight	Visiting a remote fire lookout with terrific views
Distance & Configuration	9-mile out-and-back
Elevation Gain	2,400'
Hiking Time	5 hours
Optional Map	Tom Harrison *San Jacinto Wilderness*
Best Times	April–November
Agency	San Bernardino National Forest/San Jacinto Ranger District
Difficulty	Moderately strenuous
Trail Use	Dogs allowed, suitable for backpacking
Permits	Free, self-issued San Jacinto Wilderness permit and National Forest Adventure Pass required
Google Maps	Humber Park

The name Tahquitz (pronounced by those in the know as "tak-wish") celebrates a legendary demon who, in the oral tradition of the Cahuilla Indians, used to dine on maidens and issue crackling bolts of lightning over the San Jacinto Mountains when displeased. At an elevation of 8,828 feet, the fire lookout tower perched atop the peak commands a view westward over haze

Tahquitz Peak

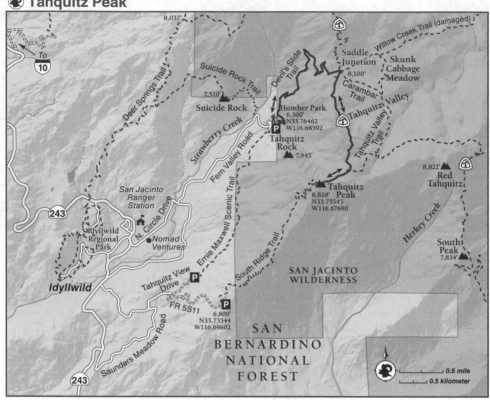

and smog to the crests of the Santa Ana and San Gabriel Mountains. On rare days of crystalline visibility, you may glimpse the coastline at Santa Monica and Malibu, as well as the offshore islands of Santa Catalina and San Clemente. This is one of the most enjoyable moderate peak climbs in Southern California.

The trip requires a San Jacinto Wilderness permit from the Idyllwild Ranger Station. There is a quota for day-use entry on the Devil's Slide Trail between Memorial Day and Labor Day. This is a great overnight trip, especially for families and youth groups, but you will need an overnight permit (quotas fill fast in the summer, so apply in advance for the Chinquipin Zone at tinyurl.com/sjwpermit).

To Reach the Trailhead: Exit I-10 at Banning, and follow Highway 243 south for 25 miles to

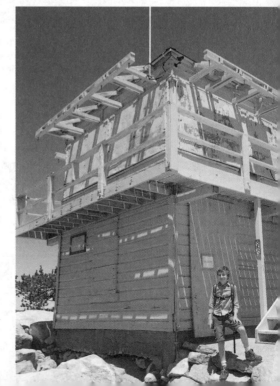

Tahquitz Peak Fire Lookout

the Idyllwild Station in Idyllwild, where you pick up your wilderness permit. Head northeast on Pine Crest Avenue. In 0.6 mile, veer right onto South Circle Drive. In 0.1 mile, turn left onto Fern Valley Road. Proceed 1.8 miles to the Humber Park Trailhead, at the road's end. A National Forest Adventure Pass is required.

Description: Hike up the Devil's Slide Trail into the San Jacinto Wilderness. The incense cedar, canyon live oak, and ponderosa pine near the start yield to sugar pine, Jeffrey pine, and white fir as you climb. In the spring and early summer, three creeks, fed by snowmelt springs, cascade down across the trail and nourish currants, which ripen later in the summer. You can savor views of Southern California's two alpine climbing meccas—Suicide Rock and Tahquitz Rock—and look at the shoulder of San Jacinto Mountain at the head of Strawberry Valley. After 2.5 miles and 1,600 feet of climbing, reach the five-way split at Saddle Junction.

Turn right (south) and take the Pacific Crest Trail toward Tahquitz Peak. Watch for faint spurs to good campsites out of sight of the trail (these are known as the Chinquapin Zone). At 3.9 miles, turn right onto the South Ridge Trail, which cuts across the north face of the peak (this steep slope can hold dangerous ice in the spring after everything else has melted out). Lodgepole and limber pines dominate the forest near the summit. Turn left at a junction just below the summit to reach the fire lookout tower atop Tahquitz Peak, which is frequently staffed between May and November. Visitors may or may not be invited to view the landscape from the tower itself. The summit view encompasses the timbered slopes of the southern San Jacinto Mountains and innumerable valleys and ridges spilling west and south toward Southern California's coast.

After taking in the view, descend from the lookout the way you came. Or, if you are seeking variety, descend the 3.5-mile South Ridge Trail. You could pre-position a car at this trailhead (high clearance sometimes required). Or you can make a great 11-mile loop with 3,200 feet of elevation gain by walking down the South Ridge Road and Tahquitz View Drive to the Ernie Maxwell Scenic Trail, which leads back to Humber Park.

HIKE 61   Mount Rubidoux

Location	City of Riverside
Highlight	Views
Distance & Configuration	3.3-mile loop
Elevation Gain	500'
Hiking Time	1.5 hours
Optional Map	USGS 7.5-minute *Riverside West*
Best Times	All year, daylight hours, but hot in the summer
Agency	City of Riverside Parks, Recreation, and Community Services
Difficulty	Moderate
Trail Use	Dogs allowed, good for kids, suitable for biking
Permit	None required
Google Maps	Ryan Bonamino Park

Mount Rubidoux is a prominent granite hill located west of downtown Riverside and south of the Santa Ana River. The mountain is named for Louis Rubidoux, who settled the area in the mid-1800s, but it was Frank Miller, one of Riverside's early promoters and the builder of the historic Mission Inn, who transformed Mount Rubidoux from an anonymous bump to a much-loved and inspirational park. Miller originally intended to develop the mountain for mansions, but his plan

🅿 Mount Rubidoux

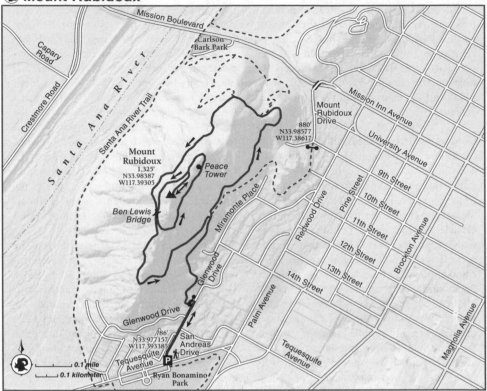

failed. Instead, Miller graded a road circling up the mountain that hikers, cyclists, joggers, and strollers enjoy today.

To Reach the Trailhead: From the 60 Freeway, take Exit 50 south onto Rubidoux Boulevard in Riverside. In 0.3 mile, turn left (east) onto Mission Boulevard. In another 1.5 miles, turn right onto Redwood Drive, and immediately stay straight on Redwood as part of the road veers left. In 0.7 mile, veer right onto Tequesquite Avenue and continue 0.3 mile to parking at Ryan Bonamino Park (5000 Tequesquite Ave.).

Description: There are two paved trails that wind up the mountain like intertwined corkscrews. The gentle route is 2 miles and loops the mountain twice, while the steeper route is 1 mile and loops the mountain only once. The two trails intersect twice.

From Bonamino Park walk northeast on San Andreas Avenue. In 0.2 mile, turn left into

Frank A. Miller Mount Rubidoux Memorial Park and follow the broad path that climbs the hillside. At 0.5 mile, stay straight at a signed four-way junction to take the longer trail up. Gnarly prickly pear cactus intermingles with coastal sage scrub and drifts downward into the backyard gardens of homes at the base of the mountain. Miller planted the yuccas, aloes, agave, and cacti that you see. As you climb, you will have views of downtown Riverside, Evergreen Memorial Cemetery, the Santa Ana River, and Flabob Airport, one of the older airports in America and a famous base for antique and home-built aircraft. Keep your eyes out for unusual planes approaching the field.

Pass the short trail a second time as you cross under the Ben Lewis Bridge and reach the Peace Tower, built by "friends of Frank Augustus Miller in recognition of his constant labor in the promotion of civic beauty, community righteousness, and world peace." Once you reach the top of the mountain, explore the amphitheater, the

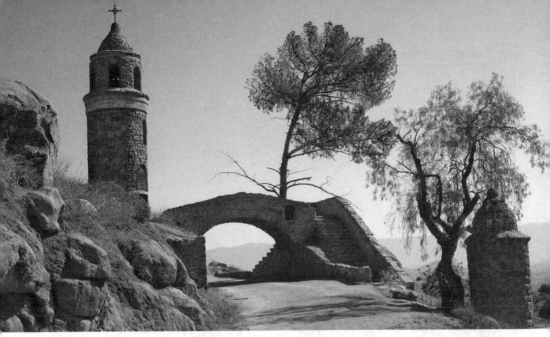

Peace Tower on Mount Rubidoux

plaque honoring Father Junipero Serra, the flagpole, and the large cross. On a clear day you will have excellent views south over Riverside.

Return along the steeper trail, which leads west along the north side of the mountain and over the Ben Lewis Bridge. When you reach the signed junction on the south side, retrace your original route east back to the trailhead.

HIKE 62   Lone Tree Point on Catalina

Location	Santa Catalina Island
Highlight	Island and sea vistas
Distance & Configuration	6-mile out-and-back
Elevation Gain	1,800'
Hiking Time	3 hours
Optional Map	Catalina Island Conservancy map (available at catalina conservancy.org, or purchase at The Trailhead Visitor Center)
Best Times	All year
Agency	Catalina Island Conservancy
Difficulty	Moderately strenuous
Trail Use	Good for kids
Permit	Day-use hiking permit required
Google Maps	Trans Catalina Trailhead

Santa Catalina Island, "26 miles across the sea," as the song goes, stretches 21 miles in length and up to 8 miles at its maximum width. The town of Avalon snuggles against a cove near the eastern end of the island, protected from prevailing winds that come out of the west and northwest. Avalon experiences the same almost-frost-free climate as the most even-tempered areas of the Southern California coastline, and it enjoys possibly the cleanest air

Lone Tree Point on Catalina

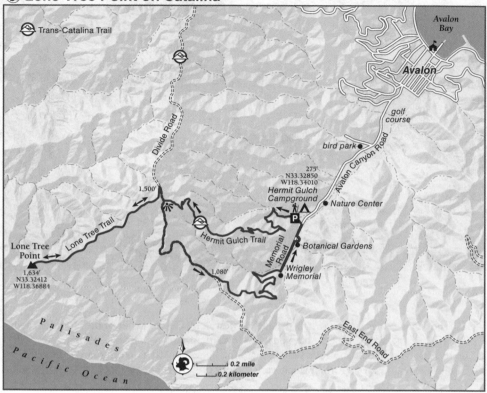

Trans-Catalina Trail

Avalon Bay

Avalon

golf course

bird park

Divide Road

Avalon Canyon Road

275'
N33.32850
W118.34010
Hermit Gulch Campground

Nature Center

1,500'

Hermit Gulch Trail

Lone Tree Trail

Memorial Road

Botanical Gardens

Wrigley Memorial

Lone Tree Point

1,634'
N33.32412
W118.36884

1,080'

East End Road

Palisades

Pacific Ocean

0.2 mile
0.2 kilometer

of any spot near the Southern California coast. In the hills above Avalon you can find wild mountainsides smothered in Catalina's own unique assemblage of chaparral, spectacular ocean views, and some of the finest hiking in all of California.

Catalina was for most of this century owned by the Wrigley family (of chewing-gum and Chicago Cubs fame). In 1972, management of most of the island passed into the hands of the Catalina Island Conservancy, whose function is to preserve and protect the island's wildlands. Recreational use, including camping, hiking, backpacking, and mountain biking (on select routes), is allowed on most of the island.

The languid pace of life on Catalina reflects its aloofness from the increasingly frantic business of living on the Southern California mainland. An overnight visit here is truly relaxing, whether you choose to lodge in Avalon or prefer to rough it at one of the several campgrounds spread around the island's coast and interior.

The hike described here, excellent during the spring wildflower season and on crisp fall or winter days, begins at Hermit Gulch Campground near Avalon and loops over the top of the hills overlooking Avalon and the ocean. (You'll need a free permit for this, available at catalinaconservancy.org or at the Trailhead Visitor Center in Avalon.) The highlight of the hike is a side trip over to Lone Tree Point, which commands an unparalleled view of the clifflike Palisades falling sheer to the ocean. You'll encounter a couple of very steep grades on the fire road leading to Lone Tree Point, so be sure to wear running shoes or boots with studs or lugs to ensure that you have plenty of traction. Small children will probably need some assistance on that stretch.

You may see bison, boar, and deer—all introduced at one time or another—on various parts of the island. Recent efforts to remove many of these non-indigenous, often destructive animals have been quite successful.

Spotting great herds of goats on the island is a thing of the past.

To Reach the Trailhead: Ferries to Catalina depart terminals at San Pedro, Long Beach, and Newport Beach. Air service is also available from Long Beach. For more information about camping, lodging, hiking, and biking on the island, as well as transportation to the island, the following phone numbers are useful: Catalina Island Conservancy, 310-510-2595, and Santa Catalina Island Company, 310-510-2800. You can also visit the conservancy's extensive website, catalinaconservancy.org, for more information and links to other websites.

From the pier in Avalon, stop at the Trailhead Visitor Center to pick up your free hiking permit, and then make your way 1.5 miles up Avalon Canyon to Hermit Gulch Campground. An inexpensive tram makes the trip hourly from the end of the pier, continuing to the canyon's end at the botanical gardens. Check with Avalon Transportation Services, 310-510-0025. Alternatively, you can walk, bring or rent bicycles, or take a taxi.

Description: From the top end of Hermit Gulch Campground, start your hike by following the well-built Hermit Gulch Trail up the ravine to the west. Before long, you leave the trickling stream in the canyon bottom and begin a twisting ascent up along a shaggy slope. During the springtime, red monkey flower, shooting star, lupine, paintbrush, and other native wildflowers dot the trailside and adorn small clearings amid the tangles of chaparral. After 1.7 miles and an elevation gain of 1,200 feet, you meet Divide Road, the fire road along the eastern spine of the island.

Turn right, walk 0.1 mile, and then turn left onto a steep fire road signed LONE TREE TRAIL. Continue over several rounded, barren hills, passing over the peaklet designated Lone Tree on most maps (2.8 miles). That's where you'll find the best view of the ocean and shoreline. Sometimes you can gaze south over shore-hugging fog and spy the low dome of San Clemente Island, some 40 miles across the glistening Pacific. When visibility's best, you can trace the mainland coast as far south as San Diego and also spy the long crest of the Peninsular Ranges, the chain of mountains running through Riverside and San Diego Counties into Baja California.

After taking in the visual feast, backtrack to Divide Road. From there you loop back to the starting point via a longer but more gradually descending route. Head south down Divide Road, then veer left on Memorial Road (4.8 miles). Easy walking down this crooked dirt road takes you along a cool, north-facing slope covered by tall and luxuriant (by mainland standards) growths of scrub oak, manzanita, and toyon.

At the bottom of the hill, you come upon Wrigley Memorial. Below that, you pass through the botanical gardens that Ada Wrigley founded in the 1920s. Because of the virtually frost-free climate, an extensive array of native and exotic plants from distant corners of the world are able to thrive here. Once you are beyond the garden gates, it's but a couple hundred yards back to the campground.

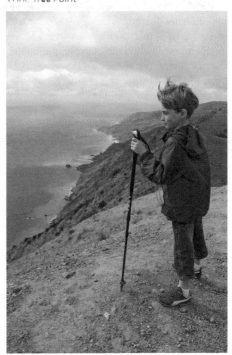

Lone Tree Point

HIKE 63   Trans-Catalina Trail

Location	Santa Catalina Island
Highlight	Classic island backpacking trip
Distance & Configuration	38.5-mile point-to-point
Elevation Gain	8,000'
Hiking Time	3–5 days
Optional Map	Catalina Island Trail Map (catalinaconservancy.org)
Best Times	October–May, closed during and after rainstorms
Agency	Catalina Island Conservancy
Difficulty	Strenuous
Trail use	Suitable for backpacking
Permits	Permit and camping reservations required (see below)
Google Maps	Trans Catalina Trailhead

The Trans-Catalina Trail is an increasingly popular backpacking trip across the length of the most visited of California's Channel Islands. The diverse scenery ranges from view-rich ridges to secluded coves to intimate woodlands. You'll likely encounter bison and deer along the trail (give them plenty of space), and you might see the Catalina Island fox and other endemic species. The campgrounds along the trail are some of the most memorable (and expensive) in California. This trip is far more than the sum of its parts. While portions involve walking dusty fire roads or weedy hillsides, the experience of hiking the entire island and seeing it from so many perspectives is unforgettable.

Go during cool weather; the beaches are appealing in the summer, but the interior is too hot for enjoyable hiking. Carry at least 3 quarts of water between campgrounds, or more on a hot day. Some portions of the trail are very steep, and trekking poles may be useful. Hiking at night is prohibited.

A free hiking permit is required and can be obtained online at the Catalina Island Conservancy website or at the visitor centers. Expensive camping permits are required in advance for each campsite and are obtained by calling Two Harbors Visitor Services (310-510-4205). Some campgrounds have two-night minimums, but these are waived for Trans-Catalina hikers. Campsites fill up, so make your reservation well in advance. Parsons Landing lacks tap water, but you can request a water jug and/ or firewood for a fee as part of your camping reservation.

To Reach the Trailhead: This trip requires a 75-minute ferry ride from San Pedro to Avalon and a return ferry from Two Harbors. The *Catalina Express* ferry schedule changes seasonally and on weekends—in winter, there may be only one ferry a day from Two Harbors and none at all on Tuesdays and Thursdays. The fare is currently $37.25 each way; check current schedules at catalinaexpress.com.

Catalina Express parking is located at Berth 95 in San Pedro. From the 110 Freeway, take Exit 1A for Highway 47. Immediately exit onto Harbor Boulevard, and then continue straight on Swinford Street to the ferry terminal. Camping fuel is prohibited on the ferry, but you can purchase all kinds of fuel at Chet's Hardware in Avalon or the General Store in Two Harbors.

Description: Start at The Trailhead, the Catalina Conservancy's visitor center, near the boat landing in Avalon. Here you can pick up your permit, buy a map, or inquire about current conditions. The first leg of the trip follows paved Avalon Canyon Road from the back of town to Hermit's Gulch Campground, at 1.5 miles. You can walk the road or take the Avalon Transit Garibaldi Bus, which loops through town. If you arrive on the afternoon ferry, you might want to spend the first night at Hermits

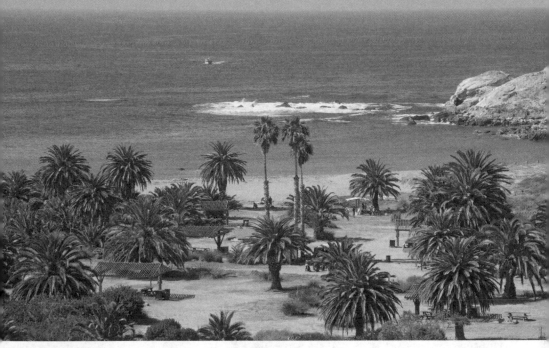

Little Harbor Campground on Catalina Island

Gulch and make a side trip to the Wrigley Memorial and Botanic Garden.

From the top of the campground, follow the Hermit Gulch Trail as it switchbacks up through chaparral and wildflowers. At 3.2 miles (from the Trailhead Visitor Center) reach Divide Road, where you turn right (north). Enjoy excellent views of Avalon Bay from the ridge. At 5.0 miles veer left onto a trail that leads to the small Haypress Reservoir. Circle around the north side of the lake to Haypress Recreation Area at 5.6 miles, where you'll find tap water, restrooms, and picnic tables beside a playground. Be sure you have plenty of water because the stretch ahead can be hot.

The trail briefly follows the reservoir before turning north and rejoining Airport Road at 6 miles. At 6.5 miles, near a viewpoint, turn left onto singletrack. The next stretch of undulating but scenic trail crosses three lightly used roads and the Skull Ridge Trail before reaching Black Jack Campground at 10.5 miles. Here you'll find tap water, restrooms, and a cold shower at the large campsite nestled in a pleasant grove of oaks and conifers.

Follow trail signs carefully as you climb through a maze of roads between Black Jack Mountain (2,010') and Mount Orizaba (2,102').

Orizaba, the highest point on the island, is easily recognized from afar by its flat summit, bulldozed to hold a white bowling pin–shaped aircraft radio beacon. At 11.5 miles beyond the saddle, the route leaves Upper Cottonwood Road and becomes a steep but scenic singletrack dropping north into Cottonwood Canyon and climbing back toward a mesa, where Airport in the Sky is situated. Turn left near the old soapstone quarry and meet Airport Road just outside the airport, at 12.8 miles. Consider stopping at the DC3 Grill at the airport for their famous buffalo burger or just to refill your water bottle.

Pass under a decorative Western arch and join the trail that circles the west end of the airport. At 13.7 miles join Empire Landing Road near Buffalo Springs Reservoir. Turn left and head west on this dull and dusty road. At 15.0 miles be sure to pick up the singletrack on the left descending Big Springs Ridge. Your long descent is rewarded by reaching Little Harbor, one of the most scenic parts of the island. At the bottom of the trail, jog right on Isthmus Road then left on the trail to reach the corner of the Little Harbor Campground, at 19.0 miles. This jewel of a campground fronting a sandy beach

continued on page 164

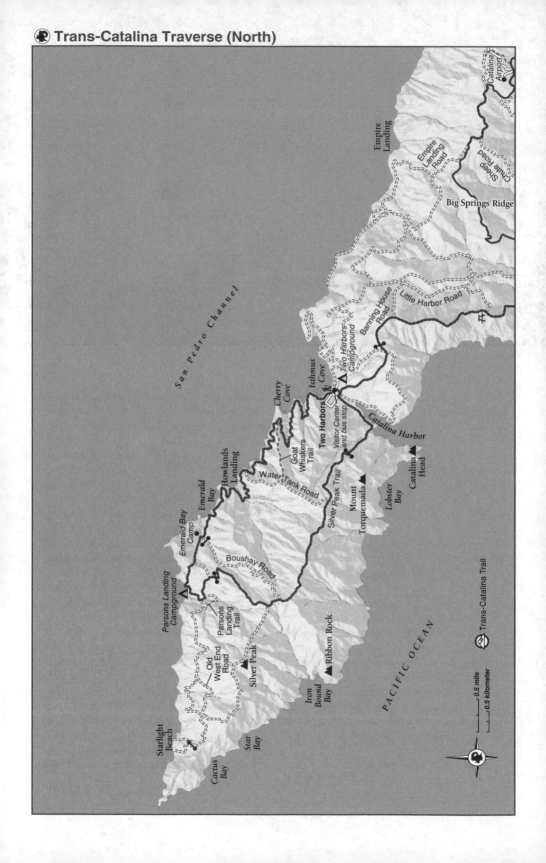

San Pedro Channel

PACIFIC OCEAN

Catalina Airport

Empire Landing

Empire Landing Road

Sheep Chute Road

Big Springs Ridge

Banning House Road

Little Harbor Road

Two Harbors Campground

Isthmus Cove

Cherry Cove

Goat Whiskers Trail

Water Tank Road

Howlands Landing

Emerald Bay

Emerald Bay Camp

Boushay Road

Parsons Landing Campground

Parsons Landing Trail

Old West End Road

Silver Peak

Starlight Beach

Cactus Bay

Star Bay

Iron Bound Bay

Ribbon Rock

Silver Peak Trail

Mount Torquemada

Lobster Bay

Catalina Head

Catalina Harbor

Two Harbors

Visitor Center and bus stop

━━━ 0.5 mile
━━━ 0.5 kilometer

🅝 Trans-Catalina Trail

Trans-Catalina Traverse (South)

San Pedro Channel
Pebbly Beach
East Peak
Avalon Bay
Trailhead Visitor Center
bus stop
Avalon
Hermit Gulch Campground
Hermit Gulch Trail
Memorial Road
Wrigley Memorial & Botanic Garden
Divide Road
Toyon Bay
HAYPRESS PARK
Grand Canyon
Lone Tree Point
White Cove
Whitleys Peak
Airport Road
Silver Canyon
PACIFIC OCEAN
Black Jack Mountain
Skull Ridge Trail
Middle Canyon Road
Black Jack Camp
Cape Canyon
Mount Orizaba
Cottonwood Canyon
Middle Canyon
Salta Verde Point
Mount Banning
Eagles Nest
Cactus Peak
Trans-Catalina Trail
Sheep Chute Road
Big Springs Canyon
Little Spring Canyon
Little Harbor
China Point
0.5 mile
0.5 kilometer
Sentinel Rock
Ben Weston Point

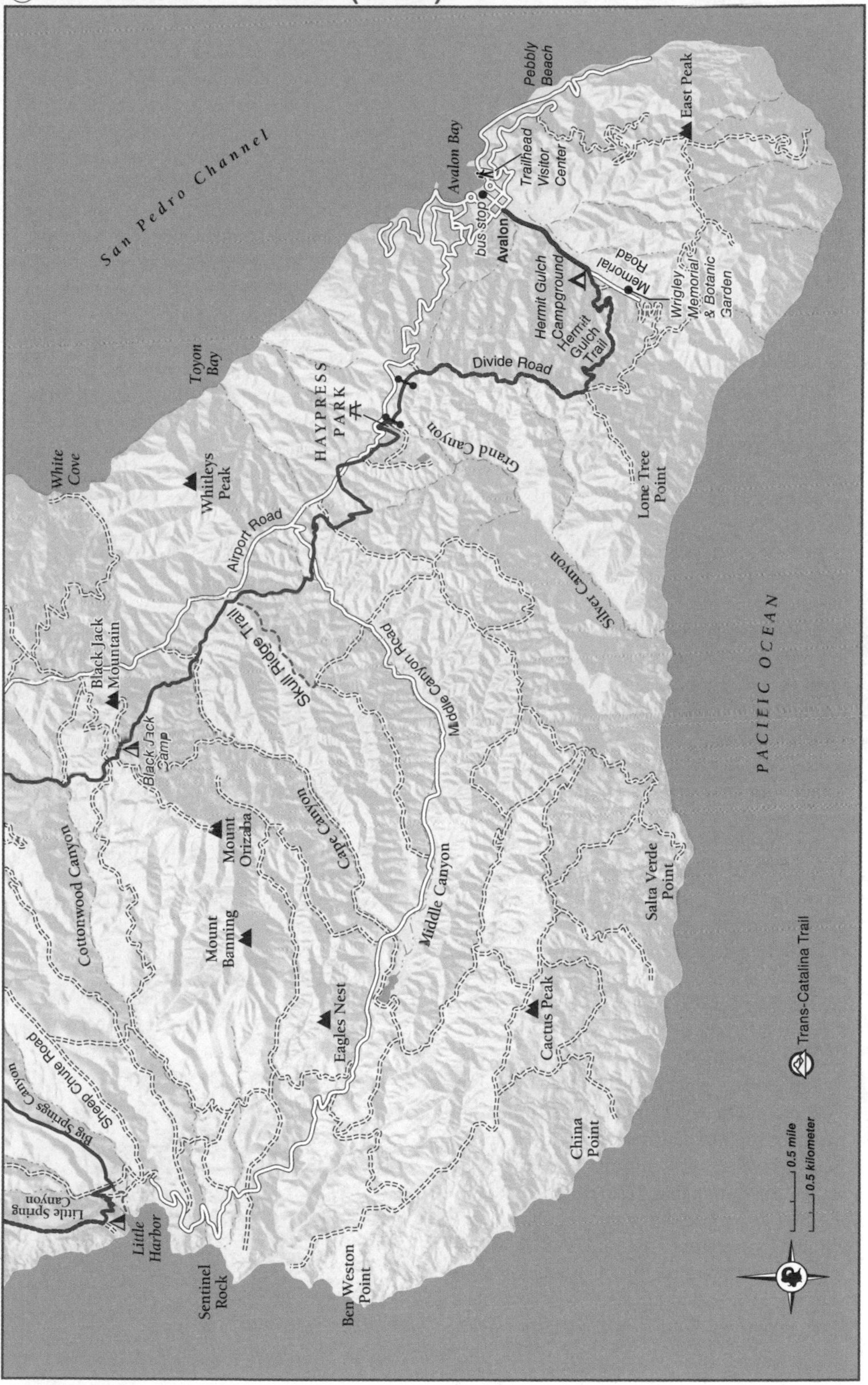

continued from page 161

is shaded by palms and has water, restrooms, and cold showers. Beware that sting rays frequent the harbor; if you go in the water, shuffle your feet to warn them you are coming and avoid stepping on one. With (expensive) advance reservations through Wet Spot Rentals (310-510-2229, wetspotrentals.com), you can rent kayaks and explore the windward side of the island on a layover day.

The signed Trans-Catalina Trail switchbacks up to the northeast above the campground. The first several hundred yards have some of the best photo opportunities on the whole trail. Send your photographer ahead to capture the rest of the group hiking up a switchback with Little Harbor in the background. The trail is steep and rough in places as it climbs to a high ridge, where you may appreciate a shade structure at a vista point at 21.7 miles. Now continuing on a dirt road, follow the ridge north to meet Banning House Road at 22.4 miles. Turn left and descend the steep road to the small town of Two Harbors (24.2 miles), on a narrow bridge of land between Isthmus Cove and Catalina Harbor.

In Two Harbors, you could enjoy a hot meal at one of several restaurants, resupply on groceries or hiking gear at the General Store, lounge on the beach, or spend a night at the Two Harbors Campground or at the historic Banning House Lodge bed-and-breakfast. The Visitor Services office at the foot of the pier is staffed by knowledgeable rangers who can help with last-minute permits (if available) or answer questions about the sights you've seen. If you want to shorten your trip, you can catch the ferry back to San Pedro from here.

Otherwise, complete the Trans-Catalina Trail around the west end of the island on fire roads by way of Parsons Landing campsite. Return to the south end of town, where the signed Trans-Catalina Trail resumes, following the west shore of Catalina Harbor before climbing steeply onto the ridge. At 28.7 miles reach a road junction. If you're looking for a side trip, you could continue west on Silver Peak Road for 1.0 mile to Silver Peak, which,

at 1,804 feet, is the highest point on the west end of the island. From Silver Peak, you could continue 2.8 miles farther to Starlight Beach on the rocky, lonely coast near the extreme west end. The Trans-Catalina Trail, however, turns north and descends Fenceline Road.

At 30.0 miles turn left; then, at 30.4 miles, turn right and descend to Parsons Landing, at 30.8 miles. This spectacular campground is right on the sandy beach. You'll hear the sea lions barking in the surf and will have spectacular sunsets followed by million-dollar views of the Palos Verdes lights across the channel. There is no tap water, but you may request as part of your reservation that the rangers leave a water jug for you in the locker. With a layover day here, you could enjoy the ocean or hike out to Starlight Beach.

When you're ready to loop back to Two Harbors, find the signed Trans-Catalina Trail leading east. At 31.3 miles it joins West End Road. Follow this road east as it contours 100–200 feet above the ocean, dipping in and out of coves and ravines and passing several youth camps. Watch for dolphins playing off the coast. The last stretch has great views of Isthmus Cove. Follow the trail into town, where your journey is complete at 38.5 miles. You may have time to stop at a restaurant or relax on the beach before your ferry back to San Pedro.

If you have more time, you can add a day at Two Harbors between Little Harbor and Parsons Landing, or a layover at Little Harbor or Parsons Landing.

POSSIBLE FOUR-DAY ITINERARY			
DAY	CAMP	MILES	ELEVATION GAIN
1	Blackjack	10.7	3,000'
2	Little Harbor	8.2	1,000'
3	Parsons Landing	11.9	3,600'
4	Two Harbors	7.7	400'

POSSIBLE FIVE-DAY ITINERARY			
DAY	CAMP	MILES	ELEVATION GAIN
1	Blackjack	10.7	3,000'
2	Little Harbor	8.2	1,000'
3	Two Harbors	5.3	1,600'
4	Parsons Landing	6.6	2,000'
5	Two Harbors	7.7	400'

HIKE 64   Lower Aliso Canyon

Location	Chino Hills State Park
Highlight	Views
Distance & Configuration	6-mile loop
Elevation Gain	800'
Hiking Time	2.5 hours
Optional Map	Chino Hills State Park brochure (free at entrance station, or download at tinyurl.com/chinohillssp)
Best Times	November–May, 8 a.m.–sunset; closed for several days after rains
Agency	Chino Hills State Park
Difficulty	Moderate
Trail Use	Suitable for mountain biking
Permit	State park entry fee
Google Maps	Bane Canyon Rd Trailhead

Chino Hills State Park was established in 1984 on the hills dividing Orange County from San Bernardino County as a critical wildlife corridor between adjoining open spaces and as an escape for humans from the endless surrounding housing developments. Now encompassing more than 14,000 acres of rolling hills, the park attracts many hikers, mountain bikers, and equestrians.

The park has dozens of choices for hikes and bike rides, both long and short, but Lower Aliso Canyon is a popular spot and a good introduction to the area. Winter and spring are the most attractive times, when the grass is green and the wildflowers emerge, but the park is enjoyable anytime it's not too hot. *Aliso* is Spanish for "sycamore," which are found along the creek, although oaks are more plentiful. Pick up a

Lower Aliso Canyon after the 2020 Blue Ridge Fire

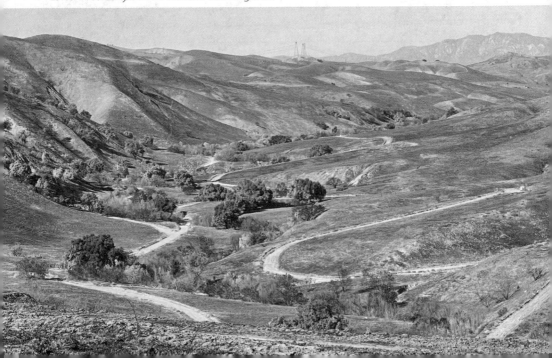

Lower Aliso Canyon

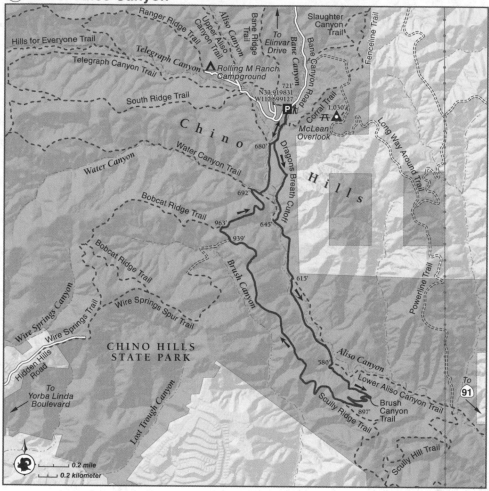

park map on your way in. The park is laced with some 100 miles of fine trails that will inevitably tempt you to return; a loop on Bane Ridge and the East Fenceline Trail is a good second visit.

The Chino Hills have been used for cattle grazing at least since the establishment of Mission San Gabriel in 1771. They are thus primarily vegetated with grasses and weeds, especially black mustard, that are prone to fire. More than 90% of the park burned in the 2008 Freeway Complex Fire, and the eastern portion burned again in the 2020 Blue Ridge Fire, but the grassy hills and oak woodlands are evolved for fire and mostly recovered quickly.

To Reach the Trailhead: From Highway 71, 7 miles north of Highway 91 and 5 miles south of Highway 60, exit west on Soquel Canyon Parkway. In 1.0 mile, turn left onto Elinvar Drive, left again after 0.2 mile, and then immediately right on Bane Canyon Road, signed CHINO HILLS STATE PARK. Drive 3 miles up the narrow park road to the Lower Aliso Canyon parking area, stopping to pay your day-use vehicle fee along the way. If you reach the historic Rolling M Ranch, you've just passed it.

Description: From the parking area, walk down the fire road signed Aliso Canyon Trail, and soon pass through a gate. Pass the signed Corral Trail on your left, then come to an unsigned trail on the left at 0.3 mile, locally known as Dragon's Breath. For variety, take this trail, which parallels the Aliso Canyon Trail and rejoins at 0.9 mile. Watch for burn marks on some of the coast live oaks telling the story of how these hardy trees survived the frequent brush fires that clear out the dead weeds.

Continue down Aliso Canyon. At 1.4 miles, come to a split. Stay right on the Aliso Canyon Trail; the Elevator Trail on the left has more ups and downs and rejoins at 2.0 miles. Just beyond, at 2.1 miles, turn right onto the signed Brush Canyon Trail, another fire road that switchbacks up the slope. You'll enjoy great views over Aliso Canyon and north toward the San Gabriel Mountains as you climb.

Reach the Scully Ridge trail at the crest (3.2 miles). Turn right and follow this undulating ridge north, passing some minor spur roads. Watch for raptors circling on the thermals. At 4.9 miles, reach the end of the ridge. The Bobcat Ridge Trail leads west, but we turn right and descend back toward Aliso Canyon. At 5.4 miles, watch for the Water Canyon Trail on the left at a hairpin turn. You could explore the singletrack up this wooded canyon for a mile if you wanted, but our route bends right and soon rejoins the Aliso Canyon Trail. Turn left and walk the last stretch back to the trailhead.

HIKE 65   Santiago Oaks Regional Park

Location	City of Orange
Highlights	Oak woodland, trickling stream
Distance & Configuration	1–3 miles (many possible loops)
Elevation Gain	100'–400', depending on exact route
Hiking Time	30 minutes–1.5 hours
Optional Map	Santiago Oaks Regional Park brochure (free at entrance station, or download at ocparks.com/parks/santiago)
Best Times	Daily, 7 a.m.–sunset; trails closed for 3 days after rains
Agency	Santiago Oaks Regional Park
Difficulty	Easy
Trail Use	Good for kids, dogs allowed, suitable for mountain biking
Permit	Park entry fee
Google Maps	Santiago Oaks Regional Park, Windes Drive

What Santiago Oaks Regional Park lacks in sheer size its rare beauty more than adequately compensates for. The core of the park is made up of two former ranch properties acquired in the mid-1970s. A small Valencia orange grove and many acres of ornamental trees planted around 1960 on these properties complement the natural riparian and oak-woodland communities along Santiago Creek.

The Canyon 2 Fire burned past the park in October 2017. The fire, which burned 9,200 acres and damaged 60 homes, was kindled from the embers of the previous month's Canyon Fire, which started when a Caltrans flare was knocked off the 91 Freeway by a passing vehicle. The park has largely recovered and draws many visitors again to its beautiful trails.

To Reach the Trailhead: From the 55 Freeway in the city of Orange, exit at Katella Avenue (Exit 15) and proceed east. Katella becomes Villa Park Road and again changes its name to Santiago Canyon Road on the eastern outskirts of Orange. Once you are 3.2 miles east of the

🅡 Santiago Oaks Regional Park

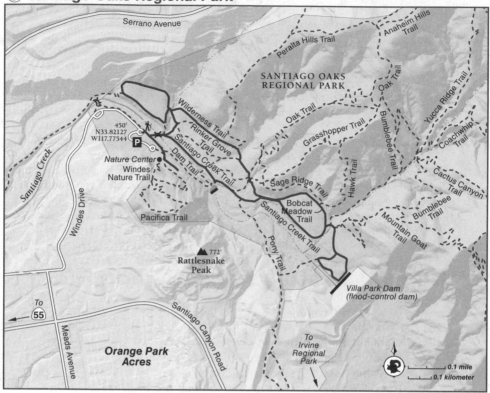

Serrano Avenue

Peralta Hills Trail

Anaheim Hills Trail

SANTIAGO OAKS
REGIONAL PARK

Oak Trail

Yucca Ridge Trail

Coachwhip Trail

Wilderness Trail

Rinker Grove Trail

Oak Trail

Grasshopper Trail

Bumblebee Trail

450'
N33.82127
W117.75544

Santiago Creek Trail

Nature Center
Windes
Nature Trail

Dam Trail

Santiago Creek

Sage Ridge Trail

Hawk Trail

Cactus Canyon Trail

Bumblebee Trail

Pacifica Trail

Bobcat Meadow Trail

Santiago Creek Trail

Mountain Goat Trail

Windes Drive

772'
Rattlesnake Peak

Pony Trail

Villa Park Dam
(flood-control dam)

To
55

Meads Avenue

Santiago Canyon Road

Orange Park
Acres

To
Irvine
Regional
Park

🅡   0.1 mile
0.1 kilometer

freeway, turn left on Windes Drive, which leads into Santiago Oaks Regional Park.

As you approach the park entrance, subdivisions quickly fade from sight, and a lush strip of riparian vegetation (willows and sycamores) comes into view on the left. Pay your day-use fee at the entry station and request the park's excellent trail map. Park in the main lot and then stroll up past some oak-shaded picnic sites to the superb nature center, which is housed in a nicely refurbished 70-year-old ranch house.

Description: The best of this park's several miles of trails stay close to the wooded bottomlands of Santiago Creek. From the nature center, make your way down to the Historic Dam Trail, the main path along the south side of the creek. Walk upstream along the shaded bank to reach a small rock-and-cement dam dating from 1892. This dam replaced an earlier one, built in 1879, that was part of one of Orange County's first irrigation systems. Today, the

surviving dam is a historical curiosity, dwarfed by the large Villa Park flood-control dam a short distance upstream and Santiago Reservoir farther upstream.

Ford Santiago Creek and stroll along several paths amid the eucalyptus, pepper, and other exotic trees rooted to the gently sloping bench on the creek's far side. Its diverse habitats make Santiago Oaks a delightful birding spot, with species ranging from the tree-dwelling western bluebird and acorn woodpecker to the water-loving great blue heron. On occasion, you may see vultures, ospreys, and some common hawks soaring overhead.

VARIATIONS

Longer-distance trails radiate outward from Santiago Oaks Regional Park toward Irvine Park to the southeast and up the slope east and northeast into Weir Canyon Park. Beware of fast-moving mountain bikers bombing down these steep trails.

HIKE 66 Crystal Cove Beach Walk

Location	Crystal Cove State Park
Highlights	Tidepools, sea cliffs, whale-watching, outstanding beach walking
Distance & Configuration	5-mile loop
Elevation Gain	100'
Hiking Time	3 hours
Optional Map	Crystal Cove State Park brochure (free at entrance station, or download at parks.ca.gov/?page_id=644)
Best Times	All year
Agency	Crystal Cove State Park
Difficulty	Moderate
Trail Use	Good for kids
Permit	State park entry fee
Google Maps	Pelican Point Entrance–Crystal Cove State Park

Hemmed in by 80-foot cliffs on one side and the restless surf on the other, Crystal Cove State Park's 3 miles of sandy beachfront seem strangely detached from the busy world above. Aside from the beachfront-cottage community at Crystal Cove, listed on the National Register of Historic Places, the midportion of the beach is largely free of encroachment by man-made structures. Come early in the morning, or anytime on a cold or rainy day, and you may have

Crystal Cove Beach Walk

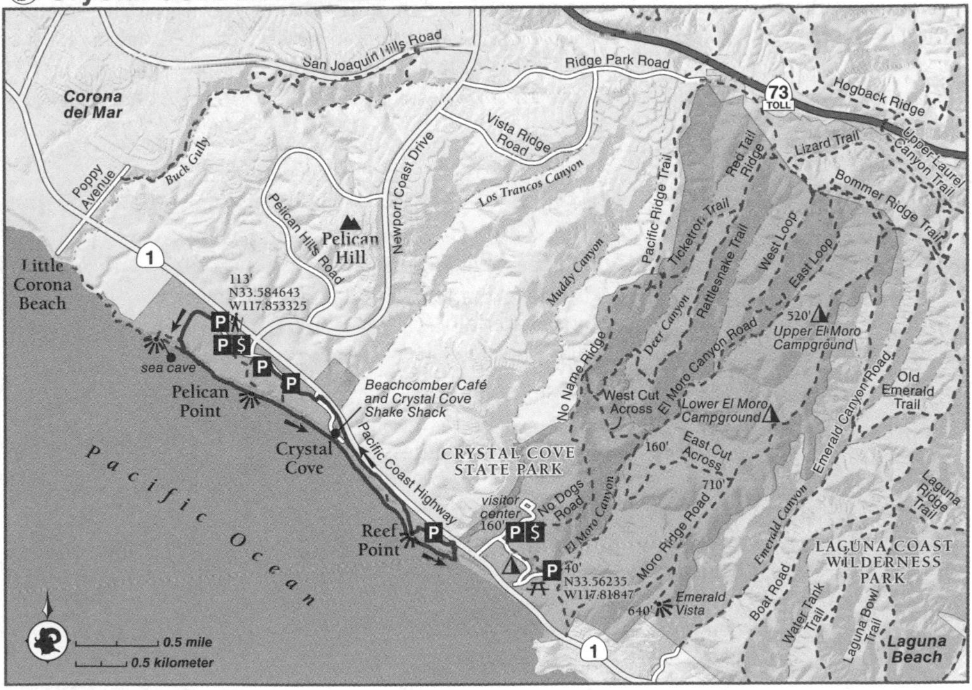

the beach all to yourself. Expect crowds on a fine summer afternoon.

To Reach the Trailhead: From the Pacific Coast Highway (Highway 1) between Corona del Mar and Laguna Beach opposite Newport Coast Drive, turn into the Pelican Point entrance of Crystal Cove State Park. Pay your admission fee ($15, or $20 on holidays). Turn right and drive to the northernmost parking area.

Description: Crystal Cove State Park has four parking entrances, so you can tailor this trip to whatever length you want. A great 5-mile hike starts at the northernmost parking area from the Pelican Point entrance.

Follow the path northwest and then down to the beach and tidepools at Treasure Cove. You can make an optional quarter-mile detour northwest to a sea cave at Little Treasure Cove, but this trip turns left and follows the beach southward past Pelican Point and more tide-pools. After 1.2 miles of walking on the sand, reach the Beachcomber Café near the Crystal Cove Historic District cottages at the mouth of Los Trancos Creek. For a shorter (3-mile) trip, you could follow the service road up to the Los Trancos entrance and loop back. For the 5-mile version, continue for another mile along the beach past Reef Point to Scotchman's

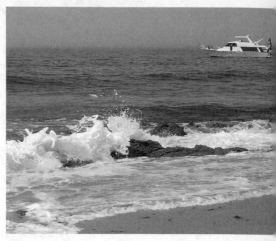

Crystal Cove

Cove, where you can climb off the beach and join the Bluff Top Trail near the Reef Point entrance.

The tops of the bluffs are excellent for watching gray whales migrate along the shore from December through February, although it's not unusual to see whales spouting just off the coast at other times of year. Using binoculars, scan the ocean surface out to a distance of 1 or 2 miles. Early- to mid-morning light (sidelight) is best for this.

HIKE 67   Laurel Canyon Loop

Location	Laguna Coast Wilderness Park
Highlights	Sandstone formations, woodlands, wildflowers, seasonal waterfall
Distance & Configuration	3.5-mile loop
Elevation Gain	700'
Hiking Time	2 hours
Optional Map	Laguna Coast Wilderness Park map (ocparks.com/parks/lagunac)
Best Times	Daily, 8 a.m.–5 p.m.
Agency	Laguna Coast Wilderness Park
Difficulty	Moderate
Trail Use	Good for kids
Permit	Parking fee
Google Maps	Willow Staging Area

® Laurel Canyon Loop

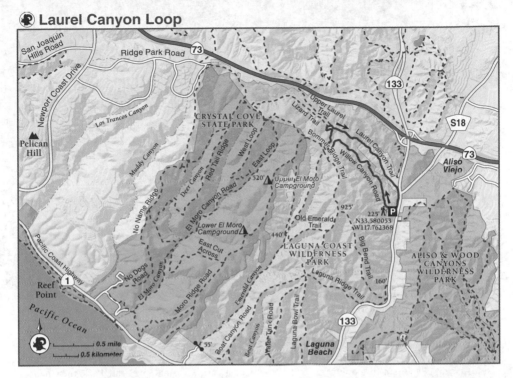

The best single hike within the Laguna Coast Wilderness Park is surely the secluded Laguna Canyon loop. Though it lies close to the San Joaquin Hills Transportation Corridor tollway, that roadway (and much of its associated urban development) is hidden from both sight and sound along most of the route. Volunteers frequently staff a booth at the Willow Staging Area, offering tips about the logistics of hiking in the park as well as the area's natural history. Park at Laguna Coast Wilderness Park's Willow Staging Area on the west side of Laguna Canyon Road, 3 miles north of Laguna Beach. This point is 5 miles south of the 405 Freeway, 0.7 mile south of the 73 Toll Road, and 0.2 mile south of the intersection of El Toro and Laguna Canyon Roads. Pay your parking fee at the machine.

Description: Start hiking on the Willow Canyon Road fire road, which gains nearly 600 feet of elevation as it climbs the ridge. Springtime wildflowers bloom in profusion along this stretch, which cuts along east- and north-facing slopes smothered in thick chaparral. At 1.5 miles, turn right on the first intersecting fire road

(Laurel Spur). Follow the trail as it plunges down through more dense growths of chaparral toward the narrow bottom of Laurel Canyon. The deeper you go, the more you gain a sense of seclusion. Just before the bottom, look for the Lizard Trail on the left. Shortly beyond, turn right onto the signed Laurel Canyon Trail (2.0 miles).

At 2.4 miles, you pass near the lip of a dramatic drop-off, a seasonal waterfall nearly 100 feet high. During most years this declivity sports only a modest trickle. Past the lip of the falls, you swing to the left side of the canyon bottom and descend along a dry, south-facing slope. Part of the canyon was designated the Laguna Laurel Ecological Reserve in 1994. This area is home to a remarkable diversity of species, including 360 kinds of plants, 146 birds, 24 mammals, 5 amphibians, and 14 snakes and lizards. By 3.0 miles you emerge in a grassy meadow, which is either green, golden, or transitional in color, depending on the season, and is flanked by cavernous sandstone outcrops. The shapes of some suggest grotesque skulls and other figures. The path through the meadow soon flanks busy Laguna Canyon Road, climbs

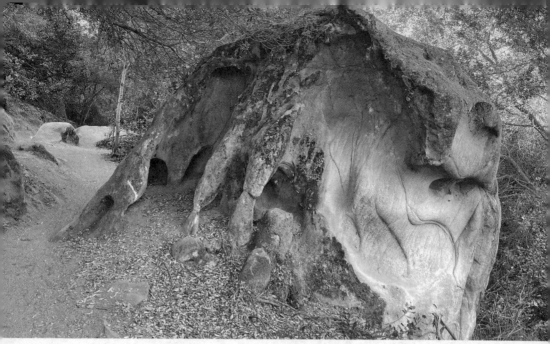

Eroded sandstone formation in Laurel Canyon

south to an exposed earthquake fault, and returns you to your starting point.

VARIATION

You can add Bommer Ridge and Upper Laurel Canyon to your hike to make a longer loop (5.6 miles with 900' of elevation gain). Instead of turning onto Laurel Spur at 1.5 miles, continue a few more yards and turn right onto the next fire road, which soon reaches Bommer Ridge.

The ridgeline offers expansive views of Laguna Coast Park, Crystal Cove State Park, the Channel Islands, the San Gabriel Mountains, and the Santa Ana Mountains. At 2.8 miles, turn right onto the signed Lizard Trail, a long-abandoned ranching road descending the beautiful upper reaches of Laurel Canyon. At 4.0 miles, make a quick left on Laurel Spur, then an immediate right onto the lower Laurel Canyon Trail to rejoin the route described above.

HIKE 68   Whiting Ranch

Location	Lake Forest and El Toro
Highlight	Red rock cliffs
Distance & Configuration	4.4-mile out-and-back
Elevation Gain	500'
Hiking Time	2 hours
Optional Map	Whiting Ranch Wilderness Park map (ocparks.com/parks/whiting)
Best Times	October–June, 7 a.m.–sunset
Agency	OC Parks
Difficulty	Moderate
Trail Use	Good for kids, suitable for mountain bikes
Permit	Parking fee
Google Maps	26701 Portola Parkway, Foothill Ranch

Whiting Ranch

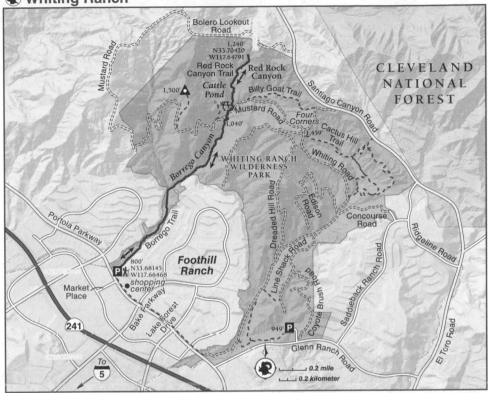

Whiting Ranch Wilderness Park was established in 1991, encompassing some 2,500 acres along the rim of the communities of Lake Forest and El Toro. Whiting Ranch's rounded hills look nondescript when viewed from the suburbs below, but they conceal some pleasant surprises, which you will discover by trekking out and back to Red Rock Canyon, the site of a spectacular erosional feature: sandstone cliffs banded with layers of ancient sand and mud. Late in the day, the sun's warm glow brings out a reddish tint in the rock.

Beware: This is mountain lion habitat, and sightings are not uncommon. In 2004, a mountain lion killed a cyclist while he was crouched down repairing his bicycle. In 2020, a lion mauled a toddler. It is safest to hike in groups. Always keep young children close to you. If threatened, respond aggressively and convince the cat you are not food. The rangers occasionally close the park due to mountain lion activity; check the park website before making the trip.

The October 2020 Silverado Fire burned to the edge of the Borrego Canyon Trail in places.

To Reach the Trailhead: To reach the park's main entrance from I-5 in southern Orange County, take Lake Forest Drive east and north for 5 miles to Portola Parkway. Turn left, and follow Portola northwest for another half mile. Turn right at Market Place. The trailhead parking is on the left, and a shopping center is on the right. The lot is open 7 a.m.–sunset. If you are using the Foothill Transportation Corridor (Highway 241) toll road, exit at either Lake Forest Drive or Alton Parkway.

Description: The trail starts at an interpretive kiosk. Take a trail map if you wish to explore the park beyond the route described here. Like most trails in the Whiting Ranch Wilderness Park, the wide dirt path ahead is open to mountain bikers and equestrians, as well as hikers. You immediately plunge into a densely shaded ravine called Borrego Canyon through which flows a trickling stream. For a while, suburbia rims the canyon on both sides, but soon enough it disappears without a trace. The trek up the canyon feels Tolkien-esque as you pass under a crooked-limb canopy of live oaks and sycamores and sniff the damp odor of the streamside willows. Often in late fall and winter, frigid air sinks into these shady recesses overnight, and by early morning, frost mantles everything below eye level.

After 1.5 miles, you come to Mustard Road, a fire road that ascends both east and west to ridgetops offering long views of the ocean on clear days. Turn right on Mustard Road, and almost immediately come to a picnic site. Two trails fork to the left; the second, signed but easily overlooked, leads into Red Rock Canyon.

Out in the sunshine now, you follow the Red Rock Trail (restricted to travelers on foot)

up the bottom of a sunny canyon that narrows and steepens. At 2.2 miles, the trail ends at the base of the eroded sandstone cliffs, formed of sediment deposited on a shallow sea bottom about 20 million years ago. This type of rock, which contains the fossilized remains of shellfish and marine mammals, underlies much of Orange County. Rarely is it as well exposed as it is here. Return the way you came.

VARIATION

After visiting Red Rock Canyon, you could return via a more roundabout and lengthy route (a 7-mile loop with 900' of elevation gain). Climb east on Mustard Road to the high point at Four Corners and then south on Whiting Road down to Serrano Canyon. The woodsy descent through Serrano Canyon takes you back to Portola Parkway, and from there you follow the sidewalk a mile back to your starting point.

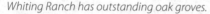

Whiting Ranch has outstanding oak groves.

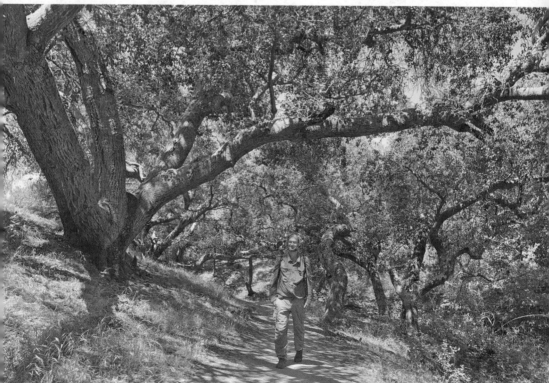

HIKE 69   Santiago Peak

Location	Santa Ana Mountains
Highlight	Best urban, mountain, and ocean views in Southern California
Distance & Configuration	16-mile out-and-back
Elevation Gain	4,000'
Hiking Time	8 hours
Optional Map	Cleveland National Forest Visitor Map–North (printed copy available at store.usgs.gov/product/207432, or download at www.avenzamaps.com/maps/839770)
Best Times	October–May
Agency	Cleveland National Forest/Trabuco Ranger District
Difficulty	Strenuous
Trail Use	Dogs allowed
Permit	National Forest Adventure Pass
Google Maps	Holy Jim Trailhead

Note: Trabuco Canyon burned in the 2018 Holy Fire. The fire, started by an arsonist, consumed 23,000 acres and burned 13 cabins in the canyon. During the subsequent winter, mudslides wiped out the Holy Jim Trail. At the time of this writing, the trail has reopened only as far as Holy Jim Falls. I've left the hike in this edition because it is a classic trip to the highest point in Orange County. Before you go, check with the Cleveland National Forest to find out whether the trail has reopened.

To the American Indians, it was Kalawpa ("a wooded place"), the lofty resting place of the deity Chiningchinish. Early settlers and surveyors named it variously Mount Downey, Trabuco Peak, Temescal Mountain, and Santiago Peak. Finally, mapmakers decided on the name that eventually stuck: Santiago. Today's bulldozer-scraped summit overrun with telecommunications antennas hardly pays sufficient homage to the peak's historic and scenic values. Witness, for example, this record of the first documented ascent of the peak in 1853, by a group of lawmen pursuing horse thieves up a canyon from the east:

After an infinite amount of scrambling, danger, and hard labor, we stood on the very summit of the Temescal mountain, now by some called Santiago . . . where we beheld with pleasure a sublime view, more than worth the journey and ascent.

In 1861, while making a geologic survey of the Santa Anas, William Brewer and Josiah Whitney reached the same summit on their second try, using a northeast ridge. Their impressions echoed the sentiments of the earlier climbers: "The view more than repaid us for all we had endured."

The view that these early climbers described so enthusiastically remains spectacular—given, perhaps, a clearer-than-average winter day. In such conditions, you can trace the coastline from Point Loma to Point Dume, spot both Santa Catalina and San Clemente Islands, and scratch your head trying to identify the plethora of mountain ranges and lesser promontories filling the landscape inland.

The major ranges on the horizon are (clockwise from northwest to southeast) the Santa Monica, San Gabriel, San Bernardino, Little San Bernardino, San Jacinto, Santa Rosa, Palomar, and Cuyamaca Mountains. To the south you might see several of the lower ranges along the Mexican border and perhaps glimpse the flat-topped summit of Table Mountain, a few miles inland from the Baja California coast. In the west and northwest, smog levels permitting, the flat urban tapestry spreads outward, spiked by the glass skyscrapers of downtown Los Angeles.

🏞 Santiago Peak

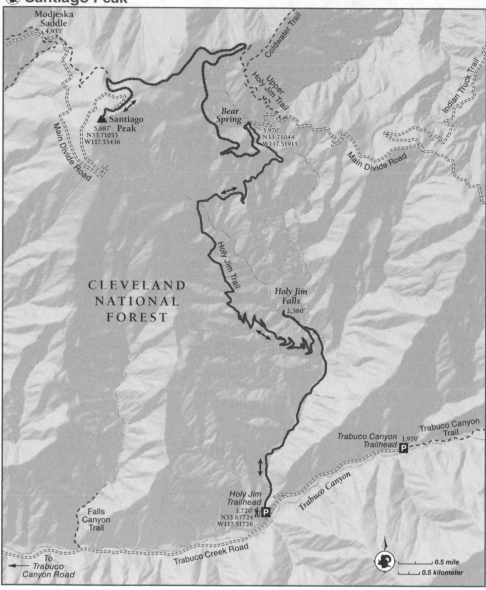

Don't underestimate the time required to bag Santiago Peak by way of today's most scenic approach, Holy Jim Trail. In winter, you'll need an early start to ensure that you return before sunset. And with summit temperatures roughly 20°F cooler than below, pack some extra clothing. Bring plenty of water too; Bear Spring, on the way to the summit, is *not* a potable water source.

To Reach the Trailhead: From the Foothill Transportation Corridor Toll Road (Highway 241) in Rancho Santa Margarita, exit onto Santa Margarita Parkway. Drive 1.5 miles east, and then turn left onto Plano Trabuco Road, which becomes Trabuco Canyon Road 0.6 mile ahead at a sharp bend to the left. Curve downward into Trabuco Canyon for 0.8 mile, and at the bottom, take a right onto unpaved Trabuco

Creek Road, which leads east toward Cleveland National Forest.

Driving this bumpy, unpaved road may be an adventure itself, but the road is generally accessible to two-wheel-drive vehicles with moderate clearance. Proceed 4.7 miles east up the canyon to the Holy Jim Trailhead on the left. You must display a National Forest Adventure Pass on your car.

Description: The first segment of the trip follows a dirt road up and to the left above the trailhead kiosk. Proceed north up along the east bank of Holy Jim Canyon's small stream, passing a number of cabins. More than a century ago this shady hollow was home to settlers who eked out a living by raising bees. Beekeeper James T. Smith became so famous for his cursing habit that he was variously nicknamed "Cussin' Jim," "Lyin' Smith," "Greasy Jim," and "Salvation Smith." Dignified government cartographers invented a new name, "Holy Jim."

In 0.5 mile a gate marks the end of the dirt road and the beginning of the trail. Continue upstream another 0.8 mile, fording the stream seven times. Just past Picnic Rock, the trail crosses the stream at a signed junction. Our route switches back sharply to the left, while a lateral trail keeps straight, going another 400 yards up along the stream to Holy Jim Falls. This little gem of a waterfall is worth the side trip if the stream is flowing decently. The Holy Jim Trail zigzags upward through dense chaparral on the west wall of Holy Jim Canyon. Well traveled but minimally cleared of encroaching vegetation, the trail offers intimate glimpses of your immediate surroundings. You have a sense of motion and accomplishment as you ascend.

Soon a few antenna structures atop Santiago Peak come into view, tantalizingly close but about 3,000 feet higher. At 3.7 miles, the trail passes a small spring dug out of the hillside and then crosses the bed of Holy Jim Canyon at an elevation of 3,500 feet, far above the falls. You might be tempted at this point to shortcut to the summit by way of the scree-covered slopes; however, the loose rock and thickets of thorny ceanothus would surely cost you more time, effort, and grief than you ever imagined. (In April 2013, a pair of teenage hikers wandered

off-trail, ran out of water, and called 911. It took four days to locate the teens.)

So continue ahead on the trail, where soon you make a delicate traverse over a section prone to landslides. After another mile on sunny, south-facing slopes, you contour around a ridge and suddenly enter a dark and shady recess filled with oaks, sycamores, big-leaf maples, and big-cone Douglas-firs. By 5 miles, you come upon Main Divide Road, opposite Bear Spring (not potable).

From now on, you simply turn left and follow the Main Divide Road (dirt road) uphill. Three more miles of steady climbing in sun and shade bring you to Santiago's summit. Alternatively, from Bear Spring, you can turn right on Main Divide Road and go 0.4 mile to the obscure, unmarked Upper Holy Jim Trail that switchbacks vigorously up to rejoin the Main Divide Road at a hairpin turn halfway up the mountain.

You must walk around the antenna installation on the summit to take in the complete panorama. Modjeska Peak, 1 mile northwest and about 200 feet lower, isn't high enough to block the view of any far-horizon features. Collectively, Santiago and Modjeska Peaks form a familiar notchlike feature visible for miles around and known as Old Saddleback. The fine-grained rock of Old Saddleback is the prototype of the "Santiago Peak volcanics" exposed on many of the coastal mountain ranges extending south through San Diego County into Baja California. These metamorphosed volcanic-rock formations were originally part of a chain of volcanic islands that collided with our continent some 80 million years ago.

Santiago Peak rises above Holy Jim Canyon.

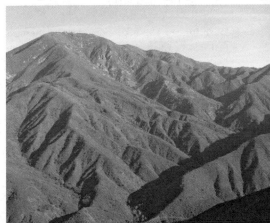

HIKE 70   Bell Canyon Loop

Location	Ronald W. Caspers Wilderness Park, Santa Ana Mountains foothills
Highlights	Interesting geologic features, wide variety of botanical features
Distance & Configuration	3.3-mile loop
Elevation Gain	400'
Hiking Time	1.5 hours
Optional Map	Ronald W. Caspers Wilderness Park brochure (ocparks.com/caspers)
Best Times	October–May
Agency	Ronald W. Caspers Wilderness Park
Difficulty	Moderate
Trail Use	Good for kids
Permit	Parking fee
Google Maps	Ronald W. Caspers Wilderness Park

The crown jewel of Orange County's regional park system, Caspers Wilderness Park is the county's largest park (8,000 acres), the least altered by human activities, and the most remote. (*Remote,* of course, is a relative term in Orange County, more than two-thirds of which is urbanized). Beware of poison oak, which grows along this trail.

To Reach the Trailhead: From I-5 at San Juan Capistrano, drive east 7.6 miles on Ortega Highway (Highway 74) to the park entrance station on the left. Pay the parking (or camping) fee here, and drive past (or visit) the park's visitor center, which houses a small museum and an open-air loft with an expansive view of the Santa Ana Mountains. Continue 1 mile to the trailhead at the site of an old windmill, your starting point for this loop.

Description: The hike touches upon the best features of Caspers Wilderness Park, starting with a rather dizzying passage across the top of some curious white sandstone formations, rather like the breaks along the upper Missouri River or the barren cliffs of the South Dakota Badlands. You'll loop up and over the main ridge that defines the west edge of the park, while enjoying views of much of Orange County's remaining rural and wild areas.

Start off on the path signed NATURE TRAIL. The trailhead is behind the equestrian parking area to the northwest and is difficult to see from the windmill. Follow the trail across the wide bed of Bell Canyon and into the dense oak woodland on the far side. After 0.3 mile, you'll spot a bench beneath a spreading oak tree. Just beyond, veer left on the Dick Loskorn Trail. This path meanders up a shallow draw and soon climbs to a sandstone ridgeline that at one point narrows to near-knife-edge width. At one point you step within a foot of a modest but unnerving abyss. The sandstone is part of a marine sedimentary formation called the Santiago Formation (roughly 45 million years old), which crops out along the coastal strip from here down to mid–San Diego County.

At 0.9 mile, after climbing about 350 feet, you reach a dirt road, the West Ridge Trail. Turn right (north), skirting the fence of Rancho Mission Viejo, a landholding that encompasses much of southern Orange County. Before World War II, it included all of Camp Pendleton as well. To the left you look down on Cañada Gobernadora ("Canyon of the Governor's Wife," though a less literal meaning refers to the invasive chamise, or greasewood, that used to fill the canyon). Luxury housing is gradually overtaking the canyon's wide floor.

At 1.6 miles, turn right on the Star Rise trail to descend into Bell Canyon. Nearing the

® Bell Canyon Loop

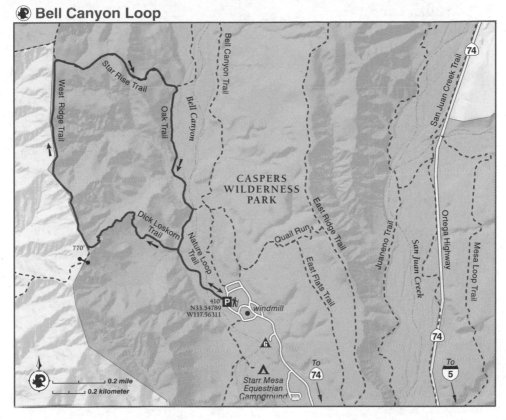

bottom, veer right on the Oak Trail (2.2 miles). On this delightful trace of a trail you meander past California sycamores and ancient coast live oaks. In late autumn, you crunch through the crispy leaf litter and watch golden sunbeams dance amid the thousands of fluttering leaves overhead. In early spring, when these leaves are emerging, the sunlight filtering through them bathes the shadows in a jungle-green luminance.

The Oak Trail returns you to a T-junction with the Nature Trail, where you turn right to reach your starting point.

HIKE 71   San Juan Loop Trail

Location	Santa Ana Mountains
Highlights	Trickling stream, small waterfall and pool
Distance & Configuration	2.1-mile loop
Elevation Gain	350'
Hiking Time	1 hour
Optional Map	Cleveland National Forest Visitor Map
Best Times	November–June
Agency	Cleveland National Forest/Trabuco Ranger District
Difficulty	Easy
Trail Use	Dogs allowed, suitable for mountain biking, good for kids
Permit	Adventure Pass
Google Maps	San Juan Loop Trailhead

🐾 San Juan Loop Trail

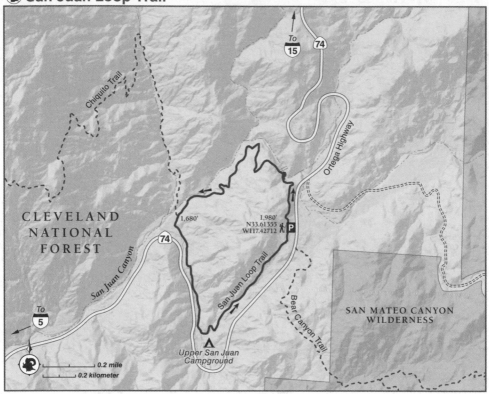

From San Juan Capistrano to Lake Elsinore, two-lane Ortega Highway stretches like a snake over the midriff of the Santa Ana Mountains, giving road warriors a taste of Orange County's wild, unfamiliar side. Even the most casual traveler can get to know the rugged and circumspect beauty of these corrugated mountains better by trying out the San Juan Loop Trail, right off the highway amid one of the most scenic spots in the range.

To Reach the Trailhead: From I-5 in San Juan Capistrano, drive 19.5 miles east on Ortega Highway (Highway 74) to reach the starting point near mile 74 RIV 2.8, the well-marked San Juan Loop Trailhead parking lot on the left. You'll need to post a National Forest Adventure Pass on your car.

Description: From the trailhead lot, a well-worn path takes off north along a slope overlooking the highway. Around a bend to the

left, the trail starts threading the side of a narrow gorge that resounds with echoes of falling water after the rainy season begins in fall or winter. A spur path leads down toward the lip of the falls; from there you can boulder-hop over to the edge of a reflecting pool. A single gnarled juniper clings sentinel-like to a rock face overlooking this pool, very far from its normal, high-desert habitat 50 miles or farther north or east. If the mood strikes you, rest your bones amid the smooth contours of the water-polished granite, and settle in for a moment of quiet meditation.

Past the falls, you descend on ramplike switchbacks through dense chaparral and presently reach the oak-dotted floodplain of San Juan Creek. Stay left at a pair of unsigned junctions with Chiquito Trail; if you cross the creek, you're off-route. Ahead, you'll plunge into a veritable thicket of centuries-old coast live oak trees. Their overarching limbs mute the glare of the sun and sky. In the soft, filtered light, the ground glows with the seasonal greens, browns, and reds of ferns, poison oak, and wild grasses. Bypass several more unsigned use paths that branch off and rejoin the main trail.

Touching briefly on the perimeter of Upper San Juan Campground, the trail veers sharply left to gain an open slope, again parallel to the highway. Continue another 0.5 mile across this sun-struck slope dotted with spring wildflowers, and arrive back at the trailhead.

HIKE 72   Sitton Peak

Location	Santa Ana Mountains
Highlight	Coast and mountain views
Distance & Configuration	9.5-mile out-and-back
Elevation Gain	2,150'
Hiking Time	5.5 hours
Optional Map	Cleveland National Forest Visitor Map
Best Times	October–May
Agency	Cleveland National Forest/Trabuco Ranger District
Difficulty	Moderately strenuous
Trail Use	Suitable for backpacking, dogs allowed
Permit	Adventure Pass; day-use sign-in at trailhead; San Mateo Canyon Wilderness permit required to stay overnight
Google Maps	San Juan Loop Trailhead

From below, Sitton Peak—a bump atop the rambling Santa Ana Mountains—looks imposing. On the summit, though, you feel decidedly on top of the world. When an east or north wind blows, cleansing the sky of water vapor and air pollution, 50-mile vistas in every direction are not uncommon. You must get a wilderness permit to camp overnight within the San Mateo Canyon Wilderness, which encompasses most of this hike.

To Reach the Trailhead: From I-5 in San Juan Capistrano, drive 19.5 miles east on Ortega Highway (Highway 74) to reach the starting point near mile 74 RIV 2.8, the well-marked San Juan Loop Trailhead parking lot on the left. You'll need to post a National Forest Adventure Pass on your car.

Description: The signed Bear Canyon Trailhead is located on the south side of the highway just west of the candy store. Sign in at the day-use register a short distance up the trail, and hike through dense chaparral, including scrub oak, chamise, sugar bush, mountain mahogany, black sage, and buckwheat. Pass the San Mateo Canyon Wilderness boundary 0.7 mile up the trail.

After 1.0 mile of moderate ascent, you come to an unsigned trail junction in a patch of oak woodland. Go right (the Morgan Trail forks left) and begin climbing more steeply along a chaparral-clothed slope. At 2.0 miles, you reach a four-way junction. The Bear Canyon Trail turns right and follows the bed of the old Verdugo Truck Trail. Note that the Bear Ridge Trail proceeds straight and rejoins the Bear Canyon Trail at Four Corners, offering an alternative return route. You soon pass oak-shaded Pigeon Spring (2.7 miles), a seasonal trickle at the head of Bear Canyon. An old horse-watering trough is here up a short spur to the left, with seeps nearby. Enjoy the shade—you won't find much more of it on the road ahead.

Continue south another half mile to reach a clearing misnamed Four Corners (3.2 miles), where four old roads and the newer Bear Ridge footpath join together. You can make an exposed camp here. Swing right on the road

🅡 Sitton Peak

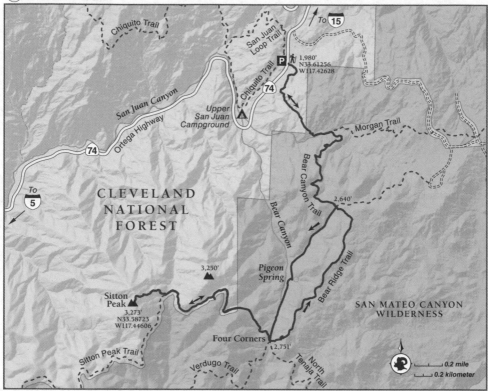

that climbs northwest, a disused section of the Sitton Peak Road. After a steady ascent of about 300 vertical feet, you reach a flat area (4.0 miles) just below a boulder-studded ridge (3,250' elevation) to the north. Easily climbed, the ridge summit offers a view somewhat similar to that from Sitton Peak. A few yards beyond, a spur leads south to a clearing by a lone oak where backpackers could camp.

Beyond the flat area, the road descends another 0.5 mile to a saddle just below Sitton Peak. From this saddle, you leave the road and follow a steep climber's trail up through scattered manzanita and chamise on the east slope of the peak.

The view from the top is especially impressive to the west. Here the foothills and western canyons of the Santa Anas merge with the creeping suburbs of southern Orange County. Beyond lies the flat, blue ocean punctuated by the profile of Santa Catalina Island. Some 2,000 feet below, toylike cars on the highway make their way down the sinuous course of San Juan Canyon.

HIKE 73   Tenaja Falls

Location	San Mateo Canyon Wilderness
Highlight	Beautiful, multilevel waterfall
Distance & Configuration	1.4-mile out-and-back
Elevation Gain	300'

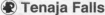

Tenaja Falls

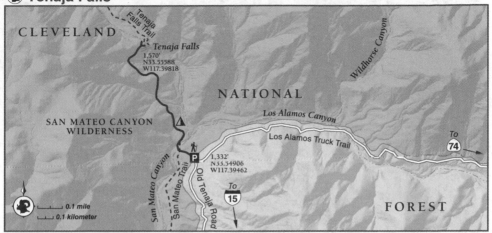

Hiking Time	1 hour
Optional Map	Cleveland National Forest Visitor Map
Best Times	December–June
Agency	Cleveland National Forest/Trabuco Ranger District
Difficulty	Easy
Trail Use	Good for kids, dogs allowed, suitable for backpacking
Permit	None required
Google Maps	Tenaja Falls Trailhead

With five tiers and a total drop of about 150 feet, Tenaja Falls is the most interesting natural feature in the San Mateo Canyon Wilderness section of Cleveland National Forest. In late winter and spring, water coursing down the polished rock produces a kind of soothing music not widely heard in this somewhat dry corner of the Santa Ana Mountains.

The only easy way to reach Tenaja Falls on foot is from the south, though the drive to that trailhead is rather lengthy by way of any approach. Beware of the plentiful poison oak growing alongside the trail.

To Reach the Trailhead (from I-5): From I-5 in San Juan Capistrano drive 23 miles east on Ortega Highway (Highway 74). Just past mile marker 74 RIV 6.50, turn right on South Main Divide Road. Proceed south to Wildomar Campground and off-road-vehicle (ORV) area. Continue a total of 16 miles (from Ortega Highway) on the paved one-lane road to a large

signed turnout on the right, overlooking the tree-covered bottom of San Mateo Canyon.

To Reach the Trailhead (from I-15): Exit I-15 at Clinton Keith Road in Murrieta. Proceed 6 miles south on Clinton Keith Road and 1.7 miles west on Tenaja Road to a marked intersection, where you must turn right to stay on Tenaja Road. Continue west on Tenaja Road another 4.2 miles, then go right on the one-lane, paved Cleveland Forest Road. Proceed another mile, passing the Tenaja Trailhead, and continue 4.6 miles farther to reach the Tenaja Falls Trailhead, a large turnout on the left, overlooking the tree-covered bottom of San Mateo Canyon.

Description: Don't forget to sign in at the self-registration box just down the trail; then head down to the canyon bottom, veer left a little, and cross the creek on remnants of an old concrete ford. Balance on rocks or wade through

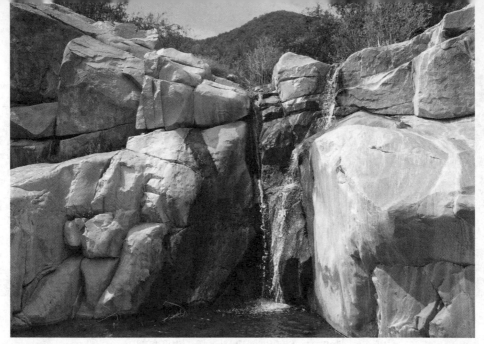

Tenaja Falls

the water. Continue north on a steadily rising old roadbed (now a wilderness trail), and you'll soon be treated to a fairly distant view of the falls. After 0.7 mile the road passes near the upper lip of the falls, where a few large oaks provide welcome shade.

Further exploration of the falls requires rock-climbing skills and extreme caution. The flow of water has worn the granitic rock almost glassy smooth. While scouting the middle tiers and pools, I found that slightly wet bare feet provided much more traction than the soles of my running shoes—don't be lured into dangerous situations though.

A somewhat safer way of approaching the lower falls is to scramble over the rough-textured rocks well away from the water. You might also backtrack down the road and then scramble down the slope into the brush-choked creekbed down near the base of the falls.

HIKE 74   Tenaja Canyon

Location	San Mateo Canyon Wilderness
Highlight	Riparian vegetation and oak woodland in a steep canyon
Distance & Configuration	7-mile out-and-back (to Fishermans Camp)
Elevation Gain	1,100'
Hiking Time	3.5 hours
Optional Map	Cleveland National Forest Visitor Map
Best Times	November–May
Agency	Cleveland National Forest/Trabuco Ranger District
Difficulty	Moderately strenuous
Trail Use	Dogs allowed, suitable for backpacking
Permit	San Mateo Canyon Wilderness permit required to stay overnight
Google Maps	Tenaja Trail Head

Tenaja Canyon

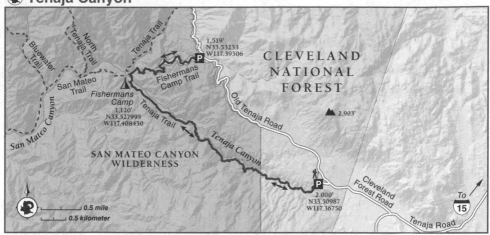

As the gloom of a late afternoon descended upon the deep-cut, linear furrow of Tenaja Canyon, dozens of orange-bellied newts waddled determinedly uphill and across the trail, oblivious to my footfalls. The cute faces and beady eyes of these little amphibians mirrored a mindless desire I cannot fathom: Sex in a bower of leaf litter and ferns? A bellyful of succulent tree-dwelling insects, ripe for the taking?

The Tenaja Trail rambles along a 10-mile stretch of the 62-square-mile San Mateo Canyon Wilderness, the largest parcel of designated wilderness near the Southern California coast. The wilderness consists mostly of steep, rough, and rocky chaparral country, softened by the strips of oak woodland and riparian vegetation that thrive along the larger canyon bottoms. This hike explores the south end of the Tenaja Trail, which follows Tenaja Canyon down to its confluence with San Mateo Canyon. The route takes you down and later all the way back up; if it's a warm day or you feel fatigued, you can always reverse your course at any time.

To Reach the Trailhead: To reach the Tenaja Trailhead, exit I-15 at Clinton Keith Road in the community of Murrieta. Proceed 5.2 miles south on Clinton Keith Road to a sharp bend where the name changes to Tenaja Road. Continue 1.7 miles west to a marked intersection,

Fishermans Camp

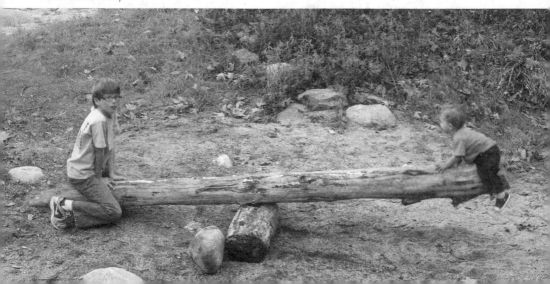

where you must turn right to stay on Tenaja Road. Go west on Tenaja Road another 4.2 miles, then turn right onto the one-lane, paved Cleveland Forest Road. Proceed another mile to the trailhead parking area.

Description: Sign in at the self-registration box, and head downhill on the trail going west. A few minutes' descent takes you to the shady bowels of V-shaped Tenaja Canyon, where huge coast live oaks and pale-barked sycamores frame a limpid, rock-dimpled seasonal stream. Mostly the trail ahead meanders alongside the stream, but for the canyon's middle stretch, it carves its way across the chaparral-blanketed south wall, 200–400 feet above the canyon bottom.

After 3.7 miles of general descent, you reach Fishermans Camp, a former drive-in campground once accessible by many miles of bad road. Today the site, distinguished by its park-like setting amid a grove of live oaks, serves as a fine wilderness campsite for an overnight backpacking trip (for which you must get a wilderness permit). Its name hints at the fishing opportunities that nearby San Mateo Canyon Creek affords during and after the rainy season. A native species of steelhead trout was discovered in this drainage, surprising experts who thought that steelhead might be extinct south of Los Angeles County.

VARIATIONS

At Fishermans Camp, three other trails diverge. The San Mateo Trail, a narrow footpath, leads southwest downstream many miles to the east boundary of Camp Pendleton. It also leads north upstream to meet Old Tenaja Road at the Tenaja Falls Trailhead. Just north of Tenaja Creek, the Fishermans Camp Trail (the old road) forks off the San Mateo Trail and climbs 1.6 miles directly up to Old Tenaja Road. If you position a vehicle at that trailhead, you can cut 2 miles and 500 feet of elevation gain off your trip by hiking out there. Otherwise, your quickest return route is back the way you came.

HIKE 75   Santa Rosa Plateau Ecological Reserve

Location	Near Temecula and Murrieta
Highlights	Green and golden hills, rare oaks, spring wildflowers, vernal pools
Distance & Configuration	6-mile loop
Elevation Gain	650'
Hiking Time	3 hours
Optional Map	Santa Rosa Plateau Ecological Reserve (rivcoparks.org/santa-rosa-plateau-visitor-center)
Best Times	November–June
Agency	Santa Rosa Plateau Ecological Reserve
Difficulty	Moderate
Trail use	Good for kids
Permit	Parking fee
Google Maps	Hidden Valley Trail Head

Note: The 2019 Tenaja Fire impacted the reserve. At the time of this writing, this trail described here is still temporarily closed.

A 200-mile-wide circle centered on the Santa Rosa Plateau Ecological Reserve in the southwest corner of Riverside County encompasses a megalopolis of some 20 million people. File this fact away in your mind, and try to fathom it while walking amid the green and golden hills of this exquisitely beautiful reserve. Here is a classic California landscape of wind-rippled grasses, swaying poppies, statuesque oak trees,

Santa Rosa Plateau Ecological Reserve

Map labels: Shivela Trail; Sylvan Meadows Multi-use Area; Engelmann Oak Loop; To 15; Tenaja Truck Trail; Mortero Trail; Hidden Valley Trailhead 1,847' N33.52704 W117.28415; Oak Tree Trail; Coyote Trail; Los Santos Trail; Hidden Valley Road; Cole Creek; Ranch Road; Lomas Trail; Monument Road; 2,046' Monument Hill; Tenaja Road; Trans Preserve Trail; SANTA ROSA PLATEAU ECOLOGICAL RESERVE; Via Volcano; Poppy Hill 1,979'; Adobe Loop; Ranch Road; 1,830' Rancho Santa Rosa Adobes; Punta Mesa Trail; Vernal Pools Trailhead 2,080'; Trans Preserve Trail; Vernal Pool Trail; Mesa de Colorado; 1,940'; vernal pool; 0.2 mile; 0.2 kilometer

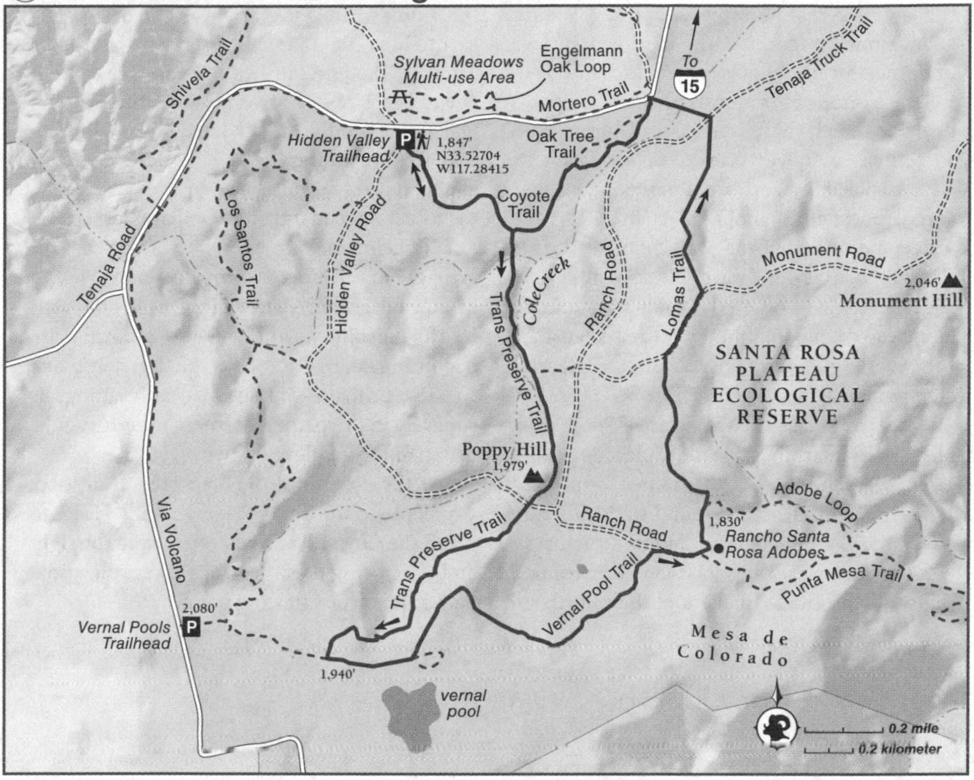

trickling streams, vernal pools, and a dazzling assortment of native plants (nearly 500 at last count) and animals. All who visit the reserve are struck by its timelessness and its insularity.

Starting with a nucleus of 3,100 acres, purchased by The Nature Conservancy in 1984, the reserve has expanded to nearly 9,000 acres (about 14 square miles) today. The west half is laced with new hiking trails as well as old ranch roads, while much of the eastern part lies off-limits to all visitation due to its ecologically sensitive nature. The 6-mile loop described here visits the major accessible highlights of the reserve, which are most beautifully presented in the green months of March and April. The 2019 Tenaja Fire burned 2,000 acres, including portions of this park.

To Reach the Trailhead: The reserve can be reached in less than 90 minutes from either central Los Angeles or San Diego. Take I-15 to the Clinton Keith Road exit in Murrieta. Drive southwest on Clinton Keith Road, passing the reserve's visitor center (open weekends) at 5 miles. At 5.2 miles, the road bends sharply right and its name changes to Tenaja Road. At 0.7 mile past this sharp bend, park at the Hidden Valley Trailhead parking area (on either side of the road). There's a small day-use fee, payable here. Trails in the reserve are open sunrise–sunset.

Description: From the Hidden Valley Trailhead, head southeast on the Coyote Trail. After 0.5 mile, turn right on the Trans Preserve Trail. Follow it over rolling and sometimes wooded terrain, passing through part of the reserve's 3,000 acres of remnant native bunchgrass prairie. Reserve managers have been implementing controlled burns to discourage the growth of nonnative grasses and promote the recovery of native plants.

The last half mile of the Trans Preserve Trail rises to a plateau called Mesa de Colorado. At the top of the mesa (2.0 miles), you turn left on the Vernal Pool Trail and soon visit one of the largest vernal pools in California (39 acres at maximum capacity). The hard-pan surface underneath vernal pools is quite impervious to water, so once winter storms fill them, the pools dry out mostly by evaporation. Unusual and sometimes unique species of flowering plants have evolved in and around this and other vernal pools throughout the state. When the watery perimeter of the pool contracts during the lengthening and warming days of spring, successive waves of annual wildflowers bloom along the drying margin. By July or August, all the water is gone, and only a desiccated depression remains.

Continue east on the Vernal Pool Trail, and descend from Mesa de Colorado to the two adobe buildings of the former Santa Rosa Ranch (3.3 miles). Built around 1845, these are Riverside County's oldest standing structures.

After a look at the adobes and a refreshing pause in the shade, make a beeline north on the Lomas Trail. Jog briefly right on Monument Road, then go left to stay on the Lomas Trail. At the junction with Tenaja Truck Trail ahead, go straight across toward the looping Oak Tree Trail. The left (streamside) branch is better, assuming the creek is flowing. Both alternatives give you a close-up look at some of the finest Engelmann oak woodland anywhere. The Engelmann oak tree, with its distinctive gray-green leaves, is endemic to a narrow strip of coastal foothills stretching from Southern California into northern Baja California. It's becoming one of the rarer of the state's oak species, primarily because its native range is squarely in the path of current and future suburban and rural development.

At the far end of the Oak Tree Trail loop, you come to the Trans Preserve Trail. Use it to reach the Coyote Trail, where a turn to the right and a retracing of earlier steps takes you a final half mile to your starting point.

Aerial view of the Santa Rosa Plateau

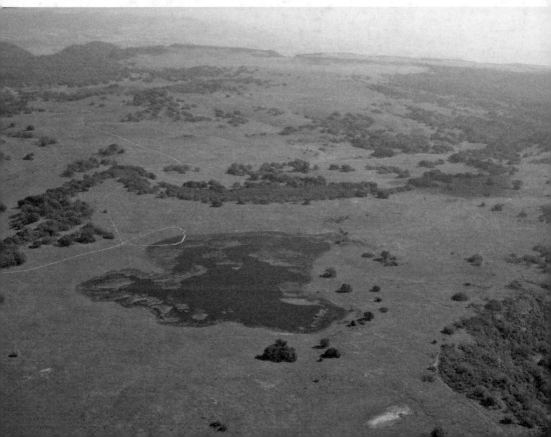

HIKE 76   Agua Tibia Mountain

Location	Agua Tibia Wilderness
Highlights	Spring wildflowers, valley and mountain views
Distance & Configuration	15-mile out-and-back
Elevation Gain	3,200'
Hiking Time	9 hours
Recommended Map	Cleveland National Forest Visitor Map
Best Times	November–May
Agency	Cleveland National Forest/Palomar Ranger District
Difficulty	Strenuous
Trail Use	Dogs allowed, suitable for backpacking
Permit	Agua Tibia Wilderness permit required to stay overnight; Adventure Pass needed to park inside or outside the campground (see details on page 190)
Google Maps	Dripping Springs Trailhead

The 18,000-acre Agua Tibia Wilderness lies northwest of Palomar Mountain, straddling the San Diego–Riverside county line in Cleveland National Forest. Agua Tibia Mountain (4,781'), one of the three distinct mountain blocks of the Palomar range, is the centerpiece of the wilderness that bears its name. Sparse groves of Coulter pine, big-cone Douglas-fir, incense-cedar, live oak, and black oak cover the highest elevations, while the lower slopes are scrub-covered and fluted by many steep canyons holding intermittent streams. The wilderness was named after one of these streams, Agua Tibia ("tepid water") Creek.

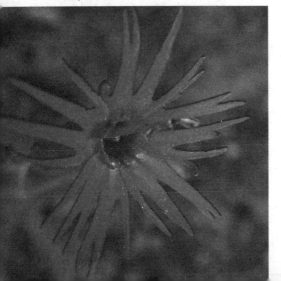

Indian pink

The Dripping Springs Trail, which is the primary route into the wilderness area, originates at Dripping Springs Campground. With only minimal interruptions, the trail ascends from the 1,620-foot elevation of the campground to a 4,400-foot crest near the high point of Agua Tibia Mountain, passing through belts of chamise chaparral, manzanita and ribbonwood chaparral, and finally oak and pine forest. The chaparral constantly encroaches on the trail and is held back only by the unending labor of trail crews; this trail is usually in good condition, but other trails in this wilderness are often overgrown. Poison oak grows close to the trail, especially near the summit. Long pants, gloves, and clippers might be helpful. In March or April of an average or better-than-average rain year, the blooming of annual wildflowers along the lower trail can be stupendous. The trail's upper part offers ever-widening, pseudo-aerial views to the north, where the distant Transverse Ranges rise out of valley mists as if they were the rim of the world.

To Reach the Trailhead: From I-15 in Temecula, drive 10 miles east on Highway 79 to Dripping Springs Campground, on the right (south) side of the road at mile marker 79 RIV 9.3. The campground lies just behind the Dripping Springs Fire Station. If the campground is closed, you can park outside the gate and

🅡 Agua Tibia Mountain

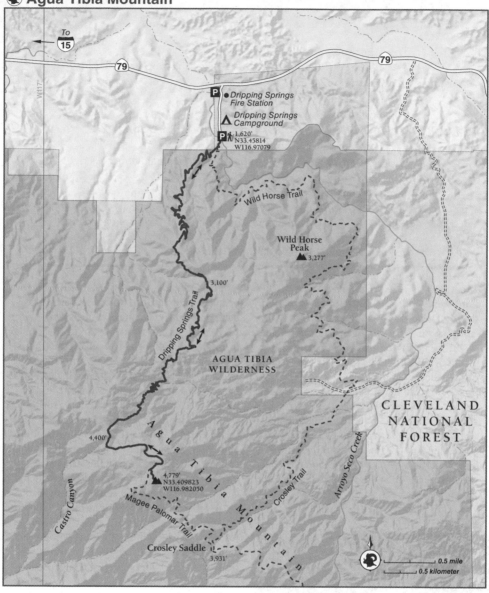

walk 0.4 mile past the campsites to reach the inner trailhead, where you sign in at a register before entering the national-forest wilderness area that lies just ahead. You'll need a National Forest Adventure Pass to park either inside or outside the campground. A limited number of spaces outside the campground are designated as free for those without an Adventure Pass, and you can also park on the highway for free.

Description: The trail mileages given below are keyed to the inner trailhead. From the campground, the Dripping Springs Trail immediately fords Arroyo Seco Creek (stay on the path to avoid disturbing the habitat of the endangered Arroyo Toad) and then begins a switchbacking ascent through sage scrub and chaparral vegetation liberally sprinkled with annual wildflowers in early spring. After only 0.1 mile, there's a trail junction. The less maintained Wild Horse Trail, on the left, gains elevation relatively slowly, sticking to the slopes overlooking Agua Tibia Creek. Your way stays right, up the Dripping Springs route that is sure to give you a solid cardiovascular workout.

After a mile, the trail gains the top of a nearly flat ridge and then continues south toward a series of 10 ascending switchbacks. Vail Lake and Southern California's four county highpoint mountains—Old Baldy, San Gorgonio, San Jacinto, and Santiago—come into view. On a clear winter day, the snow-covered summits standing bold against the blue sky are a memorable sight.

At 3.5 miles (3,100' elevation), the Dripping Springs Trail crosses the head of a small creek and continues upward amid manzanita and ribbonwood. At 4.5 miles, the trail descends a little and crosses an area of poor soil. A view opens up to the southeast and south. The white dome of the Hale Telescope at Palomar Observatory gleams on a ridge about 9 miles southeast. You can now see the pine- and oak-fringed summit ridge of Agua Tibia Mountain ahead.

Soon you follow sharp switchbacks again. At 6.5 miles, a sign indicates the end of the Dripping Springs Trail and the beginning of the Palomar-Magee Trail, an abandoned fire road, which turns left. Walk south down the Palomar-Magee Trail to a point overlooking Castro Canyon (6.6 miles). There, on most clear winter days, a clear panorama of north San Diego County, including conspicuous, undulating, linear I-15, spreads before you. On the far horizon to the west and south you can often see the Pacific Ocean and the mountains of Baja California.

At 7.5 miles, watch for a cairn marking a climbers trail on the left to Agua Tibia Mountain. Follow this short trail, squeezing around encroaching poison oak, to the summit, at 7.6 miles, where you can admire panoramic views. The true high point is a large boulder (some climbing skills required), but the summit register is by a flat rock at a great spot for a picnic lunch.

VARIATION

If the trails have been recently maintained, it might be enjoyable to make a 20-mile loop by following the Palomar-Magee, Crosley, and Wild Horse Trails. As of 2020, the loop was passable but heavily encroached by chaparral. Otherwise, return the way you came.

HIKE 77 La Jolla Shores to Torrey Pines Beach

Location	La Jolla
Highlights	Bodysurfing, remote beach backed by sheer cliffs
Distance & Configuration	5.0-mile point-to-point
Elevation Gain	Negligible (at sea level)
Hiking Time	2.5 hours
Optional Maps	USGS 7.5-minute *La Jolla* and *Del Mar*
Best Times	All year
Agency	Torrey Pines State Reserve
Difficulty	Moderate
Permit	None required
Google Maps	La Jolla Shores Beach

Del Mar

Carmel Valley Road

Torrey Pines
State Beach
N32.92981
W117.25990

$ P

P

Marsh Trail

56

5

El Camino Real

Carmel Mountain Road

Flat Rock

**TORREY PINES
STATE NATURAL
RESERVE**

North Torrey Pines Road

(Old Highway 101)

Torrey Pine
Golf Course

Black's Beach

Torrey
Pines
Scenic
Drive

Glider Port

P

805

Genesee Avenue

La Jolla
Farms
Road

North Torrey Pines Road

*University of
California
San Diego*

5

p a c i f i c   O c e a n

La Jolla Village Drive

Nobel Drive

Dike Rock
tidepools

Scripps Pier

La Jolla Shores Drive

La Jolla Scenic Drive

Gilman Drive

La Jolla
Shores Beach
N32.85731
W117.23655

P

Calle
Frescota

La Jolla
Bay

Torrey Pines Road

52

La Jolla

0.5 mile
0.5 kilometer

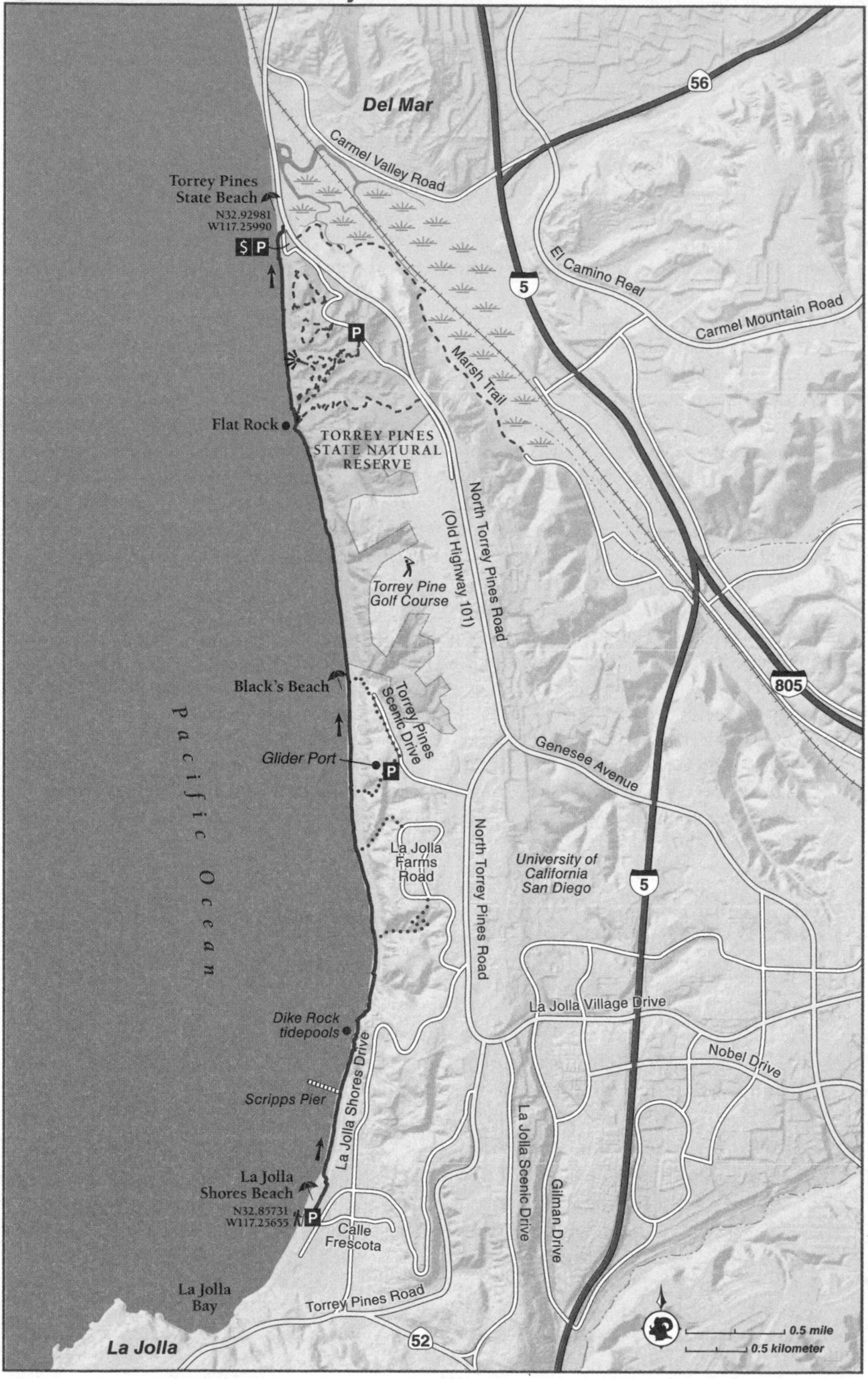

There are only a few places along the Southern California coastline where you can hike for miles and not see roads, railroad tracks, power lines, or other signs of civilization. The Torrey Pines beaches are one such place. Here, for nearly 4 miles, cliffs front the shoreline and cut off the sights and sounds of the world beyond.

Plan to do this beach walk at low tide. High tides, especially in winter, could force you to walk on cobbles at the base of the cliffs or wade in the surf. At low tide, the Dike Rock tide pools are accessible and the damp sand makes for easy walking. Beach sand is often carried away by the scouring action of the winter waves, but the currents usually replenish it as summer approaches.

To Reach the Trailhead: From I-5 north, take Exit 26A west on La Jolla Parkway (there is no exit from I-5 south, but you can also reach La Jolla from Highway 52 west). The parkway eventually becomes Torrey Pines Road. In 2.0 miles, turn right (north) on La Jolla Shores Drive. In 0.5 mile, turn left on Calle Frescota and proceed 0.2 mile into the free parking area for La Jolla Shores Beach. The grassy park alongside is known as Kellogg Park.

If you're making this a one-way trip, leave a second car along North Torrey Pines Road (the Old Coast Highway 101), next to Torrey Pines State Beach, or in the adjacent pay lot at Torrey Pines State Reserve. This is a 7-mile car shuttle. It may be easiest to have someone drop you off at the start and pick you up later at the end. Another option is to use local buses to get from the finish back to the start: At Torrey Pines State Beach you can take the 101 bus south to La Jolla Shores Drive, where a transfer to a Route 30 bus takes you to Calle Frescota near Kellogg Park. The bus drivers do not make change, so bring dollar bills and quarters.

Description: Start your hike at La Jolla Shores Beach by walking north under Scripps Pier. At 1.0 mile, reach the Dike Rock tide pools. During low tide, you may discover sea stars, sea anemones, and hermit crabs, as well as the ubiquitous mussels and limpets. This is part of the San Diego–La Jolla Underwater Park Ecological Preserve; enjoy the creatures and plant life, but do not disturb or collect anything. Once you are beyond the last of the cobbles and wave-rounded boulders, you can slip off your shoes and enjoy the feel of fine, clean

Flat Rock at Torrey Pines Beach

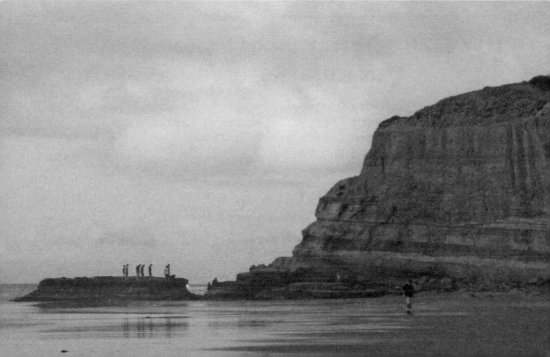

sand underfoot. On the right, you'll see the unusual Mushroom House, a guesthouse built for potato chip magnate Sam Bell in the 1960s. Guests rode a tram down the cliff to the house, but the rails are now damaged by rockfall.

You are now on Torrey Pines City Beach. At 1.5 miles, you'll see a paved road (closed to car traffic) going up through a small canyon. This is a safe way to reach (or exit) the beach. There's a limited amount of 2-hour parking at the top along La Jolla Farms Road.

At 2.2 miles, a precipitous trail ascends about 300 feet to the Torrey Pines Glider Port, where hang-gliders launch their craft. Look up to see antlike beachgoers lugging their gear up or down the zigzagging paths and hang-gliders soaring overhead. Nevertheless, the trail is signed DO NOT USE because of the unstable cliffs. You'll see a second gliderport trail at 2.8 miles.

Beyond the gliderport trail, you may notice that some people have doffed more than just shoes. You're now on Torrey Pines State Beach, also known as Black's Beach, San Diego's unofficial nude-bathing spot. The city rescinded a clothing-optional policy for this beach in the late 1970s, but old traditions have never died.

Lifeguards patrol some areas of Black's Beach during busy periods, so you can feel fairly safe about jumping into the water, which may be warmer than 70°F in July, August, and September. Shuffle your feet to alert stingrays of your presence. Elsewhere you swim at your own risk—watch out for rip currents around underwater Scripps Canyon, just offshore. This same canyon generates powerful waves that draw advanced surfers to the beach.

At 4.3 miles from Kellogg Park, you reach Flat Rock, where a protruding sandstone wall blocks easy passage. Follow the narrow path cut into the wall. If the tide is low, you can clamber onto Flat Rock and inspect an unusual tide pool on top of the rock. From a low shelf on the far side, the Beach Trail begins its ascent up a staircase to Torrey Pines State Reserve's Visitor Center.

In the fifth and last mile, the narrow beach is squeezed between sculpted sedimentary cliffs on one side and crashing surf on the other. These are the tallest cliffs in western San Diego County. A close look at the faces reveals a slice of geologic history: The greenish siltstone on the bottom, called the Del Mar Formation, is older than the buff- or rust-colored Torrey Sandstone above it. Higher still is a thin cap of reddish sandstone not easily seen from the beach—the Linda Vista Formation.

In the end, the beach widens, the cliffs fall back, and you arrive at the entrance to Torrey Pines State Natural Reserve along North Torrey Pines Road.

HIKE 78   Torrey Pines State Natural Reserve

Location	Del Mar
Highlights	Rare vegetation, wildflowers, ocean views
Distance & Configuration	Up to 4 miles total (short loops)
Elevation Gain	Up to 600'
Hiking Time	Up to 2 hours
Optional Map	Torrey Pines State Park brochure (torreypine.org)
Best Times	All year, 8 a.m.–sunset
Agency	Torrey Pines State Natural Reserve
Difficulty	Easy–moderate
Trail Use	Good for kids
Permit	Parking fee
Google Maps	Torrey Pines State Reserve

🌀 Torrey Pines State Reserve

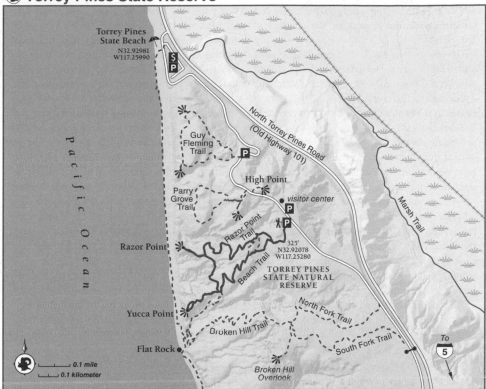

The rare and beautiful Torrey pines atop the coastal bluffs south of Del Mar are as much a symbol of the Golden State as the famed Monterey cypress trees native to central California's coast. Torrey pines grow naturally in only two places: in and around Torrey Pines State Reserve and on Santa Rosa Island, off Santa Barbara. Of the estimated 10,000 native Torrey pines now living, about a third grow within the reserve. A combination of drought and bark beetle infestation killed about 15% of the reserve's Torrey pines during the late 1980s, and the striking trees remain at risk of further decline.

Torrey Pines State Reserve would be botanically remarkable even without its pines. Three major plant communities can be found on the reserve's 1,750 acres: sage scrub, chaparral, and salt marsh. More than 330 plant species have been identified within the reserve so far. That number is approximately 20% of all the known plants native to San Diego County. This is especially noteworthy because San Diego County is

Torrey pine

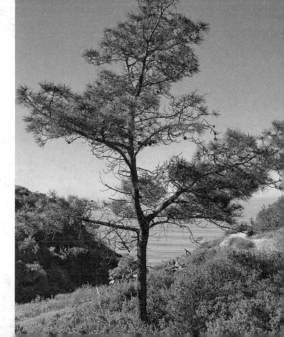

widely regarded as the most geographically and botanically diverse county in the continental United States.

If you're interested in recognizing plants and wildflowers typical of coastal and inland Southern California, come here in the spring. Excellent interpretive facilities at the reserve's museum make plant identification an easy task. Besides the exhibits, you can browse through several notebooks full of captioned photographs of common and rare plants that grow within the reserve. You can also visit the native plant gardens surrounding the museum building.

A network of trails over the eroded bluffs will take you nearly everywhere in the reserve, except into most canyon bottoms. It's important that you stick to these trails and eschew shortcuts and cross-country travel. The thin soils are easily eroded without the protection of healthy vegetation. As you'll plainly see, there are already enough instances of erosion here, due to both natural and human causes.

To Reach the Trailhead: Exit I-5 at Carmel Valley Road (Exit 33), and drive west 1.5 miles to the Old Coast Highway 101 (which is named Camino del Mar to the north and North Torrey Pines Road to the south). Turn left, drive 1 mile to the Torrey Pines State Reserve entrance on the right, and pay the day-use fee for the reserve. Past the entrance, a paved road goes up to a parking lot adjacent to the reserve office and museum. From there, you can walk to the beginning of any of the trails in 10 minutes or less. If that lot is full, you may be able to park in turnouts along the entrance road, in the beach parking lot at the reserve entrance, or along the shoulder of North Torrey Pines Road. The reserve has a finite carrying capacity. Access may be restricted on busy weekends, so get there early if you can.

Description: Pick up a handy trail map at the entrance station or the museum. After a stop at the museum for a bit of educational browsing, you might first explore nearby High Point,

The bluffs at Torrey Pines reserve are a great place to watch waves roll across the beach.

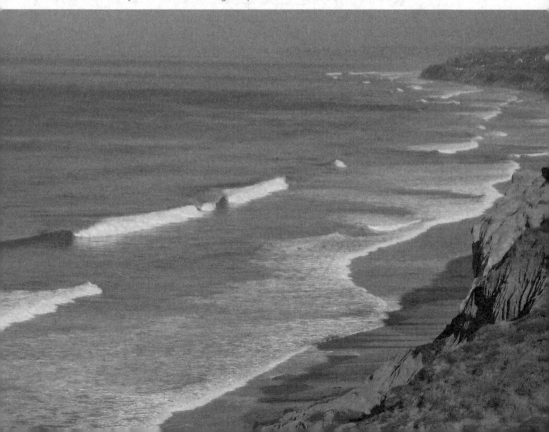

where your gaze encompasses a steep, off-limits section of the reserve known as East Grove. There, young Torrey pines are establishing a foothold on the bluffs and canyons in the aftermath of past wildfires.

Next, you might head south on the concrete roadbed of the "old" Pacific Highway (closed to car traffic) and pick up the Broken Hill Trail. The two east branches of this trail wind through thick chamise chaparral and connect with a spur trail leading to Broken Hill Overlook. You'll be able to step out (very carefully) onto a precipitous fin of sandstone and peer over to see what, except for a few Torrey pine trees here and there, looks like desert badlands. A third (west) branch of the Broken Hill Trail winds down a slope festooned with wildflowers and joins the Beach Trail at a point just above where the latter drops sharply to the beach. The popular Beach Trail originates at the parking lot across the road from the museum. It forks repeatedly, passes a sandstone outcrop called Red Butte, and intersects with trails to Yucca Point and Razor Point. Fenced viewpoints

along both of these trails offer views straight down to the sandy beach and surf. You can make a 2–3 mile loop with 300 feet of elevation change using any of these trails.

The Parry Grove and Guy Fleming loop trails wind among Torrey pine groves that were hit hard by the late-1980s drought. The 0.6-mile Guy Fleming Trail is mostly flat, while the 0.4-mile Parry Grove Trail starts with a steep descent on stairs. In spring, the sunny slopes along the Guy Fleming Trail come alive with phantasmagoric wildflower displays. Fluttering in the sea breeze, the flowers put on quite a show as several vivid shades of color dynamically intermix with the more muted tones of earth, sea, and sky. This is the best trail for families with young children to see the Torrey pines, cactus, yuccas, sage scrub, wildflowers, and ocean in a short walk.

Docent-led walks are featured on weekends. You can't picnic in the reserve, but after you hike, you can use the tables or the beach down near the entrance. Bring binoculars to watch the soaring ravens and red-tailed and sparrow hawks; you may even see hang-gliding humans.

HIKE 79   Los Peñasquitos Canyon

Location	Northern San Diego
Highlights	An oak-shaded coastal canyon and a waterfall
Distance & Configuration	6-mile out-and-back or loop
Elevation Gain	200'
Hiking Time	3 hours
Optional Map	Los Peñasquitos Canyon Preserve map (sandiego.gov /park-and-recreation/parks/osp/lospenasquitos)
Best Times	All year
Agency	Los Peñasquitos Canyon Preserve
Difficulty	Moderate
Trail Use	Good for kids, dogs allowed, suitable for mountain biking
Permit	Parking fee
Google Maps	Penasquitos Canyon Trail Head

Crickets sing, cicadas buzz, and bullfrogs groan. A sparrow hawk alights upon a sycamore limb, then launches with outstretched wings to catch a puff of sea breeze moving up the canyon. A cottontail rabbit bounds across the trail and stops to take your measure with a sidelong stare. Los

Peñasquitos Creek slips silently through placid pools and darts noisily down multiple paths in the constriction known as the falls.

Despite the noose of suburban development tightening around it, Los Peñasquitos Canyon Preserve still retains its gentle, unselfconscious

Los Peñasquitos Canyon

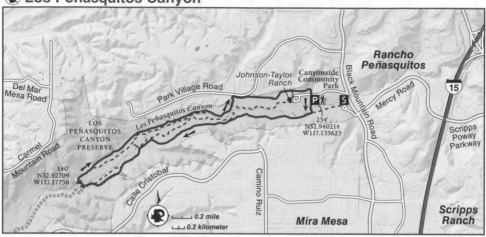

beauty. The preserve's 4,000 acres of San Diego city- and county-owned open space stretch for almost 7 miles between I-5 and I-15, encompassing much of Los Peñasquitos Creek and one of its tributaries, Lopez Canyon.

Facilities at the preserve include parking and equestrian staging areas off Black Mountain Road on the east side and next to Sorrento Valley Boulevard on the west side. Near the east entry stands the Johnson-Taylor ranch house, now the preserve's headquarters, dating from 1862. In 1991, archaeologists announced that part of the ranch house is a surviving remnant

of a residence built in 1824 for Captain Francisco María Ruiz. Ruiz was commandant of the Presidio of San Diego and the recipient of the county's first Spanish land grant. The crumbling remnants of another adobe structure, also owned by Ruiz, stand under a protective roof at the west entrance to the preserve.

Farther afield, hikers, joggers, mountain bikers, and equestrians have the run of the preserve. Take along a picnic lunch and a blanket. There are many fine places—sunny meadows, oak-shaded flats, and the sycamore-fringed streamside—to stop for an hour's relaxation.

Los Peñasquitos Falls

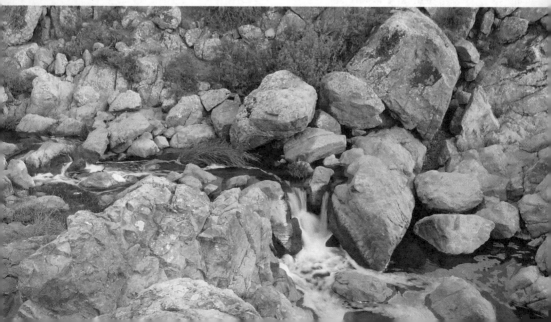

For starters, you can try the nearly level hike to the falls and back.

To Reach the Trailhead: Exit I-15 at Mercy Road/Scripps Poway Parkway (Exit 17), and go west on Mercy Road 1.3 miles to a traffic light at a T-intersection with Black Mountain Road. The main entrance to Los Peñasquitos Canyon Preserve is straight across this intersection. Drive in, pay a small day-use fee, and park in the large parking lot. Alternatively, there is a free entrance available at the west end of Canyonside Community Park; follow signs toward the ranch house and look for a gate on the left.

Description: On foot (or on wheels—the preserve sometimes swarms with mountain bikers), head west on a dirt road. In the first mile the road hugs Los Peñasquitos Canyon's south wall, a steep, chaparral-covered hillside (*peñasquitos* means "little cliffs"). Various paths fork off in both directions, but stay on the main dirt road.

As you pass near the Johnson-Taylor Ranch (screened from view by willows and dense vegetation along the creek), you'll notice several nonnative plants, such as eucalyptus, fan palms, feather-duster palms, and fennel, introduced to this area over the past century. Efforts to remove these exotic species are ongoing. Next, you enter a long and beautiful canopy of intertwined live oaks accompanied by a lush understory of mostly poison oak. You can stay on the road or take some narrower no-bike paths closer to the creek. Remain on signed trails; don't create new social paths.

Mileposts along the roadside help you gauge your progress. At mile 2 the trail winds out of the dense cover of oaks and continues through grassland dotted with a few small elderberry trees. Wildflowers such as wild radish, mustard, California poppies, bush mallow, blue-eyed grass, and violets put on quite a show here in March and April. Look, too, for the fuchsia-flowered gooseberry, quite unmistakable when in bloom.

At the 3-mile marker the road starts winding up onto a chaparral slope to detour around a narrow, rocky section of the canyon. At a signed junction for the waterfall viewpoint, make your way down to a narrow, rocky constriction along the canyon bottom. During winter and early spring, water in decent quantity tumbles through here. Polished rock 10 feet up on either side and deep, circular potholes testify to its sometimes violent flow. The outcrops of greenish-gray rock have been identified as Santiago Peak volcanics—the same hardened metavolcanic rock found farther north at Santiago Peak in the Santa Ana Mountains and farther south into Baja California.

You can make a loop by returning along a path on the north side of the canyon.

HIKE 80   Bernardo Mountain

Location	Escondido
Highlights	Wildflower-dotted hillsides, lake views, bird-watching
Distance & Configuration	7-mile out-and-back
Elevation Gain	1,000'
Hiking Time	3.5 hours
Optional Map	USGS 7.5-minute *Escondido*
Best Times	All year
Agency	San Dieguito River Park
Difficulty	Moderately strenuous
Trail Use	Dogs allowed, suitable for mountain biking
Permit	None required
Google Maps	Bernardo Mountain Summit Trail–Access Road

🏃 Bernardo Mountain

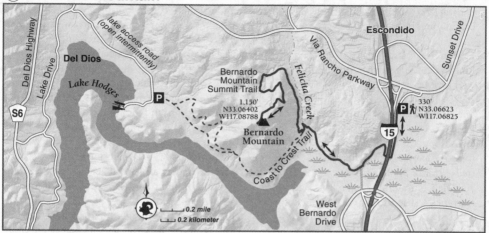

Imagine a hiking, biking, and equestrian trail extending from the coast at Del Mar to the crest of the mountains in central San Diego County. Today, certain sections of this 55-mile-long route, known as the Coast to Crest Trail, are already open. These and other future sections of the trail will define the main axis of the San Dieguito River Park, now taking shape along the watersheds of the San Dieguito River and its main tributary, Santa Ysabel Creek. Many pieces of the proposed park are in place today and open to the public, but fleshing out the entire 60,000 acres of parkland promises to involve much wrangling with landowners and long-term efforts by interested citizens and various local governments.

On this hike you'll travel one of the more accessible and scenic segments of the Coast to Crest Trail, overlooking scenic Lake Hodges, and you'll climb to the summit of Bernardo Mountain, which was purchased in 2002 for inclusion in San Dieguito River Park. Bird lovers will enjoy the diversity of birds that live on and near the lake.

To Reach the Trailhead: Exit I-15 at Via Rancho Parkway (Exit 27), and go east 0.2 mile to the first southbound street on the right, Sunset Drive. Drive to the end of Sunset Drive and park (free).

Description: From the parking area, continue south on the Coast to Crest Trail, initially a concrete path paralleling the freeway. In 0.4 mile, the path turns sharply right and passes under the I-15 bridge that goes over the east arm of Lake Hodges. Depending on the amount of rainfall over the past year or two, the lake (a San Diego city reservoir) could be brimming with water at this spot or be completely dry, as it has been during recent droughts.

After swinging north on the far (west) side of the freeway, the Coast to Crest Trail for a short time joins the crumbling pavement of the long-abandoned Highway 395, the former inland highway running north from San Diego into Riverside County and beyond. Soon, however, the pavement disappears, and you're on a dirt trail following the shoreline west. Pass the David Kreitzer Lake Hodges bridge, the world's longest stress-ribbon structure, completed in 2009. Take a short detour onto the bridge for fine views of the lake and mountain.

At 1.5 miles from the start, you cross Felicita Creek, a small perennial brook deeply shaded by oaks, sycamores, palms, and other water-loving vegetation. Rise out of the creek and ascend moderately, wrapping around the broad flank of Bernardo Mountain. The sunny slope on the right hosts an eye-popping assortment of wildflowers from March through May. On the left, look for snowy egrets parasailing over the wind-rippled surface of the lake. Overhead, hawks and ravens can often be seen patrolling the afternoon skies, riding on thermals. Ospreys and golden eagles have been seen in this area as well—not to mention

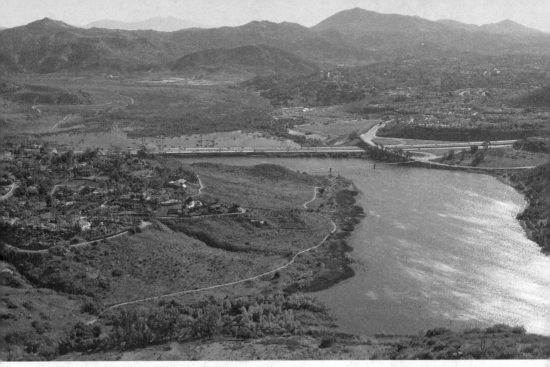

Lake Hodges from Bernardo Mountain

small and circumspect California gnatcatchers, which are classified as an endangered species.

At 1.7 miles, a few minutes past the creek crossing, make a very sharp right turn on the Bernardo Mountain Summit Trail, heading north. You ascend slowly, with the oaks and sycamores of Felicita Creek just below you on the right and Bernardo Mountain rising on the left. By about 2.5 miles, you've swung around to the north side of the mountain. This area was burned bare by wildfire in October 2007, but the chaparral is rapidly regenerating as it has evolved to do. As the ascent quickens, stay left (uphill) at the next two trail intersections. Note the poorly marked junctions carefully so that you take the correct trail on your return.

You continue either rising or contouring in a zigzag pattern, passing a large water tank at 3.2 miles and finally reaching the rocky summit at 3.6 miles. From this lofty vantage point you can clearly see the patchwork of urban, suburban, and wildland that inland north San Diego County has become. The white noise of traffic on I-15 wafts upward to you, but peering in certain other directions you see little apparent human impact on the landscape. Westward, down the valley below Lake Hodges, a slice of Pacific Ocean is visible on clear days.

HIKE 81   Cowles Mountain

Location	Mission Trails Regional Park
Highlight	Best view of urban San Diego County
Distance & Configuration	2.8-mile out-and-back
Elevation Gain	950'
Hiking Time	2 hours
Optional Map	Mission Trails Regional Park brochure (mtrp.org)
Best Times	All year
Agency	Mission Trails Regional Park

Difficulty Moderate
Trail Use Good for kids, dogs allowed
Permit None required
Google Maps Cowles Mountain Trailhead, Golfcrest Drive

Touted as one of the largest urban parks in the country, Mission Trails Regional Park, in San Diego's San Carlos district, preserves some of the last remaining open space close to the heart of this sprawling city. Cowles Mountain, centerpiece of the park, stands 1,591 feet above sea level and is recognized as the highest point within San Diego's city limits. Hundreds of people walk the main south trail to its summit daily. Hikers can choose from among several summit routes. We describe the ever-popular south route, which consistently offers vistas stretching from the Pacific Ocean to Mexico.

To Reach the Trailhead: Exit I-8 at College Avenue (Exit 10), go north 1.3 miles, and turn right (east) on Navajo Road. Continue 2 miles to the Cowles Mountain Trailhead (which has a parking lot and restrooms) on the northeast corner of Navajo Road and Golfcrest Drive. The lot is often full; additional parking is available along Golfcrest Drive.

Description: From the trailhead, you ascend steadily, zigzagging almost constantly up through low-growing chaparral punctuated by outcrops

of granitic rock. Because the trail was cut into decomposed granite, it is quite susceptible to erosion. Don't shortcut the switchbacks, tempting as it may be, as this tramples plants and tends to destabilize the trail.

Nearly 1 mile up, a spur trail branches right toward a flat spot on the mountain's south shoulder. This site of ancient winter-solstice ceremonies by the ancestral Kumeyaay Indians has become a popular place to visit at dawn on or near the solstice (usually December 21). If you view it from the right spot, the sun's disk, just peeping over the mountains to the east, gets momentarily split into two brilliant points of light by a large outcrop atop a distant ridge.

Just beyond the spur trail, another trail branches right and eventually descends the east slope. Stay left and continue up the slope on the series of long switchbacks leading to the rocky summit. A cluster of antennas somewhat obstructs the northward view, but otherwise the panorama is complete. With binoculars and the help of a large interpretive panel that identifies nearby and distant landmarks, you could spend a lot of time getting to know the region. In the rift between the mesas to the west,

☻ Cowles Mountain

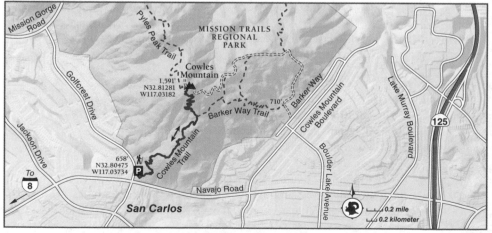

there's a good view of Mission Valley and the tangle of freeways that pass over and through it. Southwest, the towers of downtown San Diego stand against Point Loma, Coronado, and sparkling San Diego Bay. Lake Murray shimmers to the south. The chain of Santee Lakes contrasts darkly with pale hills to the north. In all directions, you look out over the abodes of the nearly 5 million people now living in the combined metropolis of San Diego and Tijuana.

On the clearest days, the higher peaks of San Diego County stand in bold relief against the sky. Southward into Baja, you should spot the flat-topped Table Mountain behind Tijuana and the Coronado Islands offshore. Try looking for the dusky profiles of Santa Catalina and San Clemente Islands to the northwest and west, respectively.

Here's a suggestion for romantics and adventurers who don't mind descending the trail by flashlight: Catch the sunset from Cowles' summit when the moon is full. After the sun slides into the Pacific, turn around and enjoy the moonrise over the El Cajon valley!

HIKE 82   Woodson Mountain

Location	Poway–Ramona
Highlights	Giant boulders, superb views
Distance & Configuration	7-mile out-and-back
Elevation Gain	2,000'
Hiking Time	4 hours
Optional Map	poway.org/502/trails-hiking
Best Times	October–June
Agency	Lake Poway Recreation Area
Difficulty	Moderate
Trail Use	Dogs allowed, suitable for mountain biking
Permit	Parking fee
Google Maps	Mount Woodson Trailhead

The native Kumeyaay people called it Mountain of Moonlit Rocks, an appropriate name for a landmark visible over great distances, even at night. Early white settlers dubbed it Cobbleback Peak, a name utterly descriptive of its rugged, boulder-strewn slopes. For the past 100 years, however, it has appeared on maps simply as Woodson Mountain, in honor of a Dr. Woodson who homesteaded some property nearby well over a century ago.

The light-colored bedrock of Woodson Mountain and several of its neighboring peaks in the Poway–Ramona area is a type geologists call Woodson Mountain granodiorite. When exposed at the surface, it weathers into huge spherical or ellipsoidal boulders with smooth surfaces. The largest boulders have a tendency to cleave apart along remarkably flat planes, forming "chimneys" from several inches to

several feet wide. Sometimes, one half of a split boulder will roll away, leaving a vertical and almost seamless face behind. It's no wonder that Woodson Mountain (or Mount Woodson, as it is popularly called) is regarded as one of the finest places to practice the craft of bouldering in Southern California.

The most unforgettable rock formation on the mountain is an enormous thin flake, cantilevered over a big drop. This Potato Chip Rock has become a major tourist attraction in the San Diego area. On a busy weekend, you might have a 2-hour wait behind a crowd waiting to take social-media profile pictures on the rock, so go early on a cool morning if you have the choice.

Woodson can be approached from the east via a loop on a service road and the Fry-Koegel Trail, or from the west via Lake Poway. This trip

🜂 Woodson Mountain

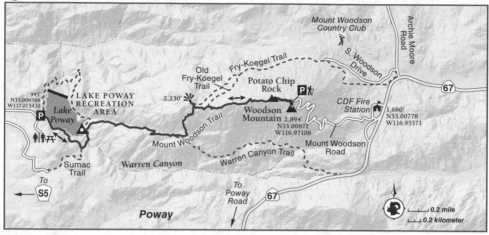

describes the Lake Poway approach, which is the most scenic option.

To Reach the Trailhead: From I-15, take Exit 24 east on Rancho Bernardo Road, which eventually becomes Espola Road and then veers right. In 4.0 miles, turn left onto Lake Poway Road. Drive past the entrance station (fee for nonresidents on weekends and holidays), and park at the end near the concession building.

Description: The signed start of the Lake Poway Trail is on the left side of the concession building, but it's better to start on the

right side and pick up a footpath circling the lake counterclockwise. At 0.6 mile, pass a sign for the Sumac Trail, and then at 0.8 mile, reach a four-way junction on the east side of Lake Poway. A short trail on the left leads to a picnic bench and excellent viewpoint over the lake. Straight ahead, the Lake Poway Trail circles the north side of the lake, a longer (1.9 miles) and less attractive return option. Your trip turns right onto the Mount Woodson Trail, which begins an unrelenting ascent of the chaparral-covered slopes.

At 1.8 miles, pass the Warren Canyon Cutoff Trail on the right, a little-used undulating trail

Potato Chip Rock

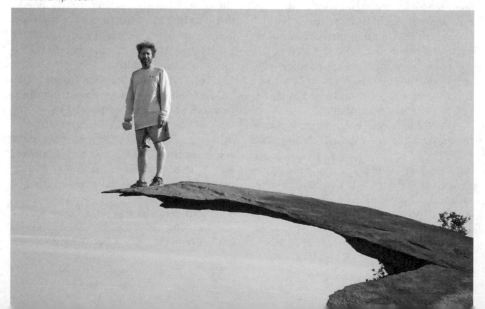

leading to Highway 67. At 2.4 miles, reach the Fry-Koegel Trail on the left, which also leads to Highway 67. A sign here indicates a 100-yard spur trail to a brushy hilltop offering the best panoramic views of the entire trip. Soon after, you'll see a post marking the Old Fry-Koegel Trail, which soon joins the main Fry-Koegel. The rock formations become larger and more interesting, including The Ogre, a 30-foot over-hanging monster with a challenging off-width crack considered a local testpiece.

At 3.4 miles, reach the unmistakable Potato Chip Rock on the left, the result of exfoliation and weathering. From the right camera angle,

you can get a dramatic photo of your friend standing on what appears to be a horrifyingly thin flake. Shortly thereafter, reach a paved ser-vice road leading through an antenna farm to the highest point on the mountain (3.6 miles). Unless you want a high dose of radio frequency radiation, it's best to retreat from the summit before taking a long snack break.

VARIATION

You could also take the service road 1.7 miles down the east side, eventually joining a trail that emerges on Highway 67 by the Ramona Fire Station.

HIKE 83 Iron Mountain

Location	Near Poway
Highlights	Panoramic views
Distance & Configuration	6-mile out-and-back
Elevation Gain	1,200'
Hiking Time	3 hours
Optional Map	poway.org/502/Trails-Hiking
Best Times	October–June
Agency	Lake Poway Recreation Area
Difficulty	Moderate
Trail Use	Good for kids, dogs allowed, suitable for mountain biking
Permit	None required
Google Maps	Iron Mountain Trailhead

North San Diego County's Iron Mountain thrusts its conical summit nearly 2,700 feet above sea level, frequently well above the low-lying coastal haze. On many a crystalline winter day, the summit offers a sweeping, 360-degree panorama from glistening ocean to blue moun-tains and back to the ocean again. Access to the summit—by foot, horse, or mountain bike—is now afforded by a key link in the city of Poway's ever-expanding multiuse trail system. Expect to have plenty of company on this extremely popular trail. Parking fills early on weekends.

To Reach the Trailhead: The large and popu-lar Iron Mountain Trailhead is located at the intersection of Highway 67 and Poway Road at mile marker 67 SD 15.00, 8.7 miles east of

I 15 by way of Poway Road or 15.0 miles north of I-8 by way of Highway 67. There's a second-ary trailhead on Ellie Lane, 0.7 mile north on Highway 67 from the main trailhead, in case you want to try the extended route noted at the end of the description.

Description: From the main trailhead, the shortest way up the mountain (3 miles one-way) takes you along signed pathways. Thick stands of chaparral along the trail burned in 1995 and again in the 2003 Cedar Fire but are adapted to periodic fire and have fully regen-erated. Pass a four-way junction with paths leading left to Ellie Lane and right to loop and rejoin the main Iron Mountain Trail. At 1.0 mile, where the trail briefly veers north on the

Iron Mountain

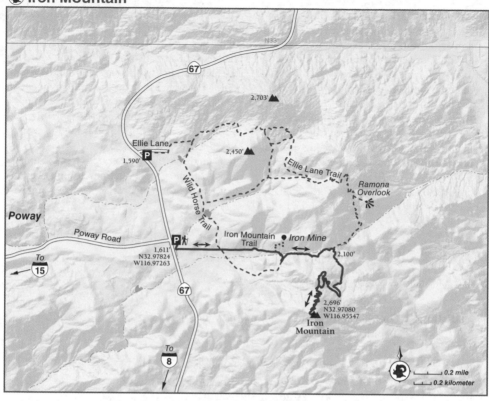

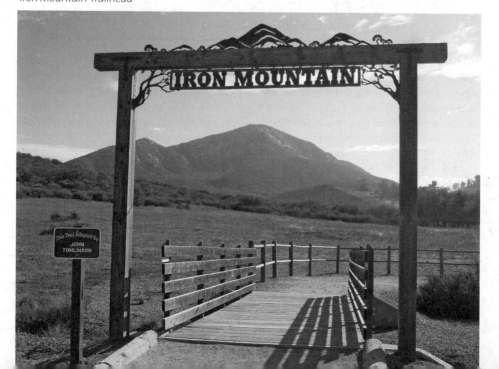

Iron Mountain Trailhead

side of a hill, look up for some gray rock out-crops. Iron was once extracted from a small pit mine up the hill, giving the nearby mountain its name.

You soon commence a steeper ascent. At 1.4 miles you reach a trail junction in a saddle, where you turn right to head for Iron Mountain's summit, 1.5 meandering trail miles away. Numerous switchbacks on the trail's final half mile take you back and forth across the ever-narrowing summit cone. On the summit you'll find a massive, pier-mounted free telescope thoughtfully provided for the purpose of scanning the near and far horizons.

VARIATION

If you don't want to retrace your steps, you can opt for a more challenging traverse over hill and dale to the north. The northern loop, which passes Table Rock and two old cattle ponds, adds 3 additional miles to the round-trip and involves several severe up-and-down pitches. You could also emerge at the Ellie Lane Trailhead, 0.7 mile north of the main trailhead.

HIKE 84   El Capitan County Preserve

Location	Near Lakeside
Highlights	Frequent vistas of coastal lowlands and ocean
Distance & Configuration	12-mile out-and-back
Elevation Gain	4,000'
Hiking Time	8 hours
Optional Maps	USGS 7.5-minute *San Vicente Reservoir* and *El Cajon Mtn.*
Best Times	November–April, 8 a.m.–sunset
Agency	County of San Diego Department of Parks and Recreation
Difficulty	Strenuous
Trail Use	Suitable for mountain biking, dogs allowed
Permit	None required
Google Maps	El Cajon Mountain Trailhead Parking

As you walk along the granite-ribbed ridgeline, down the middle of the El Capitan County Preserve, a binational panorama of ocean, islands, and innumerable mountain peaks lies in view. The broad San Diego River valley below curves beneath the sheer south face of El Cajon Mountain, informally known as El Capitan. This 2,800-acre preserve was pieced together out of former Bureau of Land Management (BLM) lands adjacent to the Cleveland National Forest. If you have the determination to tackle some really severe uphills and downhills and get the benefit of a serious cardiovascular workout, try following the preserve's main route, an old, sometimes precariously steep road bulldozed by miners years ago. It twists and turns over a scrubby, boulder-punctuated landscape that in spring comes alive with a blue frosting of ceanothus (wild lilac) blossoms. Parts of this mining road are gradually being bypassed or improved and incorporated into the fledgling Trans-County Trail—a major multiuse pathway that will stretch east–west across San Diego County from Del Mar on the coast to Borrego Springs in the desert. Its ups and downs and lack of abundant shade make this hike surprisingly difficult. Many hikers underestimate the amount of drinking water they will need. Bring at least 3 quarts on a cool winter day and more when it's hot. The trails close at sunset, necessitating a reasonably early start and a steady pace.

To Reach the Trailhead: From I-8, take Highway 67 north 5.8 miles, then turn east on Mapleview Street where the freeway portion of the highway ends. In 0.3 mile turn left (north) on Ashwood Street. Ashwood soon becomes Wildcat Canyon Road. Proceed north on it a total of 4.4 miles to a signed parking lot for the preserve on the right. (You can use the green

🦌 El Capitan County Preserve

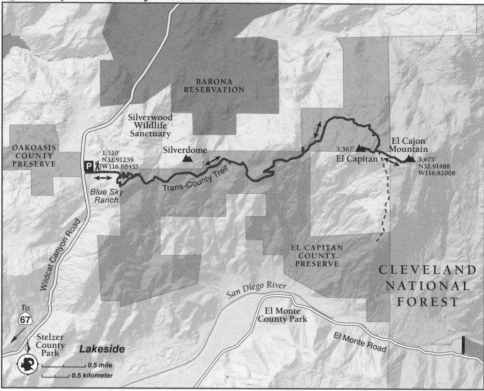

mile markers by the roadside as your guide; slow down after mile marker 4.0.)

Description: From the lot, walk east 0.4 mile on the entry road to the private Blue Sky Ranch, and pass the ranch to reach a trailhead with a large outhouse. The dirt road continues to the south, but it is more scenic to pick up the narrow trail, which starts a steep, zigzagging ascent up a cool, north-facing slope. You soon rejoin the old mining road, and the going gets easier for a while. (*Note:* These directions may change once a planned bypass trail is completed between the trailhead and the old mining road. You may observe a variety of side roads and trails, but stay on the main road all the way.)

As you reach a small summit (about 1.2 miles from the start) and start descending on the old mining road, the round top and sheer south brow of El Cajon Mountain (El Capitan) become visible in the middle distance. A

very steep uphill pitch, commencing at about 3 miles, will surely reduce you to painfully slow uphill scrambling, if only for a few minutes. At a little less than 4 miles, you reach another significant summit. From this spot, a short side road leads north to some abandoned mines, shallow tunnels cut into a chalky hillside.

Similar to Sisyphus' struggle, your elevation gain is tragically interrupted just ahead. You sink 300 feet in less than half a mile on slippery, decomposing granite and then resume your uphill progress. At 4.7 miles there's a rock-lined spring on the left, either brimming with iron-rich, nonpotable water or possibly dry. At 5.5 miles, the road arrives on a saddle between El Cajon Mountain's summit on the left (east) and a smaller 3,367-foot peak on the right (west).

Turn left and follow a narrow path that threads 0.5 mile through thick chaparral and around jumbo-size granitic boulders to El Cajon Mountain's summit. (The route is slated to be improved and incorporated into the San Diego Sea to Sea Trail.) Although the summit is rounded and clogged with boulders, the view is panoramic in all directions. On a clear day, as your gaze turns counterclockwise, you will be able to see San Jacinto, Palomar Mountain, Mount Baldy, Santiago Peak, Woodson Mountain, Iron Mountain, Black Mountain, Catalina and San Clemente Islands, Miramar Airfield, downtown San Diego and Point Loma, peaks of northern Baja, the El Capitan reservoir, and the Cuyamaca and Laguna Mountains.

Return to the saddle. Most hikers are satisfied at this point and return the way they came. If you are feeling energetic, however, you have two more options to explore. By turning right (west) and walking 0.2 mile, you reach a 3,367-foot summit, with evident remnants of a radio antenna installation. This rocky peaklet offers a nice panoramic view west and south.

The most difficult alternative is a 1.4-mile trek straight ahead (south) from the saddle, using a severely eroded and partially overgrown roadbed. This route takes you to the sheer brow of El Capitan. Walk out to the edge, beyond the end of the old roadbed, and descend over boulders 50 or 100 yards for a pseudoaerial view of the San Diego River valley and El Capitan Reservoir, complete with toylike boats floating on its blue surface.

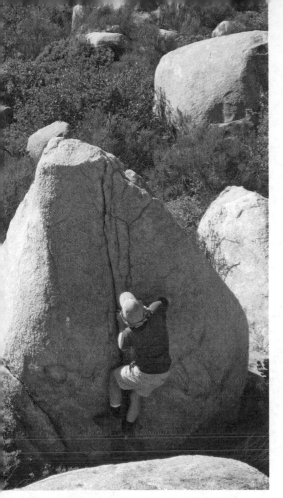

Working a boulder problem on El Cajon

HIKE 85   Doane Valley

Location	Palomar Mountain State Park
Highlights	Verdant meadows, bubbling streams
Distance & Configuration	3.3-mile loop
Elevation Gain	300'
Hiking Time	1.5 hours
Optional Map	Palomar Mountain State Park brochure (parks.ca.gov/?page_id=637)
Best Times	All year, 6 a.m.–sunset
Agency	Palomar Mountain State Park
Difficulty	Moderate
Trail Use	Good for kids
Permit	State park fee
Google Maps	Palomar Mountain State Park

Doane Valley

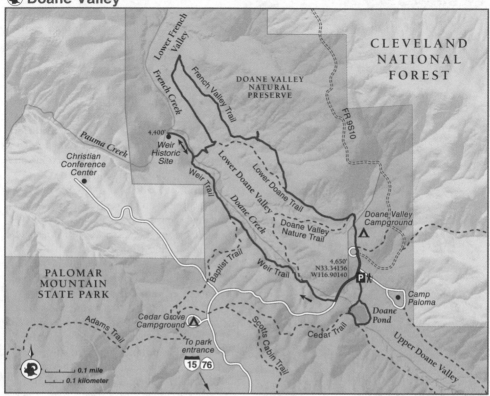

This is a hike for inspiration. Here, at Palomar Mountain State Park, you'll find some of Southern California's finest montane scenery, complete with trickling streams; rolling meadows; and mixed forests of pine, cedar, and oak. The long, stomach-churning drive up the mountain's slopes is well worth the trouble once you get out of the car and start breathing in Palomar's sweet, tangy air.

Palomar Mountain is wonderful in every season. In summer, the mountain air and shady trails offer a respite from the heat of the valley. In fall, the black oaks turn brilliant gold before shedding their leaves. In the winter, a dusting of snow can turn the mountain into a winter wonderland. And in spring, the creeks run strong, and the flowers and new buds emerge.

To Reach the Trailhead: Palomar Mountain State Park lies in far-north San Diego County, about 20 miles east of I-15. From most parts

of San Diego County, it's fastest to use County Route S6 (Valley Center Road), which heads north from Escondido, to reach a T-intersection with Highway 76 near the foot of Palomar Mountain. Turn right (east) onto Highway 76 and continue about 5 miles to mile marker 76 SD 38.00, where you turn left back onto S6. Upon reaching the crest in 6.9 miles, turn left and immediately left again onto County Route S7, which becomes State Park Road. After paying your day-use or camping fee at the park entrance in 3.0 miles, continue 1.7 miles farther to the Doane Pond parking area at the end of the road, following signs for School Camp and staying right at all junctions. A restroom is available a few yards down the Cedar Trail.

Description: You begin your hike at the signed Doane Valley Nature Trail in the corner of the parking area. The trail leads across the road and downstream along Doane Creek. Along

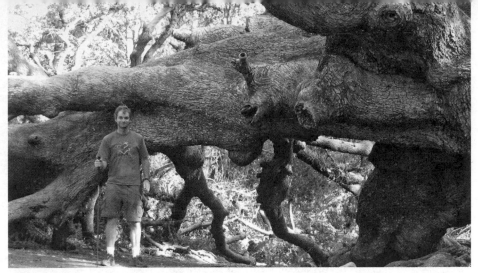

A massive live oak that toppled in 2009 at the age of about 1,000 years

the bank grow box elder trees, creek dogwood, wild strawberry, mountain currant, and Sierra gooseberry. You pass a massive incense-cedar tree towering more than 100 feet high. If you weren't informed of its true identity, you might think it was a giant sequoia.

After 0.3 mile, the nature trail curves and climbs around a hill to connect with Doane Valley Campground. At a trail junction here, bear left on the Weir Trail, following Doane Creek through stately groves of white fir and incense-cedar. Walk all the way down to the weir at the end of the trail, and admire the stone-and-mortar structure above it. This small dam and gauging station were built in 1926 to test the stream's hydroelectric potential. The tests proved there was not enough flow to justify construction of a power plant. Today, the silted-in dam holds barely enough water to soak your feet in. Some years ago, park rangers were surprised to discover banana slugs (like those in California's central and northern Coast Ranges) in this drainage.

From the weir, backtrack 0.2 mile and take the Lower Doane Trail left across the valley to the French Valley Trail. Go left (north), passing into Lower French Valley. The setting is idyllic: rolling grasslands dotted with statuesque ponderosa pines and surrounded by hillsides clothed in oaks and tall conifers. The 2007 Poomacha Fire whipped across the park and cleared out the underbrush but left most of the mature trees intact. Land managers are coming to recognize

that wildfire serves an essential natural role in the ecosystem and that decades of aggressive fire suppression have disrupted this role.

Several of the pine trees are riddled with holes, some of which are plugged with acorns. This is the handiwork of the acorn woodpecker, which uses the holes to store acorns filled with larvae. The birds retrieve these acorns and the grubs in leaner times. Listen for this woodpecker's repetitive, guttural call, and observe the distinctive red patch on its head and its white wing patch when it's in flight.

The trail abruptly turns sharply right and leads back above the meadow. Hike as far as the bank of French Creek, and then head back toward your starting point along the upper part of the French Valley Trail. A shady glade beneath a grove of enormous live oaks invites you to rest your feet and contemplate the majestic trees. Beyond, you walk beneath the trunk of a massive live oak. Until this tree toppled in 2009 at the age of about 1,000 years, it was the largest oak in San Diego County. Join Lower Doane Trail, pass a junction with the Nature Trail, arrive at Doane Valley Campground, and then turn right and walk through the campground to the parking lot where you began.

VARIATIONS

Doane Pond is located south of the parking area and is well worth the quarter-mile stroll. If you have more time to enjoy the park, there are many more miles of scenic trails.

HIKE 86   Eagle Rock

Location	Near Warner Springs
Highlight	Unusual rock formation
Distance & Configuration	6-mile out-and-back
Elevation Gain	700'
Hiking Time	3 hours
Optional Map	Tom Harrison *San Diego Backcountry*
Best Times	October–June
Agency	Vista Irrigation District (grants an easement but does not field questions from hikers)
Difficulty	Moderate
Trail Use	Good for kids, dogs allowed
Permit	None required
Google Maps	Eagle Rock Trailhead

Eagle Rock, perched on a hill overlooking Warner Springs Ranch, bears a stunning likeness to its namesake raptor. In April, the surrounding meadows explode with wildflowers. A walk along the oak-lined banks of Cañada Verde Creek caps off this magnificent hike.

To Reach the Trailhead: From I-15, take Exit 58, and follow Highway 79 east for 38.6 miles to the south end of Warner Springs. Park in a turnout across from the California Department of Forestry fire station, 0.3 mile south of mile marker 79 SD 34.50.

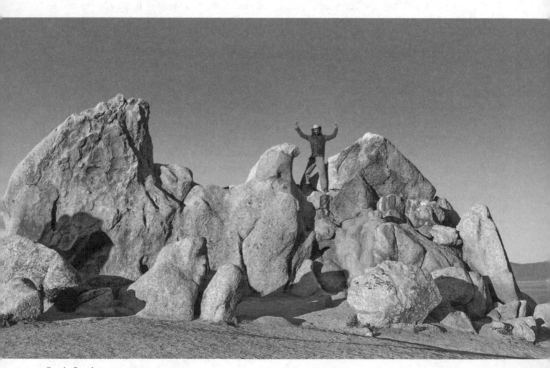

Eagle Rock   Benjamin Harris

🦅 Eagle Rock

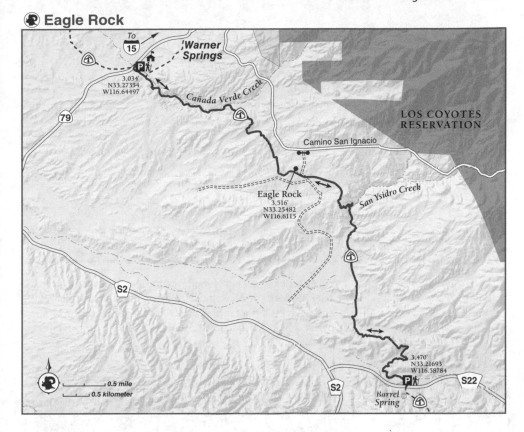

If you wish to make a one-way trip with a shuttle (see variation), drop your second vehicle at the Pacific Crest Trail's Barrel Spring Trailhead: Continue south on Highway 79 for 2.5 miles to turn left onto San Felipe Road (County Route S2). In 4.7 miles, turn left onto Montezuma Valley Road (County Route S22). In 1.0 mile, park at the Barrel Spring Trailhead in a large dirt lot on the right, near a Pacific Crest Trail (PCT) sign.

Description: Cross to the southeast side of the highway, and pass through a gate at a sign for the PCT. Cross Cañada Verde ("green ravine") Creek, and pass through a second gate. The California Riding and Hiking Trail veers left toward Warner Springs, but your trip continues straight on the PCT.

In 0.1 mile, pass a third gate, and hike up the oak-lined canyon. At 1.2 miles, the trail departs the canyon and veers south across rangeland. At 3.0 miles, reach a cluster of granite rocks. A trail curves around to the back side, where Eagle Rock is clearly recognizable.

VARIATION

If you set up a car or bicycle shuttle, you could continue on the PCT another 5 miles to its intersection with County Route S22 at Barrel Spring. In the springtime, San Ysidro Creek flows through a scenic canyon and delightful wildflowers carpet the meadows.

HIKE 87   Cedar Creek Falls

Location	Near Ramona
Highlights	Beautiful cascade and punchbowl
Distance & Configuration	6-mile out-and-back
Elevation Gain	1,100'
Hiking Time	3 hours
Optional Maps	USGS 7.5-minute *El Cajon Mountain* and *Tule Springs*
Best Times	November–June
Agency	Cleveland National Forest/Palomar Ranger District
Difficulty	Moderate
Trail Use	Good for kids, dogs allowed
Permit	Day-use permit required; reserve at recreation.gov
Google Maps	Cedar Creek Falls Trailhead, Thornbush Road

The San Diego River and its upper tributaries drain the pastoral valleys and forested hillsides around Julian and the rugged western slopes of the Cuyamaca Mountains. The water flows generally southwest through V-shaped canyons and eventually reaches El Capitan Reservoir, not far from San Diego's eastern suburbs. Quite frequently the water encounters resistant layers

Cedar Creek Falls

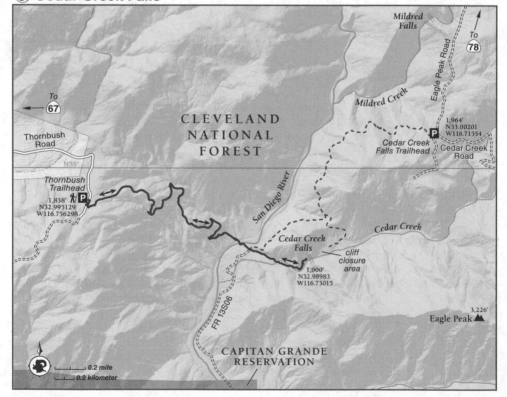

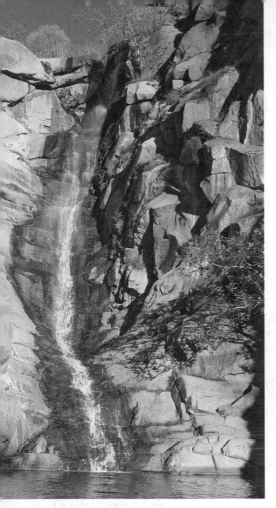

Cedar Creek Falls

in the underlying igneous and metamorphic rocks. In several places it tumbles over cataracts up to 100 feet high. The grinding of stones trapped in pockets below these falls has created deep pools, or punchbowls. Cedar Creek Falls, along with its punchbowl, is one of the more attractive and accessible of these wonders.

Before the construction of El Capitan Dam in the early 1930s, the falls were a popular destination for Sunday outings and could be reached relatively easily on a road up the San Diego River Valley from Lakeside. Now, the drive to the Cedar Creek Falls trailhead, which is more circuitous but scenic nonetheless.

This seemingly innocuous trail holds the dubious distinction of requiring more rescues and body removals than any other in San Diego

County. It is dry and shadeless until Cedar Creek and can be extremely hot, resulting in regular incidents of heatstroke. Many dogs have died on the trail as well. Wear appropriate clothing and a wide-brimmed hat; bring more water than you think you'll need; and, if it is hot, leave your pet behind. Go in the winter or spring; avoid this trail on days warmer than 90°F. Several visitors have fallen to their death from the slippery cliffs above the falls, including a teenager in 2011. The falls also developed a reputation as a party spot, and thoughtless visitors trashed the canyon.

Because of these factors, the falls were temporarily closed in 2011–12 and are now open with a strict permit system. You must reserve your permit through recreation.gov for a modest fee, carry a printed copy, and sign in at the trailhead. There is a quota on permits that usually fills up in advance, so plan ahead. Alcohol is prohibited, and you must stay on the trail. The area is habitat for the endangered arroyo toad and California gnatcatcher, so protect these species by staying on the trail and taking care not to leave any trash. Violators face hefty fines.

To Reach the Trailhead: Most visitors now approach from Thornbush Road in Ramona. From Highway 67 in Lakeview, turn east on Mapleview Street. In 0.3 mile, turn left on Ashwood Street, which becomes Wildcat Canyon Road. In 13.2 miles, turn right on San Vicente Road, and go 2.6 miles to turn left on Ramona Oaks Road. In 2.9 miles, turn right on Thornbush Road, and follow it 0.4 mile to the trailhead. The small lot fills early, so you will likely need to park on the road; be sure not to obstruct the residents of the neighborhood below.

Description: Sign in with your permit number at the trailhead and top off your water at the spigot. The rather unremarkable trail leads along slopes covered in chamise chaparral with California sagebrush, laurel sumac, Mission manzanita, occasional yucca and cactus, and spring wildflowers. In 0.5 mile, views of the San Diego River Gorge open up as you round a bend. Well-graded switchbacks lead you down to the river crossing (2.5 miles). At a junction on the far side, take the signed trail to Cedar

Creek Falls, which crosses the creek twice before reaching the spectacular punchbowl at the falls.

You can picnic on the rocks and swim in the pool at the base of the falls, but remember to save some energy for the uphill return hike.

VARIATION

The falls can also be reached from the northeast with about the same hiking distance and elevation change but a much longer drive from San Diego. From the town of Julian, drive west 1 mile on combined Highway 78/79. Near mile marker 78 SD 57.0, turn south on Pine Hills Road. After 1.5 miles, bear right on Eagle Peak Road. In another 1.4 miles, pass Boulder Creek Road on the left and continue 8.2 miles on a dirt road to an intersection called Saddleback.

This is the trailhead for an abandoned road now called the Cedar Creek Falls Hiking and Equestrian Trail. Descend the road 2.3 miles to the aforementioned junction by the San Diego River, then turn left to the falls.

HIKE 88   Three Sisters Falls

Location	North of Descanso
Highlights	Three-tiered waterfall
Distance & Configuration	4-mile out-and-back
Elevation Gain	1,000'
Hiking Time	2.5 hours
Optional Maps	USGS 7.5-minute *Tule Springs*
Best Times	November–June
Agency	Cleveland National Forest/Palomar Ranger District
Difficulty	Moderate
Trail Use	Good for kids, dogs allowed
Permit	None required
Google Maps	Three Sisters Falls Trailhead, Boulder Creek Road

Little known until recently, Three Sisters Falls became popular after the temporary closure of nearby Cedar Creek Falls. The U.S. Forest Service built a proper trail and established trailhead parking in 2018, and now this remote but stunning hike teems with visitors every weekend.

Even with the improvements, this trail continues to be the site of frequent rescues and occasional deaths of hikers and dogs, particularly on account of near-daily incidents of heatstroke in the warmer months. The trail draws a disproportionate number of inexperienced hikers who neglect to bring enough water. Carry 2 quarts of water on a cool day and more if it will be warm. Avoid this hike if temperatures are forecast to exceed 90°F. Leave your dog at home unless it has plenty of experience on rocky backcountry trails. Remember that the return hike is all uphill and shadeless.

To Reach the Trailhead: From I-8 at Descanso, take Highway 79 north. In 1.3 miles, turn left on Riverside Drive. In 0.6 mile at the complex main intersection of Descanso, veer left onto Oak Grove Drive. Go 1.6 miles and then turn right onto Boulder Creek Road. Follow this road, initially paved and soon graded dirt, 13 miles to the obvious trailhead parking area. Unless the road has deteriorated, it is normally passable by carefully driven low-clearance vehicles.

Description: From the parking area, hike west on a former ranching road, now a trail, toward Eagle Peak. At 0.6 mile, reach a post on a saddle where you get your first view of the waterfalls. The Eagle Peak Trail continues west, but Three Sisters hikers turn left and circle the Sheep Camp Creek valley. Traverse a tunnel-like section beneath arching chaparral before

🅟 Three Sisters Falls

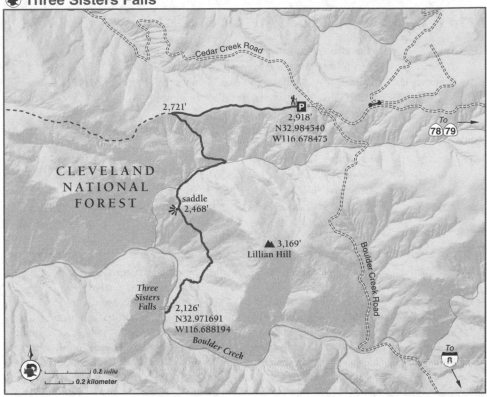

Cedar Creek Road

2,721'

2,918'
N32.984540
W116.678475

P

To
78 79

CLEVELAND
NATIONAL
FOREST

saddle
2,468'

▲ 3,169'
Lillian Hill

Boulder Creek Road

*Three
Sisters
Falls*

2,126'
N32.971691
W116.688194

Boulder Creek

To
8

0.2 mile
0.2 kilometer

reaching a saddle at 1.2 miles. This spot is a great place to take a break and enjoy the best views of the waterfalls.

The newly constructed trail then descends into Boulder Creek Canyon. The last stretch is rocky. Reach a gorgeous pool at the base of the middle waterfall. If the rock is dry, picking a path down to the lower waterfall is usually straightforward. Reaching the upper waterfall involves exposed scrambling. Exercise good judgment to stay safe while enjoying the cascade.

VARIATION

You can add 3 miles round-trip and another 1,000 feet of elevation gain by making a side trip to Eagle Peak on your return. The summit has terrific views from atop a dramatic cliff. Be aware that the Forest Service sometimes closes the peak to protect raptor nesting sites; look for signs, or check the Forest Service website (www.fs.fed.us/r5/cleveland) before you go.

Three Sisters Falls

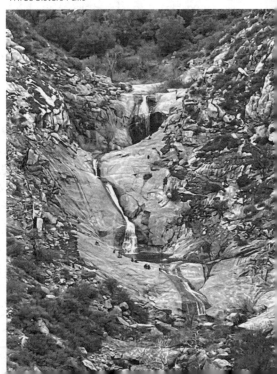

HIKE 89   Volcan Mountain

Location	Near Julian
Highlights	Pastoral mountain landscapes
Distance & Configuration	3.2 miles to gate or 5.0 miles to summit (out-and-back)
Elevation Gain	900' (to gate) or 1,300' (to summit)
Hiking Time	2–2.5 hours
Optional Map	sdparks.org/content/sdparks/en/park-pages /VolcanMountain.html
Best Times	October–June
Agency	County of San Diego Parks and Recreation
Difficulty	Moderate
Trail Use	Good for kids, dogs allowed, suitable for mountain biking
Permit	None required
Google Maps	Volcan Mountain Trailhead

Rising boldly above the apple orchards outside Julian, Volcan Mountain's oak- and pine-dotted slopes are swept by some of the freshest breezes found anywhere. Soughing through the trees like waves spending themselves against a sandy beach, these gusts bear the astringent dryness of the nearby desert, as well as the volatile scents of pine needles and sun-baked grass.

Named by early Spanish-speaking travelers for its dubious resemblance to a volcano, Volcan Mountain (called the Volcan Mountains on topographic maps) is really a fault-block mountain, like many others in the Peninsular Ranges. The Elsinore and Earthquake Valley Faults bracket the mountain on its southwest and northeast sides, respectively.

Off-limits to public use for the past century, Volcan Mountain is gradually falling into the public domain today. As funding becomes available, San Diego County and the San Dieguito River Park Joint Powers Authority are purchasing privately owned land on the mountain. One such parcel, Volcan Mountain Wilderness Preserve—has already become an unsung crown jewel in the county parks system.

To Reach the Trailhead: From the center of Julian (on Highway 78/79, 50 miles northeast

🅟 Volcan Mountain

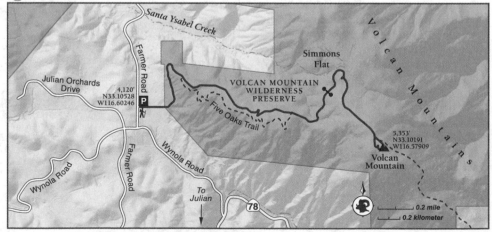

of San Diego), drive 2.3 miles north on Main Street (which soon becomes Farmer Road) to Wynola Road. Jog right briefly, and then go left on the continuation of Farmer Road. Just ahead, on the right, a wooden sign announces the preserve. Park alongside Farmer Road.

Description: From your parked car, walk east on a dirt access road. After 0.2 mile, you come upon a carved entry structure and stonework designed by noted Julian artist James Hubbell. There's also a small, open-air kiva with a compass rose embedded in the floor, used during interpretive programs. The Elsinore Fault, a major splinter of the San Andreas, passes almost directly under this spot.

Just beyond this formal entrance, your wide path leads sharply up a hill overlooking an apple orchard. You soon swing sharply right and continue climbing in earnest along a rounded ridgeline leading toward the Volcan Mountain crest. Along the ridge, wind-rippled expanses of grassland alternate with dense coppices of live oak and black oak. The rust-red bark of the many manzanita shrubs along the way perpetually peels, revealing a green undercoat. Look for the manzanitas (Spanish for "little apples"), the ripe, reddish-brown berries that look and taste a bit like the apples hanging from the trees down in the valley below.

In 0.4 mile, a sign indicates the start of the Five Oaks Trail on the right. This delightful trail, named for the five oaks—black, canyon, coast live, scrub, and poison—found in abundance along its course, is open only to hikers. It is slightly longer, but it offers better views and a more intimate experience and is the recommended route on the way up if you are on foot. It parallels the main path and rejoins it in 1.1 miles.

As you climb higher, the view expands to include parts of Julian, the dusky Cuyamaca Mountains to the south, and—on the clearest days—the blue arc of the Pacific Ocean to the west and southwest.

After 1.5 miles and 900 feet of climbing, reach the Midsummit Gate. The gate may be closed in the winter, making this your turnaround point.

If the gate is open, you can continue up the road. Shortly before reaching the ridgeline, pass through a splendid grove of incense-cedar and live oak. The path veers right upon reaching the ridge. Watch for a stone chimney on the right. This is a remnant of a cabin used from 1928 to 1932 by astronomers who were evaluating sites for the Hale Telescope, which was eventually constructed on Palomar Mountain instead.

The road makes a final climb to a loop on the summit of Volcan Mountain. Atop the mountain are the ruins of an airway beacon built in 1928. Such beacons, spaced about 10 miles apart, were used to light the way for airmail pilots flying at night; the beacons became obsolete with the development of radio navigation aids. On your descent, look for a white tower on a mountaintop to the north; this is a very high frequency omnidirectional radio (VOR) beacon, which became the preferred means of navigation in the 1950s. The Global Positioning System (GPS) is gradually rendering VORs obsolete.

HIKE 90   Cuyamaca Peak

Location	Cuyamaca Rancho State Park
Highlights	Panoramic views and lessons in fire ecology
Distance & Configuration	5.5-mile out-and-back
Elevation Gain	1,650'
Hiking Time	3 hours
Optional Maps	Cuyamaca Rancho State Park map (parks.ca.gov/667) or Tom Harrison *San Diego Backcountry*
Best Times	All year
Agency	Cuyamaca Rancho State Park

Difficulty Moderately strenuous
Trail Use Dogs allowed, suitable for mountain biking
Permit Parking fee
Google Maps Paso Picacho Picnic and Campground

Cuyamaca Peak, San Diego County's second-highest summit after Hot Spring Mountain, lies only a few miles from the county's geographical center. Its unique position and height make it the best land-based vantage point for studying the topography of the southernmost section of California. The 2003 Cedar Fire improved the view from the top by effectively removing most of the trees that used to block the panorama.

The one-lane, paved Lookout Road (called Cuyamaca Peak Fire Road on some maps) is closed to public vehicles but provides a straightforward passage to the top of the peak for self-propelled travelers, including hikers, runners, cyclists, and (rarely) cross-country skiers.

To Reach the Trailhead: You begin this hike at Paso Picacho Campground and Picnic Area on Highway 79, 0.2 mile north of mile marker 79 SD 9.00, about 12 miles north of I-8 near Descanso and about 11 miles south of Julian. Day-use parking is available here for a fee, next to the picnic sites. Walk through the campground to find the Lookout Road Trailhead near the southernmost campsites.

Description: Once you are on Lookout Road, you will find the initial uphill grade to be only moderately steep. The dense pine, fir, cedar, and oak forest that grew on these Cuyamaca slopes before October 2003 was hard-hit by the fire.

After you cross the California Riding and Hiking Trail (1.2 miles), which is called Fern Flat Fire Road to the south and Azalea Spring Fire Road to the north, the paved road gets seriously steep and remains so for most of the remainder of the climb. The widening vista to the north and east includes Cuyamaca Reservoir and several desert mountain ranges. Notice how the aptly named Stonewall Peak to the east

(just across Highway 79) appears to shrink in stature as you continue your climb. In the final steep stretch, you climb past timber snags and suddenly arrive at the antenna-cluttered summit of the peak. A fire-lookout structure stood here until the late 1980s, when it was removed for lack of use.

After the air has been cleared by Santa Ana winds or by major winter storms, Cuyamaca Peak becomes a grandstand seat for views stretching into at least five counties and one foreign state. Features visible within San Diego County include the Palomar Mountains (look for the tiny white speck, the Hale Telescope dome, on the summit ridge), over 30 miles northwest; Hot Springs Mountain, 26 miles almost due north over the summit of nearby Middle Peak; Granite Mountain, 11 miles northeast; the south end of the Santa Rosa Mountains, 40 miles northeast; and Whale Peak and the Vallecito Mountains, 18 miles east/northeast.

Closer in, just 10 or so miles to the southeast, are the wooded Laguna Mountains. South and southwest along the international border are Tecate Peak and Otay Mountain, 25–30 miles away. The Pacific Ocean gleams in the west, with Point Loma, the Silver Strand, San Diego Bay, and Mission Bay visible at distances of about 35–40 miles. Along an arc from west to southwest, you'll spot coastal peaks such as Black Mountain, Soledad Mountain, Fortuna Mountain, Cowles Mountain, Mount Helix, and San Miguel Mountain. Along a west-to-south arc but closer in, you'll see El Cajon Mountain, Viejas Mountain, Lyons Peak, and Corte Madera Mountain.

To enhance your resting time on the peak, bring along binoculars and a map of regional features, such as the Tom Harrison map listed in the key information.

⊕ Cuyamaca Peak

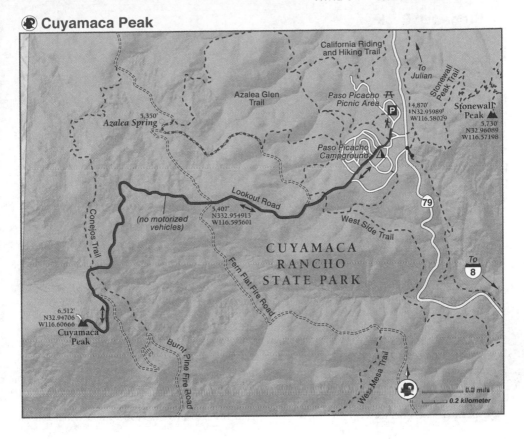

HIKE 91   Stonewall Peak

Location	Cuyamaca Rancho State Park
Highlights	Outstanding summit views
Distance & Configuration	4.5-mile out-and-back
Elevation Gain	850'
Hiking Time	2.5 hours
Optional Maps	Cuyamaca Rancho State Park map (parks.ca.gov/667) or Tom Harrison *San Diego Backcountry*
Best Times	All year
Agency	Cuyamaca Rancho State Park
Difficulty	Moderate
Trail Use	Good for kids
Permit	Parking fee
Google Maps	Stonewall Peak Trailhead

Stonewall Peak

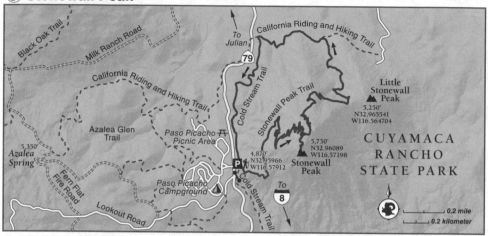

Stonewall Peak's angular summit of white granitic rock is a conspicuous landmark throughout Cuyamaca Rancho State Park. Although Stonewall stands some 800 feet lower than nearby Cuyamaca Peak (see previous hike), its unique position and steep southern exposure provide a more inclusive view of the park area itself. The peak was named for the lucrative Stonewall Jackson mine that William Skidmore established on its northeast slope in 1870.

To Reach the Trailhead: You'll begin this hike at Paso Picacho Campground and Picnic Area on Highway 79, 0.2 mile north of mile marker 79 SD 9.00, about 12 miles north of I-8 near Descanso and about 11 miles south of Julian. Day-use parking is available for a fee next to the picnic sites.

Description: Beginning across the highway from the entrance to Paso Picacho, the trail

Aerial view of Cuyamaca and Stonewall Peaks

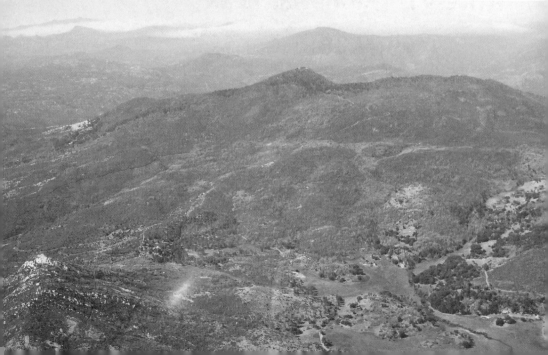

climbs steadily on a set of well-graded switchbacks up the west slope of Stonewall Peak. For many years to come, it will offer a fairly unobstructed view, since the majority of trees that grew here prior to the 2003 Cedar Fire did not survive.

About halfway up the trail, you can gaze down on Cuyamaca Reservoir to the north, its water level and extent varying according to the season and the year's precipitation. When it is full, water covers nearly 1,000 acres.

When you reach the top of the switchbacks, turn right and continue south toward the summit. Soon you arrive at the base of the granite cap that crowns the peak. The trail veers right onto that rock and goes up some rough steps (with a guardrail) to the top. Small children may need assistance on this last airy segment.

The main Cuyamaca massif stands taller in the west, blocking views of the coastline, but the foreground panorama of the park's rolling topography is impressive enough. Patches of meadow along the streamcourses and the bald grassland areas below change color with the seasons: green in spring, yellow in summer, brown or gray in fall, and occasionally white with fallen snow in winter. The recovering forests below will probably appear different from year to year as they mature.

Swallows or swifts may buzz the Stonewall summit like miniature fighter jets, and larger birds, such as ravens, hawks, and even bald eagles, may cruise by. Eagles, along with egrets, herons, and ospreys, are sometimes attracted to the shoreline of nearby Cuyamaca Reservoir, especially in winter.

Descend 0.2 mile to the junction you passed on the way up. The way you came is the shortest way down.

VARIATION

If you would like to make an enjoyable loop that's a mile longer, go straight on a trail that descends to the Los Caballos equestrian camp. Turn left onto the California Riding and Hiking Trail and then left again onto the Cold Stream Trail, which will lead you back to the Stonewall Trailhead.

HIKE 92   Horsethief Canyon

Location	Pine Creek Wilderness
Highlights	Cascades and shallow pools
Distance & Configuration	3.2-mile out-and-back (to Pine Valley Creek)
Elevation Gain	500'
Hiking Time	2 hours
Optional Map	Tom Harrison *San Diego Backcountry* or Cleveland National Forest Visitor Map
Best Times	November–June
Agency	Cleveland National Forest/Descanso Ranger District
Difficulty	Moderate
Trail Use	Good for kids, dogs allowed, suitable for backpacking
Permit	Pine Creek Wilderness permit required to stay overnight
Google Maps	Horsethief Canyon Trailhead

The croak of a raven cracks the stillness as we saunter down the green-fringed path. A groggy dragonfly flits through a beam of morning sunlight. Cool air, slinking down the night-chilled slopes, caresses our faces and sets aflutter the papery sycamore leaves. Approaching the pools and cascades of Pine Valley Creek, we smell the moist exudations of willow trees and mule-fat (a willow look-alike). We cup the clear, cold water in our palms and dash it across our heads.

If you want this kind of escape from the city—and you want it relatively quickly—Pine

📷 Horsethief Canyon

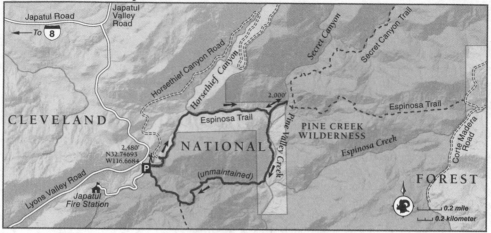

Creek Wilderness, east of San Diego, is a great place to find it. The 13,000-acre wilderness, in the Cleveland National Forest, was created by an act of Congress in 1984 and now includes about 25 miles of hiking trails within its borders. Hiking in this wilderness does not require a permit, though you must obtain one to stay overnight. The quickest and most impressive route into it is by way of Horsethief Canyon.

Average or better winter rains followed by spring sunshine transform the place into a foothill garden, with water dancing down the larger ravines and careening off boulders in Pine Valley Creek, the large drainage bisecting the wilderness. The tough chaparral vegetation coating the slopes gets to looking temporarily soft; the green of emerging annual grasses turns positively lurid; and the live oaks, sycamores, and cottonwoods send out new leaves and branches in a burst of growth.

Pine Creek Wilderness is only a dozen miles from the Mexican border. Migrants and smugglers sometimes pass through the area. The U.S. Forest Service recommends hiking in a group and staying on designated trails.

To Reach the Trailhead: From I-8 at Alpine (Exit 30), follow Tavern Road 2.7 miles south, Japatul Road 7.3 miles east, and Lyons Valley Road 1.5 miles south to the trailhead. The large lot is adjacent to a sign for the Japatul Fire Station. From Jamul, in south San Diego County,

drive east and north, using Skyline Truck Trail and Lyons Valley Road to get to the same point.

Description: From the trailhead parking lot, hike east and then north along a gated dirt road for 0.25 mile. You then veer right down a ravine on the signed Espinosa Trail. After a fast 400-foot elevation loss over 0.5 mile, the path reaches an unsigned junction on the canyon bottom with a side trail leading north into the canyon. Turn right (east) to stay on the main path into the oak- and sycamore-lined Horsethief Canyon, named for the horse thieves who stashed stolen horses in this corral-like cavern in the late 1800s in preparation for their passage across the international border.

The canyon bottom is dry most of the year. In July 2006, 16,000 acres in and around the Pine Creek Wilderness burned in the Horse Fire, which was started by an abandoned campfire. The chaparral has largely recovered, but charred limbs beneath the new growth offer a reminder of the conflagration. In September 2020, the Valley Fire burned another 16,000 acres south of the Espinosa Trail. At 1.2 miles, pass an unsigned side trail on the right near Pine Valley Creek. Shortly thereafter, you arrive at the creek, which in winter and early spring brims with runoff from its headwaters in the Laguna Mountains. Here you'll find flat, durable ground where you could camp; avoid trampling the grass.

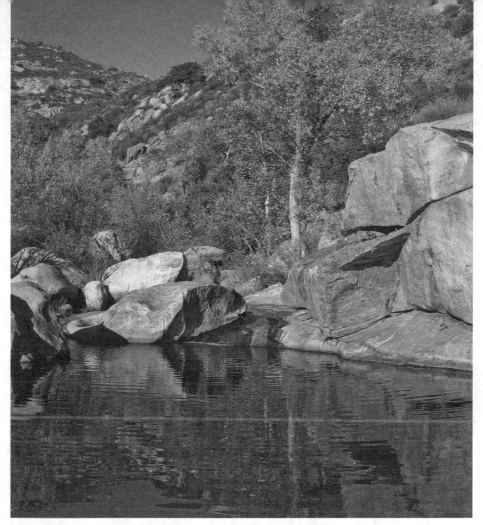
Horsethief Creek

VARIATIONS

Upstream from the pool, you can make your way alongside or over a jumble of car-size boulders and past several small cascades. Tangled willows and mule fat impede your progress. Watch your step on slippery slabs of rock, and be aware of thickets of poison oak, possible rattlesnakes, and fast water if your visit comes immediately on the heels of a big storm. You can continue in this manner—straight up the canyon bottom—for 3 or more picturesque miles. The Secret Canyon Trail leads 14 miles all the way to the Pine Creek Trailhead, a popular backpacking route.

If you would rather make a loop hike, you can return to the junction you just passed and follow the unmarked trail south along Pine Valley Creek. This is not an official U.S. Forest Service trail and is unmaintained, so be prepared to turn back if it has become overgrown. In 0.8 mile, after rounding the hill on the right, the trail starts to veer away from the creek. You may notice a lightly used track on the left returning toward the creek, but stay right and begin climbing the drainage on a long-abandoned roadbed. In 0.5 mile, cross the usually dry wash, then stay left at a junction with a faint, now-closed trail. Upon reaching the ridgeline, the trail turns right and returns to the parking area. This variation is 4 miles for the complete loop.

HIKE 93   Garnet Peak Loop

Location	Laguna Mountains
Highlight	Outstanding desert views
Distance & Configuration	12-mile loop
Elevation Gain	1,700'
Hiking Time	5 hours
Optional Maps	Laguna Mountain Recreation Area map or Tom Harrison *San Diego Backcountry*
Best Times	All year
Agency	Cleveland National Forest/Descanso Ranger District
Difficulty	Strenuous
Trail Use	Dogs allowed
Permit	Adventure Pass required
Google Maps	Pioneer Mail Picnic Site

Laced with a web of trails, Laguna Mountain National Recreation Area in Cleveland National Forest is a playground for San Diego–area outdoor lovers. Perched atop a mile-high ridge, the trails are usually enjoyable year-round, although they may be hot in midsummer or icy after a winter storm. This popular route combines the Noble Canyon and Indian Creek Trails with the Pacific Crest Trail (PCT) to form an appealing loop through many different ecosystems. A highlight is Garnet Peak, perched on the rim of the Laguna Mountains, from

Garnet Mountain

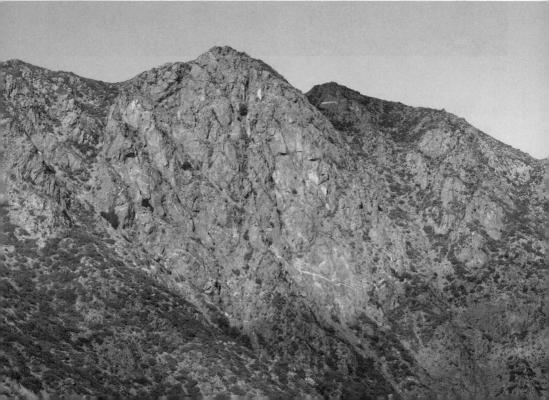

🅡 Garnet Peak Loop

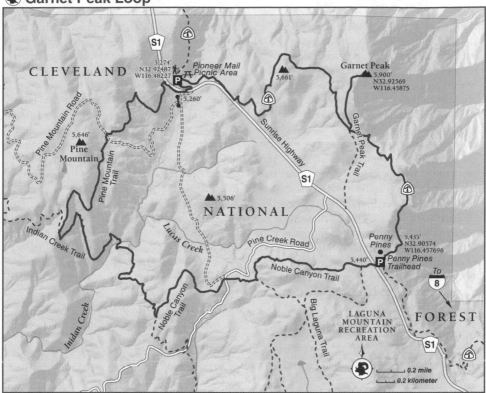

which you can see both the pine-clad Laguna plateau and the raw desert below.

Especially rewarding is a predawn pilgrimage to observe the sunrise from the summit of Garnet Peak. Around the winter solstice, the sun's flattened disk peeps up over the desert wastes of northwestern Sonora, Mexico, some 150 miles away. On the clearest mornings at that time of year, you might witness the famed green flash, an event occasionally seen on the horizon at sunset on the coast but seldom seen at sunrise anywhere.

To Reach the Trailhead: This trip starts at the Pioneer Mail Picnic Area on Sunrise Highway (County Route S1) between mile markers 29 and 29.5. Post an Adventure Pass on your vehicle.

Description: This hike begins on the Pacific Crest Trail at the Pioneer Mail Picnic Area. The trailhead was incorrectly named in the 1930s to commemorate the first transcontinental mail

service from 1857. At the time, it was believed that the mail route crossed this saddle coming up Cottonwood Canyon, but historians later concluded the route ascended Oriflamme Canyon, farther north. Stagecoaches carried the mail and passengers as far as the Colorado River, and then mules continued across the desert to San Diego. Officially known as the San Antonio and San Diego Mail Line, it was derogatorily renamed Jackass Mail by a San Francisco newspaper that believed the line should end in Northern California, and the name stuck. The Jackass Mail was soon superseded by the Butterfield Stage Line.

Follow the PCT southbound on the shoulder of Garnet Peak. This area has been scoured by the 2002 Pines Fire, the immense 2003 Cedar Fire, and the 2013 Chariot Fire, but the ceanothus, manzanita, and yucca are accustomed to the never-ending cycle of fire and regeneration. In 2.3 miles, meet the Garnet Peak Trail coming up from Sunrise Highway near mile marker 27.8. At 2.8 miles, turn left and take the Garnet Peak Trail, which slants north up the peak. Garnet Peak's summit is crowned by a jagged cluster of layered, tan-colored metasedimentary rock, the type seen along much of the Laguna escarpment. The peak falls away abruptly to the east and south, revealing a vertiginous panorama of Storm Canyon and its distant alluvial fan. Along the horizon lie the Salton Sea and Baja's Laguna Salada, both desert sinks. To the south and west, the Laguna crest, dusky with patches of pine and oak trees and chaparral, seems to roll like a frozen wave to the edge of the escarpment.

Return to the PCT and follow it to the Penny Pines Trailhead (4.9 miles), where the trail crosses to the west side of Sunrise Highway at mile marker 27.3. This trailhead was named for the Penny Pines program, established in California in 1941 to support replanting burned-over areas through private donations. Leave the PCT and take the signed Noble Canyon Trail west. This trail is popular with mountain bikers, who consider the lower segment to be a Southern California technical classic.

Stay right at an immediate fork where a branch of the Big Laguna Trail departs. Hike across a pleasant area with pines, ribbonwood, and chaparral. At 6.0 miles, cross paved Pine Creek Road. Climb onto the edge of a hill, then descend to meet the Indian Creek Trail at 7.2 miles. Turn right and follow the Indian Creek Trail. Cross the grass-lined creek at 8.2 miles and switchback up the hill to the northwest, reaching Champagne Pass at 9.4 miles.

Turn right onto the Pine Mountain Trail, and follow the ridge northeast. At 10.5 miles, cross Pine Mountain Road, then make the zigzagging descent to Sunrise Highway across from Pioneer Mail.

HIKE 94   Sunset Trail

Location	Laguna Mountains
Highlight	Colorful spring and autumn vegetation and views
Distance & Configuration	7-mile loop
Elevation Gain	700'
Hiking Time	3.5 hours
Optional Map	Laguna Mountain Recreation Area map or Tom Harrison *San Diego Backcountry*
Best Times	September–June
Agency	Cleveland National Forest/Descanso Ranger District
Difficulty	Moderately strenuous
Trail Use	Good for kids, dogs allowed
Permit	Adventure Pass required
Google Maps	Sunset Trailhead, Sunrise Highway

The Sunset Trail, opened in 1993, permits easy access by foot along the western rim of the high Laguna Mountain plateau. Like the sunrise-facing Pacific Crest Trail, its analogue a few miles east, the Sunset Trail offers fine panoramas but on the sunset side of the mountain. Early mornings are by far the best time (certainly during the warm summer season) to take advantage of cool temperatures and clear, tangy air. In the hour or two after sunrise, you can often look down upon a white and frothy ocean of stratus clouds hugging a 100-mile strip of coastline.

To Reach the Trailhead: From I-8 just east of Pine Valley, drive 5 miles up Sunrise Highway. At mile 19.1, park along the shoulder, which is wide enough in this area to accommodate parking for the hundreds of visitors who come in winter to play in the snow. Post an Adventure Pass on your vehicle.

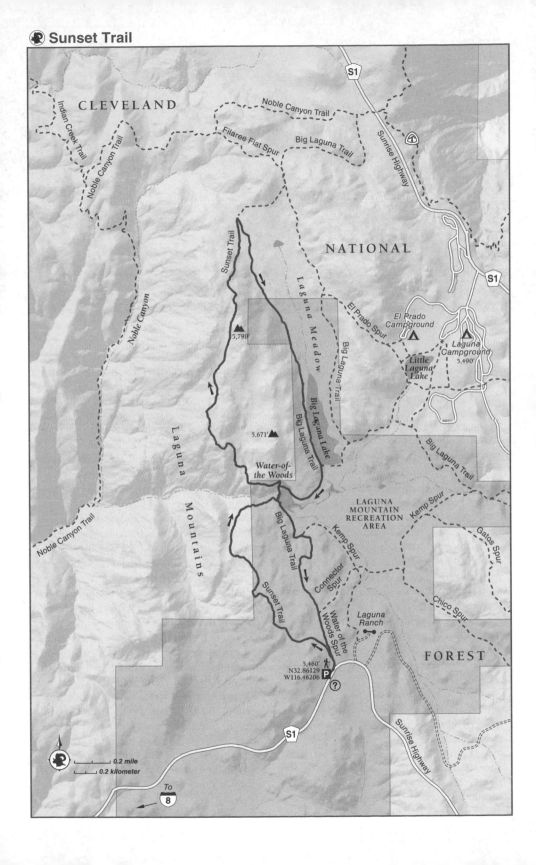

Sunset Trail

CLEVELAND

Indian Creek Trail

Noble Canyon Trail

Noble Canyon Trail

Filaree Flat Spur

Big Laguna Trail

Noble Canyon Trail

NATIONAL

S1

S1

Sunrise Highway

Sunset Trail

Laguna Meadow

El Prado Spur

El Prado Campground

Big Laguna Trail

Little Laguna Lake

Laguna Campground
5,490'

5,798'

Noble Canyon

5,671'

Big Laguna Lake

Big Laguna Trail

Water-of-the Woods

Laguna

Noble Canyon Trail

Mountains

Big Laguna Trail

LAGUNA MOUNTAIN RECREATION AREA

Kemp Spur

Kemp Spur

Gatos Spur

Big Laguna Trail

Connector Spur

Chico Spur

Sunset Trail

Water of the Woods Spur

Laguna Ranch

FOREST

5,460'
N32.86129
W116.46206

S1

Sunrise Highway

0.2 mile
0.2 kilometer

To
8

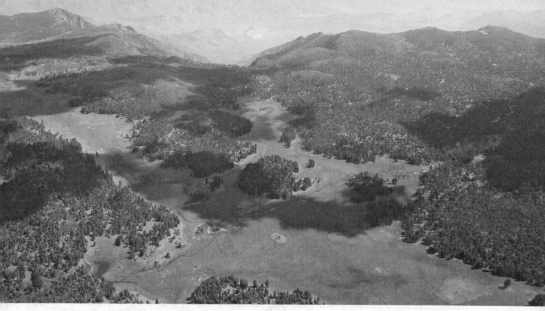

Aerial view of Big Laguna Meadow

Description: Pass through a gate at the signed Meadows Trailhead. In 80 yards stay left on the main trail at an unmarked fork. In 0.1 mile, stay left again at a junction with the Big Laguna Trail. You will loop back to this junction when you return.

Gradually climb toward a gently undulating ridgecrest dotted with vanilla-scented Jeffrey pines and black oaks. After nearly a mile, the trail suddenly veers left to circle a rocky outcrop. There, a view opens of velvet-smooth Crouch Valley, some 500 feet below, and much of coastal San Diego County whenever clear air prevails at lower altitudes. The view is certainly worth the trivial effort you have invested so far.

Onward, you descend gradually for a while, then rise again, reaching, at 1.7 miles, the lowermost edge of Laguna Meadow and a beautiful pond called Water-of-the-Woods. Veering left, the Sunset Trail follows the edge of the pond for a short while and then slants up the ridge to the left (northwest).

You climb back up to the viewful crest, with more opportunities to scan the broad western horizon, including Cuyamaca and Stonewall Peaks. Farther north, you pass over a hilltop with views to Garnet Peak, Toro Peak, San Jacinto, and San Gorgonio. Descend to the northernmost arm of Laguna Meadow. Turning east, the trail meets, at 3.7 miles, the Big Laguna Trail. Beware that the Big Laguna Trail is not a single path but a complex network of trails in the vicinity of Laguna Meadow. Pay attention to the map to take the proper forks.

Turn right on the Big Laguna Trail, and follow it south to Big Laguna Lake, the biggest of several shallow, ephemeral lakes in the meadow. In an average rainy season, these lakes begin to fill with water or snow by December or January. By April or May, as the meadow dries, carpets of wildflowers—tidy tips, buttercups, goldfields, dandelions, wild onions, and western irises—begin to appear. Summer heat causes water levels in the lakes to decline rapidly.

Just past Big Laguna Lake, the Big Laguna Trail forks (5.2 miles). The left fork leads to the far side of the lake, but you continue straight on the path that returns to Water-of-the-Woods. At the southwest corner of the lake, where you originally arrived by the Sunset Trail, turn left to stay on the Big Laguna Trail.

When you reach the south end of the meadow, the Big Laguna Trail forks again. Segment 6 leads left (east), but you continue straight on Segment 1 toward Sunrise Highway. Continue straight again at another fork where Segment 7 turns left. Soon you will arrive back at the junction with the Sunset Trail near where you began your hike.

HIKE 95   Hellhole Canyon

Location	Northern Anza-Borrego Desert State Park
Highlight	Hidden waterfall in desert canyon
Distance & Configuration	5.5-mile out-and-back
Elevation Gain	900'
Hiking Time	3.5 hours
Optional Map	USGS 7.5-minute *Tubb Canyon*
Best Times	December–May
Agency	Anza-Borrego Desert State Park
Difficulty	Moderately strenuous
Trail Use	Suitable for backpacking, good for kids
Permit	Parking fee
Google Maps	Hellhole Canyon Trail

In the midst of one of the hottest and driest deserts in the United States, it feels surprising to find a place where mosses, ferns, sycamores, and cottonwoods flourish around a sparkling waterfall in a palm oasis. Maidenhair Falls is such a place, and it lies not far from Borrego Springs and the popular Anza-Borrego Desert State Park Visitor Center.

Hellhole Canyon

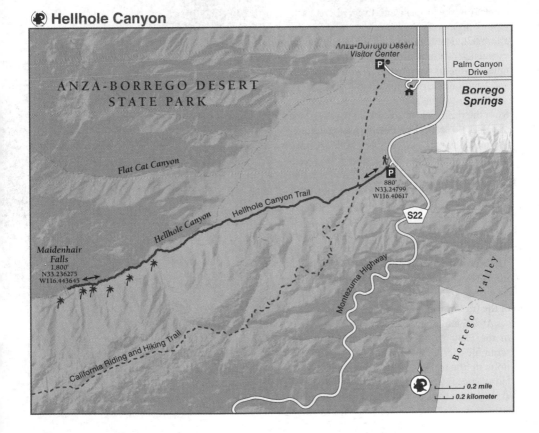

To Reach the Trailhead: From Christmas Circle (the traffic circle in the center of Borrego Springs), drive 1.3 miles west on Palm Canyon Drive to Montezuma Highway (County Route S22), and go south 0.7 mile to the large trailhead parking area on the west side of Montezuma Highway. Pay the day-use parking fee.

Description: From the parking lot, head west on a wide trail (an old roadbed) straight across and up an alluvial fan toward the gaping mouth of Hellhole Canyon. In 0.2 mile, pass a four-way junction. The California Riding and Hiking Trail goes left toward Culp Valley, and a 0.8-mile trail goes right to the visitor center.

The sandy surface of the fan supports a variety of vegetation, stratified according to elevation. Some common plant species of the lower fan are burroweed, cheesebush, Indigo bush, chuparosa, creosote bush, desert lavender, and Gander cholla. These are largely replaced by jojoba, brittlebush, ocotillo, and teddy bear cholla on the upper fan. Everywhere, jackrabbits flit among the bushes, startled by your approach. Families with children should be especially cautious around the cholla, whose fallen segments seem to jump from the ground and latch onto careless passersby!

As you approach the canyon mouth, a mile from the trailhead, you may hear (in a wet year at least) the sound of flowing water. Usually the water doesn't get very far on the surface; it quickly sinks into porous sand as it spreads out and slows on the fan below. At 1.9 miles, cross the wash for the second time where the canyon walls pinch in. You soon find yourself threading a path near the flowing water. Watch for cat's claw acacia that still grows close to the path. Fan palms—the signature tree of the Anza-Borrego Desert—begin to appear. Watch for a deep *mortero* (a grinding hole used by the American Indians) in a granite slab 2 feet left of the trail near the first palms.

At 2.5 miles, reach the main palm grove in the Hellhole Canyon oasis. You'll have to scramble over boulders here and there to continue up the trail. You may find a small waterfall at a headwall on the right side of the canyon at the top of the oasis, but this is not the main attraction. Stay left and continue up the rocky

canyon about 200 yards to the grotto containing Maidenhair Falls, which plunge about 25 feet into a shallow pool. Tiers of maidenhair fern adorn the grotto, and sopping-wet mosses cover the places the ferns don't.

VARIATION

Traveling upcanyon from Maidenhair Falls involves battling with boulders and the underbrush—slow going on a day hike and slower if you're carrying a backpack. Ambitious hikers can explore the canyon's remote higher reaches. Some hikers have traveled up the canyon's South Fork tributary, which leads to Pena Spring near Culp Valley, and some have reached San Ysidro Peak, a strenuous day for sure.

Hellhole Oasis

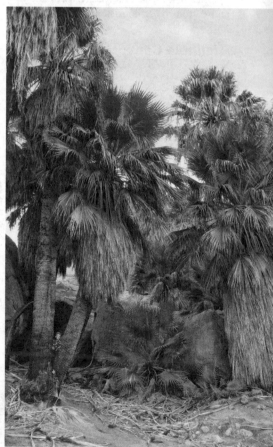

HIKE 96 Borrego Palm Canyon

Location	Northern Anza-Borrego Desert State Park
Highlights	Spring wildflowers, the most dramatic display of native palms in California
Distance & Configuration	2.9-mile out-and-back
Elevation Gain	450'
Hiking Time	1.5 hours
Optional Map	Tom Harrison *San Diego Backcountry*
Best Times	October–May
Agency	Anza-Borrego Desert State Park
Difficulty	Easy
Trail Use	Good for kids
Permit	Parking fee
Google Maps	Borrego Palm Canyon Trailhead & Parking

Borrego Palm Canyon has long been famous for harboring many hundreds of native palm trees in an otherwise austere setting of rock and sun-blasted vegetation. This popular hike starts near the busy Borrego Palm Canyon Campground and Anza-Borrego State Park

Borrego Palm Canyon

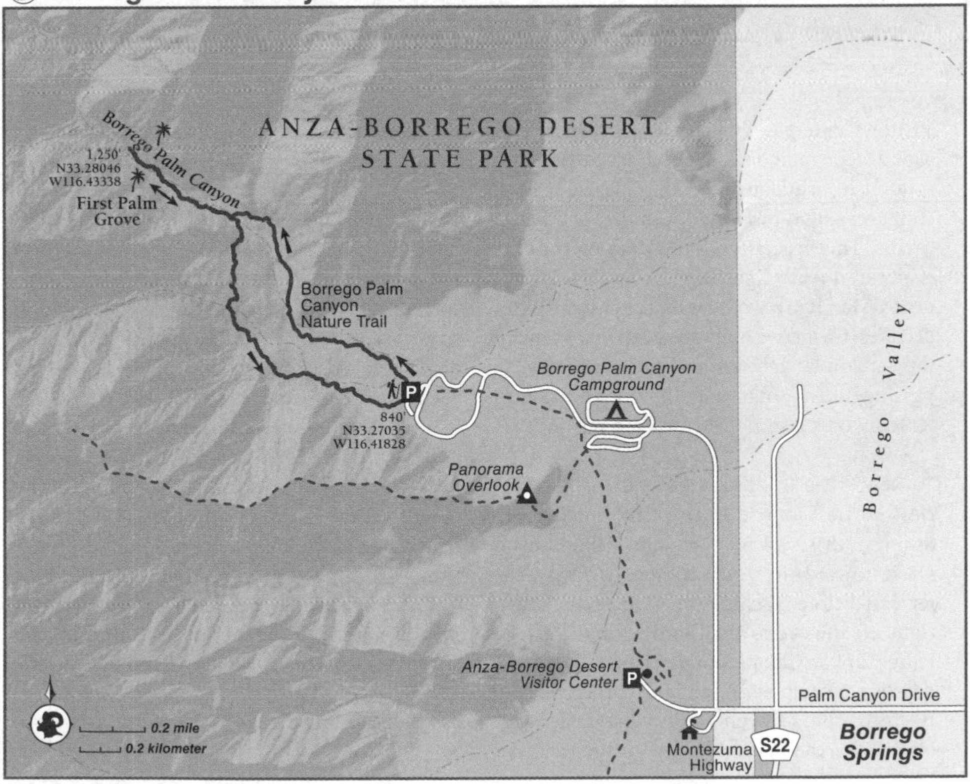

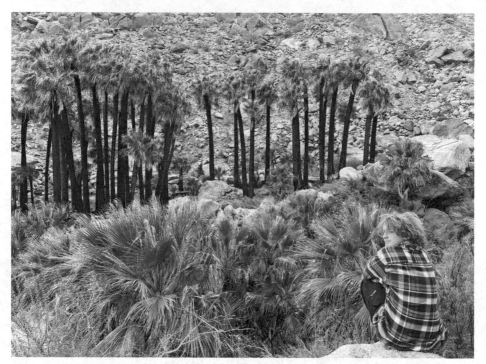

Borrego Palms Oasis survived a 2020 wildfire.

Visitor Center. You'll see mesquite; sage; cat's claw acacia; indigo bush; desert lavender; creosote bush; brittlebush; ocotillo; desert-willow; chuparosa; and beavertail, Gander, and barrel cactus. This vegetation looks drab most of the year, but it really lights up in a rainbow of colors by March in a wet year. In the past couple of decades, the native bighorn sheep that frequent the canyon have become quite accustomed to passing hikers. Sometimes they may graze contentedly only a stone's throw from the trail.

To Reach the Trailhead: From Christmas Circle (the traffic circle in the center of Borrego Springs), drive 1.4 miles west on Palm Canyon Drive toward the Anza-Borrego Visitor Center. Just before reaching the visitor center, turn right on the access road leading into Borrego Palm Canyon Campground. At the gate, pay the day-use or camping fee, and then proceed to the Borrego Palm Canyon Trailhead at the far west end of the campground. Next to the trailhead

are restrooms, a drinking fountain, and a pond holding transplanted desert pupfish.

Description: Pick up a brochure at the trailhead with the key to the numbered interpretive markers lining the main nature trail. The trail roughly parallels the canyon bottom and measures about 1.5 miles along its revised alignment. Also, bring plenty of water; the trail is continuously exposed to the sun.

Follow the trail up the canyon bottom. As you approach the canyon's narrow mouth, desert-varnished rock walls soar dramatically 3,000 feet upward on both sides. Cross to the south side of the creek, where you find a junction with an alternate trail at 1.0 mile. Stay out of the alluring creekbed to give the vegetation a chance to regenerate. The trail climbs some steps (believed to have been built in the 1930s by the Civilian Conservation Corps), crosses the creek twice more, and arrives at First Grove.

Perhaps 80% of these palms, which have surprised and delighted thousands of visitors over several decades, were summarily evicted from the canyon at 4:45 p.m. on September 10, 2004. On that afternoon an isolated, intense summer thunderstorm dumped buckets of rain over a relatively small area of the San Ysidro Mountains above. Sheets of water falling down the steep slopes gathered strength and speed as they joined forces in the narrow constriction of the canyon. A wall of water perhaps 30 feet high tore away nearly everything in its path. Borrego Palm Canyon Campground was hit soon after with a roiling mass of muddy water about 100 feet wide and moving at least 40 miles per hour, carrying palm trunks and other debris. Witnesses ran for higher ground or escaped down the campground's entrance road in speeding cars. Ironically, not a drop of rain fell that day in Borrego Springs, just 3 miles away.

Although a ghost of its former self, the grove remains quite attractive, with a cluster of large palms and many young ones sprouting nearby. They are of one variety, *Washingtonia filifera,* the only palm indigenous to California. You'll notice that most of the palms have green fronds at the top but are now missing their skirts of dead fronds on the trunks. In 2020, a fire burned through the grove and burned away the skirts but did not kill any of the trees. Remain on the trail to avoid disturbing new vegetation growing after the fire.

The Borrego Palm Canyon Nature Trail ends at First Grove. Further exploration of the canyon ahead is not for casual tourists. The game is to work your way upward on sketchy paths high above the canyon bed or, more often, along the flood-scoured bed itself, which is paved unevenly with sand and flood-tossed rocks and granitic or metamorphic bedrock slabs. As riparian vegetation returns to the canyon bottom in the years to come, it will increasingly slow the pace of intrepid hikers.

At 3.3 miles from the trailhead, the South Fork of Borrego Palm Canyon branches obviously to the left (southwest), its discharge of water less than that of the main fork. A spectacular double cascade of water lies 0.4 mile ahead up this rough gorge and makes a worthy destination for motivated hikers willing to clamber over angular rocks.

VARIATION

On your return, you might choose to take the less crowded alternate trail, which follows the ocotillo-dotted slopes above the wash. Watch for quail and raisin-size bighorn sheep pellets along this trail.

HIKE 97   Villager Peak

Location	Northern Anza-Borrego Desert State Park
Highlights	Ever-present dramatic views
Distance & Configuration	14-mile out-and-back
Elevation Gain	5,000'
Hiking Time	11 hours
Recommended Maps	USGS 7.5-minute *Fonts Point* and *Rabbit Peak*
Best Times	October–May
Agency	Anza-Borrego Desert State Park
Difficulty	Very strenuous
Trail Use	Suitable for backpacking
Permit	None required
Google Maps	(Unofficial) Trailhead for Villager Peak

Villager Peak

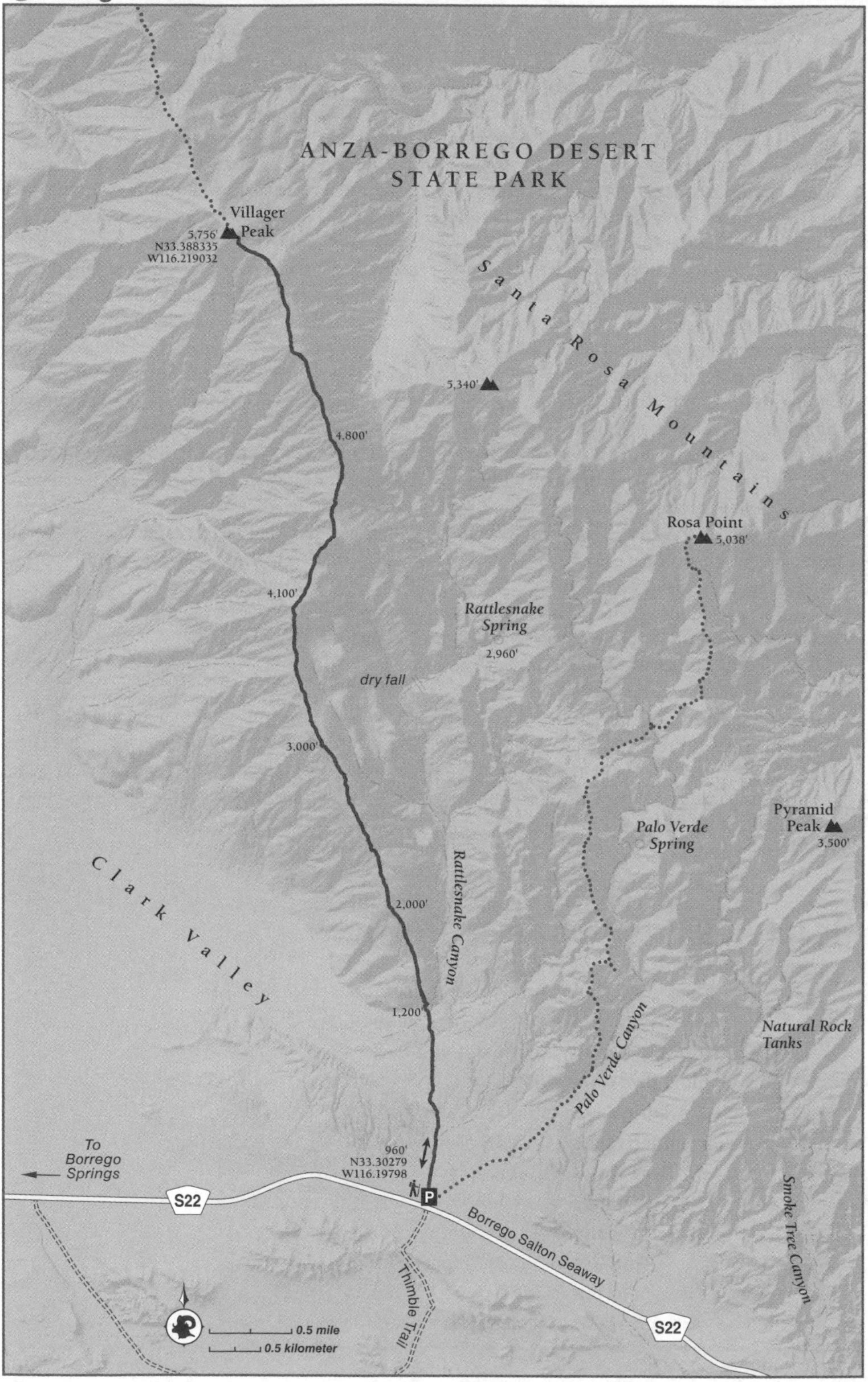

ANZA-BORREGO DESERT STATE PARK
Villager Peak
5,756'
N33.388335
W116.219032
Santa Rosa Mountains
5,340'
4,800'
Rosa Point
5,038'
4,100'
Rattlesnake Spring
2,960'
dry fall
3,000'
Pyramid Peak
3,500'
Palo Verde Spring
Clark Valley
Rattlesnake Canyon
2,000'
1,200'
Natural Rock Tanks
Palo Verde Canyon
960'
N33.30279
W116.19798
To Borrego Springs
S22
P
Borrego Salton Seaway
Smoke Tree Canyon
Thimble Trail
S22
0.5 mile
0.5 kilometer

Despite its remoteness, Villager Peak is one of the more popular destinations for "serious" Southern California peak baggers. Hundreds of people every year reach the summit, and the box containing the peak register is often overflowing with business cards and other mementos. Many people backpack the route, but others, who must start at or before sunrise, manage to complete the round-trip as a day hike. The importance of taking plenty of water on this waterless route cannot be overemphasized.

The approach to Villager Peak is straightforwardly up, using a single north-trending ridge of the Santa Rosa Mountains. One or more paralleling trails follow this ridge—the result of recent use by hikers, prehistoric use by desert-dwelling American Indians, and more or less continuous use by bighorn sheep. On the way down, however, you may encounter navigational difficulties where watershed divides split and go their separate ways. Bighorn sheep don't necessarily stick to the main route, and their trails may lure you off the main ridge onto some steeply plunging side ridge. Get a good sense of your surroundings at the trailhead or bring a GPS receiver because It can be difficult to find your way back cross-country if you are caught out past dark.

To Reach the Trailhead: From Borrego Springs, drive 13 miles northeast on Borrego Salton Seaway (County Route S22). Park in the northside turnout at mile 31.8, opposite a dirt road called Thimble Trail.

Description: Locate a good use trail leading north from the parking area. On foot, proceed north toward the east end of a long, sandy ridge 0.5 mile away. The north face of this ridge is a huge scarp along the San Jacinto Fault—said to be one of the largest fault scarps in unconsolidated earth material in North America. North of this ridge, flash floods exiting Rattlesnake Canyon have cut a series of braided washes in a swath about 0.6 mile wide. A surprisingly good path takes you over this dissected terrain to the base of the long, ramplike ridge leading to Villager Peak.

The use trail switchbacks up the steep toe of the ridge and soon levels off to a rather steady gradient averaging about 1,000 feet per mile.

Stay on the highest part of the ridge to remain on the route. Creosote bush, ocotillo, and glistening specimens of teddy bear and silver cholla cactus, barrel cactus, and hedgehog cactus grace the slopes below 3,000 feet. Thread a spiny gauntlet of wicked-looking agave at 3,000–4,000 feet.

At 4,100 feet and 4.3 miles, you pass along the edge of a spectacular crumbling drop-off overlooking Clark Valley. The white band of rock prominently displayed along the face of this escarpment is marble, or metamorphosed limestone. Thought to be some of the oldest rock exposed in San Diego County, it originated from ocean-floor sediments deposited about half a billion years ago. Just beyond the 4,800-foot contour, at 5.0 miles, the ridge descends a little to a small, exposed campsite with airy views both east and west.

Villager Peak has thorny defenses.

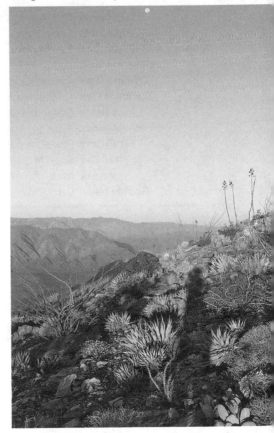

In the next mile, the ridgeline becomes quite jagged. Pinyon, juniper, Mojave yucca, and nolina (a cousin of the yucca) now dominate. At 7 miles, you reach the rounded, 5,756-foot summit of Villager Peak, which offers good campsites amid a sparse forest of weather-beaten pinyon pines. The views are practically aerial all around the compass. A clear, calm, moonless night spent here is an unforgettable experience. Despite the horizon glows of cities from Los Angeles to Mexicali, the stars above shine fiercely in a charcoal sky. At dawn, the silvery surface of the Salton Sea mirrors the red glow spreading across the east horizon.

VARIATIONS

Those looking for an even more grueling expedition have been known to continue along the undulating ridge to Rabbit Peak, the 6,640-foot hogback looming to the north. This monster climb involves a total of 23 miles and 7,900 feet of elevation gain.

Rosa Point (5,083') is another excellent desert peak that is accessed from the same trailhead and is similar in difficulty to Villager. Follow a ridge west of Palo Verde Canyon, then cross the upper reaches of the canyon and hike up the south ridge of Rosa Point. This is a 12-mile round-trip with 5,500 feet of gain. The views of the Salton Sea from the summit are unsurpassed. It is also possible to make a very strenuous loop, climbing Rosa, traversing northeast over Mile High Peak and down to a saddle, and then climbing Villager and descending the south ridge of Villager. This is 17 miles with 7,300 feet of gain.

HIKE 98   Calcite Mine

Location	Northern Anza-Borrego Desert State Park
Highlights	Slot canyons, historical interest
Distance & Configuration	4.2-mile loop
Elevation Gain	800'
Hiking Time	2 hours
Optional Map	Tom Harrison *San Diego Backcountry*
Best Times	November–April
Agency	Anza-Borrego Desert State Park
Difficulty	Moderate
Trail Use	Good for kids, suitable for mountain biking
Permit	None required
Google Maps	Calcite Mine Slot Canyon Trailhead

Thousands of years of cutting and polishing by water and wind erosion have produced the chaotic rock formations and slotlike ravines you'll discover in the Calcite Mine area. The highlight of this hike is, of course, the mine itself. During World War II, this was an important site—indeed the only site in the United States—for the extraction of optical-grade calcite crystals for use in gunsights. Trench-mining operations throughout the area left deep scars upon the earth, seemingly as fresh today as when they were made. The road to the mine is still passable by jeeps and other high-clearance four-wheel-drive vehicles, so you may encounter occasional traffic on your hike.

To Reach the Trailhead: From Borrego Springs, drive 19 miles northeast on Borrego-Salton Seaway (County Highway S22). Park at the Calcite jeep road intersection, 0.1 mile east of mile marker 38.0.

Description: An interpretive panel at the trailhead gives some details about the history of the mine. Walk up the jeep road as it dips into and out of South Fork Palm Wash and continues northwest toward the southern spurs of the Santa Rosa Mountains. Ahead you will see an intricately honeycombed, whitish slab of sandstone, called Locomotive Rock, which lies behind (northeast of) the mine area.

Calcite Mine

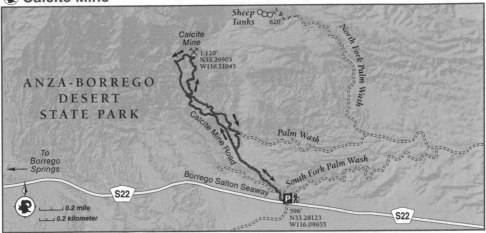

Sheep Tanks 820'
Calcite Mine 1,120'
N33.29903
W116.11045
North Fork Palm Wash

ANZA-BORREGO
DESERT
STATE PARK

Calcite Mine Road

Palm Wash

To Borrego Springs

South Fork Palm Wash

Borrego Salton Seaway

S22

P 596'
N33.28123
W116.09653

S22

0.2 mile
0.2 kilometer

About 1.4 miles from S22, the road dips sharply to cross a deep ravine. You'll have the option of exploring it on your way back. At the mine at road's end, you may find bits of calcite crystal strewn about on the ground, glittering in the sunlight. You could spend a lot of time exploring the mining trenches and the pocked slabs of sandstone nearby. Palm Wash, a frightening gash in the earth, precludes travel to the east.

Adventurous hikers may enjoy making a partial loop back through the ravine, which contains one of the best slot canyons in Anza-Borrego. From the upper trench of the mine, look for a use trail curving left and down toward a canyon. The canyon is deep, with

Slot canyon below Calcite Mine

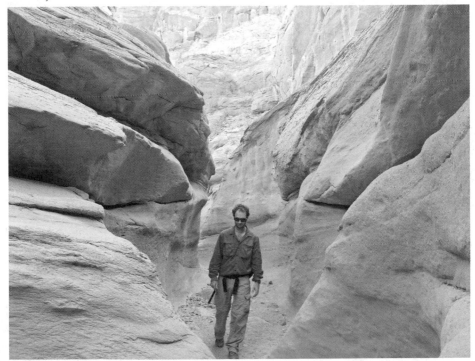

vertical walls, but look for a trench slicing down a weakness that offers a way to scramble to the bottom. If you turn right, you will soon find the canyon blocked by a 20-foot drop jammed with two huge chockstones; only technical climbers with proper gear could head that way. Instead, turn left and walk down the canyon. You will have to scramble down two interesting drops and several more easy ones while descending the gorgeous slot to rejoin the jeep road.

Whether you explored the upper ravine or backtracked on the road, you'll likely enjoy leaving the road here and descending the lower portion of the ravine. As you pass through deeper and deeper layers of sandstone strata, the ravine narrows until it allows only one person at a time to pass. When you reach the jumbled blocks of sandstone in Palm Wash at the bottom of the ravine, turn right, walk 0.3 mile downstream, and exit via a short link of jeep trail that leads back to the Calcite road.

HIKE 99   Moonlight Canyon Loop

Location	Agua Caliente Regional Park (Southern Anza-Borrego)
Highlights	Desert views, geological interest
Distance & Configuration	1.5-mile loop
Elevation Gain	350'
Hiking Time	1 hour
Optional Map	USGS 7.5-minute *Agua Caliente Springs*
Best Times	October–May
Agency	County of San Diego Parks and Recreation
Difficulty	Easy
Trail Use	Good for kids
Permit	Parking fee, access fee for hot springs
Google Maps	Agua Caliente County Park

Take in a deep breath of clean, dry air. Bask in the larger-than-life brilliance of the desert sun. Sink into the womblike comfort of warm spring water. At Agua Caliente Springs you can have your cake and eat it too—hike first, then enjoy a relaxing soak in the hot springs. A San Diego County park has been established here in the midst of state park lands at the foot of the Tierra Blanca Mountains.

A splinter of the Elsinore Fault is responsible for the upwelling of warm, mineral-rich water here. The same fault passes through the Lake Elsinore area and Warner Springs, where hot springs are also found. You have two options for soaking at Agua Caliente Springs: a shallow outdoor pool with spring water flowing through at an ambient temperature of about 95°F and a large indoor Jacuzzi pool where the water's temperature is boosted to more than

100°F. The pools are open 9:30 a.m.–5 p.m., and there is a small fee for day use. Overnight campers should make reservations well in advance for the popular sites.

To Reach the Trailhead: You'll find Agua Caliente along County Highway S2, 27 miles northwest of I-8 at Ocotillo and 22 miles southeast of Highway 78 at Scissors Crossing. Currently, the park is open September–May and closed during the hot summer months. Pay your day-use fee.

Description: As for hiking, the Moonlight Canyon Trail (one of several short trails in the area) is a good one to start on. This well-marked but somewhat steep and rugged trail starts at the south end of the campground, climbs over a rock-strewn saddle, drops into a small wash mysteriously named Moonlight

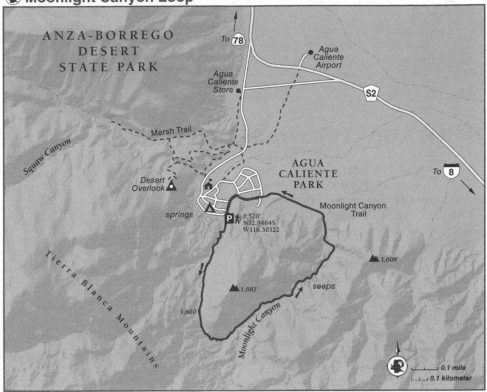 Moonlight Canyon Loop

Canyon, descends past some seeps and a little oasis of willows in the wash bottom, and finally circles back to the campground. Kids will enjoy scrambling up the rocks. The canyon is rich with spiky desert vegetation, including barrel and teddy bear cholla cactus, desert agave, and ocotillo. Bighorn sheep roam the area; scan the ridgetops near the canyon mouth for the well-camouflaged animals. Although moonlight treks around this trail are possible, a good flashlight wouldn't hurt after dark.

True to their name, which means "white earth," the Tierra Blanca Mountains are composed of light-colored granitic rock. In some areas, this type of rock gradually acquires a patina of oxidized iron and manganese called desert varnish. Right here, however, the rock has been pounded and fractured by movements along the Elsinore Fault. It easily decomposes into the light-colored mineral crystals that make up the coarse sand you are walking on.

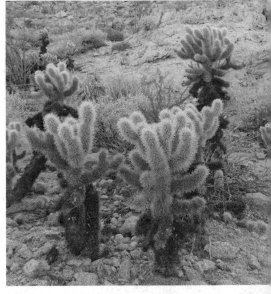

Teddy bear cholla cacti

VARIATIONS

From the high point on the Moonlight Canyon Trail, 300 feet above the campground, you can climb off-trail an additional 250 feet to reach Peak 1,882', which offers a superb view of Carrizo Valley and the Vallecito Mountains, including Whale Peak. If you would like, you could take on another, longer side trip, again cross-country and upcanyon (south), in Moonlight Canyon to a point overlooking the Inner Pasture, an isolated valley ringed by the boulder-punctuated Tierra Blanca and Sawtooth Mountains.

HIKE 100   Mountain Palm Springs

Location	Southern Anza-Borrego Desert State Park
Highlights	Groves of native palms
Distance & Configuration	2.1-mile loop
Elevation Gain	350'
Hiking Time	1.5 hours
Optional Map	Tom Harrison *San Diego Backcountry*
Best Times	October–May
Agency	Anza-Borrego Desert State Park
Difficulty	Moderate
Trail Use	Good for kids
Permit	None required
Google Maps	Mtn. Palm Springs Loop Trailhead

If you like the contrast between palm-tree oases and a raw landscape of sand and eroded rock, you'll love Mountain Palm Springs. The palms here are gregarious, growing in dense clusters, often with pools of water at their feet. Some have never been burned: they still hold full skirts of dead fronds around their trunks, the better to serve the local population of

Mountain Palm Springs Oasis

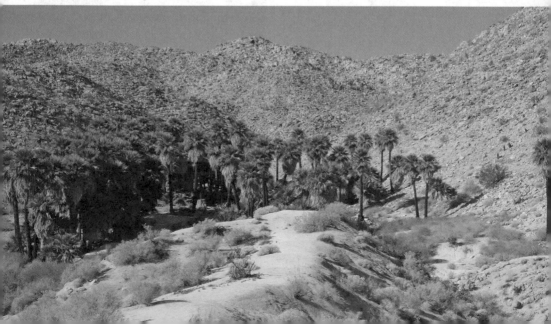

Mountain Palm Springs

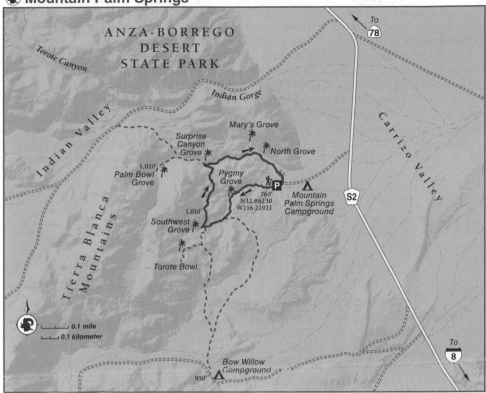

rodents and snakes. In late fall and early winter, the sticky, sweet fruit of the palms hangs in great swaying clusters, sought after by birds and the sleek coyotes that prowl up and down the washes. The palm groves are distributed along several small washes that drain roughly a square-mile area on the east side of the Tierra Blanca Mountains near the south end of Anza-Borrego Desert State Park.

The trails in this area are often faint and unsigned. Don't hike here unless you have a good sense of direction, and pay close attention to your surroundings. When a trail becomes faint, watch for cairns marking the way. Consider the loop hike described here as a fairly complete tour of the area, but be enticed to extend your explorations in the form of side trips or extended loop trips if the spirit moves you.

To Reach the Trailhead: From County Highway S2 at mile 47.1 (20 miles north of Ocotillo or 29 miles south of Scissors Crossing), take a signed dirt road going 0.7 mile west, passing the Mountain Palm Springs primitive camping area and ending at a bowl at the foot of the mountain range.

Description: Two canyon mouths open near the road's end. Start up the small canyon to the left (southwest) behind an interpretive panel. Past some small seeps, you'll come upon the first groups of palms, Pygmy Grove. Some of these smaller but statuesque palms grow out of nothing more than rock piles.

Follow the canyon as it veers left, then follow the trail onto the low ridge to the left, where you reach a junction with a trail coming up from Bow Willow Campground. Continue west on the ridge to Southwest Grove, a restful retreat shaded by a vaulted canopy of shimmering fronds. A rock-lined catch basin fashioned for the benefit of the local wildlife mirrors the silhouettes of the palms. A couple of elephant trees cling to the slopes just above the grove, but for a better look at these curious plants, you can climb a spur trail to Torote Bowl, which has a larger group of elephant trees.

From Southwest Grove, pick up the well-worn but obscure trail that leads north over a rock-strewn ridge to Surprise Canyon Grove in Surprise Canyon. Upcanyon from this small grove lies Palm Bowl, filled with tangled patches of mesquite and fringed on its western edge by more than 100 tall palms. On warm winter days, the molasses-like odor of ripe palm fruit wafts upon the breeze, and phaino-peplas hoot and flit among the palm crowns, their white wing patches flashing.

North of Palm Bowl, an old American Indian pathway leads over a low pass to Indian Gorge and Torote Canyon, where many more elephant trees thrive—another possible diversion. To conclude your loop, however, return to Surprise Canyon Grove and continue downcanyon to the campground. On the way, you pass North Grove, hidden in a side drainage on the left.

HIKE 101 Mortero Palms to Goat Canyon

Location	Southern Anza-Borrego Desert State Park
Highlights	Rugged, palm-filled canyon; view of a historic railroad
Distance & Configuration	6-mile out-and-back
Elevation Gain	2,400'
Hiking Time	5 hours
Recommended Map	USGS 7.5-minute *Jacumba*
Best Times	November–April
Agency	Anza-Borrego Desert State Park
Difficulty	Moderately strenuous
Trail Use	Suitable for backpacking
Permit	None required
Google Maps	Goat Canyon Trestle Trailhead, Jacumba Hot Springs

The 200-foot-high, 600-foot-long trestle over Goat Canyon on the San Diego & Arizona Eastern rail line is revered among railroad buffs everywhere. It has been called the longest curved railroad trestle and is one of the highest wooden trestles in the world.

Dubbed the impossible railroad, the San Diego & Arizona Eastern tracks were laid through southern Anza-Borrego's Carrizo Gorge in the second decade of the 20th century. Starting in 1919, the railroad carried freight and, for a time, passengers between San Diego and the Imperial Valley. The gorge section features 11 miles of twisting track, 17 tunnels, and numerous trestles. The current Goat Canyon trestle, built over a tributary of Carrizo Gorge, was completed in 1933 as part of a realignment of the original route. In 1976 Hurricane Kathleen churned northward up along the Gulf of California, dropped about 10 inches of rain on southern Anza-Borrego, and severely mangled the gorge section of the railroad, rendering it impassable for almost five years. After reopening in 1981, the line was quickly severed again, this time by a fire that burned several trestles. The line did not open again until 2004, and even then it was restricted to limited freight service. At the time of this writing, it is inactive yet again.

Walking the tracks is expressly forbidden. This hike makes a beeline approach over rough terrain to get a fine view of the magnificent Goat Canyon trestle, which lies in the middle and most remote section of Carrizo Gorge. This

ⓟ Mortero Palms to Goat Canyon

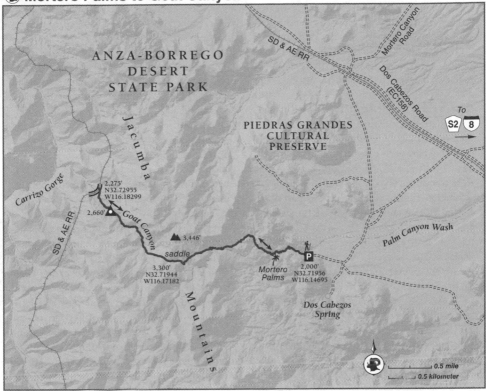

ANZA-BORREGO
DESERT
STATE PARK

Jacumba

PIEDRAS GRANDES
CULTURAL
PRESERVE

SD & AE RR

Mortero Canyon Road

Dos Cabezos Road (EC158)

To
S2 8

Carrizo Gorge

2,275'
N32.72955
W116.18299

2,660'

Goat Canyon

SD & AE RR

▲ 3,446'

saddle

3,300'
N32.71944
W116.17182

Mountains

Mortero
Palms

🄿
2,000'
N32.71956
W116.14695

Palm Canyon Wash

Dos Cabezos
Spring

0.5 mile
0.5 kilometer

is a trip for those who enjoy rock-hopping and cross-country navigation; it is not for the faint of heart.

To Reach the Trailhead: Reaching the remote trailhead is an adventure in itself. A high-clearance vehicle is required, but when the road is in good shape, four-wheel-drive is not essential. These directions assume you have a detailed topographic map of the area. Don't rely on having cell coverage. You start hiking at the Mortero Palms Trailhead, close to the rock outcrop known as Dos Cabezos ("two heads"). To get there from I-8 at Ocotillo, proceed north and west on County Route S2 for 4.1 miles to Dos Cabezos Road on the left, unsigned but marked with a post labeled EC119. This road leads through the Ocotillo Wind Energy Facility, a 265-megawatt energy project, and becomes dirt.

In 1.1 miles, stay right; the road is now signed EC158. Continue west another 4.6 miles, passing many intersections on the wind

farm, some of which are confusing. Turn left across the railroad tracks on a paved crossover. Go right, continue another 0.1 mile, and then veer left, away from the tracks. Go another

Cholla flowers

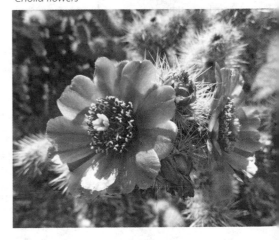

0.9 mile to a Y-junction at a sign for Piedras Grandes Cultural Preserve, where you stay left. Cross Palm Canyon Wash, and pass spurs on both sides. In 0.7 mile, go right at a second signed Y-junction, and reach the end of the road in 0.4 mile, where you can park or camp.

Description: A wide wash lies below the road's end. The Mortero Palms grove, your first destination, is hidden in Palm Canyon to the west (not the narrower canyon to the south). So head northwest along the south side of that west-trending canyon for a while, avoiding the vegetation-choked streambed. This part of the Jacumba Mountains is home to all things sharp and thorny, including at least six species of cactus, cat's claw acacia, honey mesquite, Mojave yucca, nolina, desert agave, and ocotillo—don't stumble! Late April is a promising time to see cacti, agave, and ocotillo in bloom.

In 0.3 mile, you may notice a concrete guzzler on the right. Beware of a trail marked by cairns that may tempt you to veer north; instead, continue straight (west) up the bouldery canyon, watching for a use trail on the north side. After you've climbed the steep slope, look for a half dozen *morteros* (American Indian mortars), namesakes of the palm grove, in the center of the drainage 100 yards below the lower end of the grove.

Groundwater close to the surface supports the dense cluster of palms amid an otherwise dramatically desolate scene of rounded granitic boulders set against the deep-blue sky. On warm days the grove is a seductively cool spot,

and it takes some willpower to get moving again to tackle the short but steep stretch of canyon ahead. Traverse left or right, or climb the water-polished rocks directly if you're a real daredevil. Any way you choose, you'll get briefly involved in at least one difficult rock-climbing maneuver.

Watch for cairns and a surprisingly good use trail heading up the canyon. At the 2,400-foot contour, it's easier to leave the watercourse temporarily and go up on the slope to the north through stands of cholla cactus and Mojave yucca. Drop back in at about 2,750 feet, but leave the wash again at the 2,840-foot contour. Proceed west and southwest across a small saddle, and continue west over a divide into the Goat Canyon drainage, 2.0 miles from the start.

Descend to a delightful, juniper-dotted bowl at about 3,200 feet, a pleasant spot to spend the night if you are backpacking. Goat Canyon descends steeply farther west of here. Down at about 2,700 feet in the canyon, where you reach a sudden drop (3 miles), there's an excellent, though somewhat distant, view of the curved trestle, framed by the steep walls of the canyon. If you don't mind more steep rock scrambling, you can descend the slopes to the left of the dry waterfall and pick a path another 0.3 mile down to the trestle, which is bracketed by tunnels at both ends.

VARIATION

Further exploration in the area might include a visit to 4,512-foot Jacumba Peak, the high point of the Jacumba Mountains, which lies some 2 miles south.

Goat Canyon Trestle

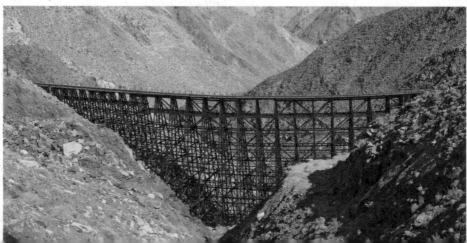

Agencies and Information Sources

Agua Caliente Band of Cahuilla Indians 760-699-6800, aguacaliente.org

Big Morongo Canyon Preserve 760-363-7190, bigmorongo.org

Bureau of Land Management, Palm Springs–South Coast Field Office 760-833-7100,
 blm.gov/office/palm-springs-south-coast-field-office

Catalina Island Conservancy 310-510-2595, catalinaconservancy.org

Chino Hills State Park 951-780-6222, parks.ca.gov/?page_id=648

City of Riverside Parks and Recreation 951-826-2000, riversideca.gov/park_rec/welcome

Cleveland National Forest fs.usda.gov/cleveland

   Descanso District 619-445-6235

   Palomar District 760-788-0250

   Trabuco District 951-736-1811

Coachella Valley Preserve 760-833-7100, blm.gov/visit/coachella-valley-preserve

Conejo Recreation and Park District 805-495-6471, crpd.org

County of San Diego Parks and Recreation Department 858-565-3600, sdparks.org

Crystal Cove State Park 949-494-3539, crystalcovestatepark.org

Cuyamaca Rancho State Park 760-765-3023, parks.ca.gov/?page_id=667

Devil's Punchbowl Natural Area 661-944-2743,
 parks.lacounty.gov/devils-punchbowl-natural-area-and-nature-center

Eaton Canyon Natural Area 626-398-5420,
 parks.lacounty.gov/eaton-canyon-natural-area-and-nature-center

Glendale Parks and Recreation 818-548-2000,
 glendaleca.gov/government/departments/community-services-parks

Griffith Park 323-644-2050, laparks.org/griffithpark

Joshua Tree National Park 760-367-5500, nps.gov/jotr

Lake Poway Recreation Area 858-668-4772, poway.org/401/Lake-Poway

Los Peñasquitos Canyon Preserve 858-484-7504,
 sdparks.org/content/sdparks/en/park-pages/LosPenasquitos.html

Mission Trails Regional Park 619-668-3281, mtrp.org

Mount San Jacinto State Park 951-659-2607, parks.ca.gov/?page_id=636

Orange County Parks 714-973-6865, ocparks.com

Palomar Mountain State Park 760-742-3462, parks.ca.gov/?page_id=637

continued on next page

Palos Verdes Estates Shoreline Preserve 310-378-0383, pvestates.org

Placerita Canyon State Park 661-259-7721, parks.lacounty.gov/placerita-canyon-state-park

Point Mugu State Park 805-488-1827, parks.ca.gov/?page_id=630

Ronald W. Caspers Wilderness Park 949-923-2210, ocparks.com/caspers

San Bernardino National Forest fs.usda.gov/sbnf

   Mountaintop District 909-382-2790

   Mill Creek Visitor Center 909-382-2882

   San Jacinto District 909-382-2921

   Front Country Ranger District 909-382-2851

San Dieguito River Park 858-674-2270, sdrp.org

Santa Monica Mountains Conservancy 310-589-3200, smmc.ca.gov

Santa Monica Mountains National Recreation Area 805-370-2301, nps.gov/samo

Santa Rosa and San Jacinto Mountains National Monument 760-862-9984,
tinyurl.com/srsjnationalmonument

Santa Rosa Plateau Ecological Reserve 800-234-7275,
rivcoparks.org/santa-rosa-plateau-wildlife-area

Santiago Oaks Regional Park 714-973-6620, ocparks.com/santiagooaks

Torrey Pines State Natural Reserve torreypine.org

The Wildlands Conservancy 760-325-7222, wildlandsconservancy.org/preserves/whitewater

Will Rogers State Historic Park 310-230-2017, parks.ca.gov/?page_id=626

Recommended Reading

Anderson, Kristi, and Tavernier, Arleen (eds.), *Wilderness Basics,* 4th edition, The Mountaineers Books, 2013.

Bakker, Elna, *An Island Called California,* 2nd edition, University of California Press, 1984.

Belzer, Thomas J., *Roadside Plants of Southern California,* Mountain Press Publishing Company, 1984.

California Coastal Commission, *California Coastal Access Guide,* 7th edition, Berkeley: University of California Press, 2014.

Clarke, Herbert, *An Introduction to Southern California Birds,* Mountain Press Publishing Company, 1989.

Dale, Nancy, *Flowering Plants: The Santa Monica Mountains, Coastal and Chaparral Regions of Southern California,* Consortium Book Sales and Distributing, 1986.

Ferranti, Philip, *140 Great Hikes in and near Palm Springs,* Westcliffe Publishers, 2014.

Furbush, Patty A., *On Foot in Joshua Tree National Park: A Comprehensive Hiking Guide,* 5th edition, M. I. Adventure Publications, 2005.

Harris, David, and Robinson, John W., *Trails of the Angeles,* 10th edition, Wilderness Press, 2021.

Lightner, James, *San Diego County Native Plants,* 3rd edition, San Diego Flora, 2011.

Lindsay, Diana, and Lowell Lindsay, *The Anza-Borrego Desert Region,* 6th edition, Wilderness Press, 2017.

McAuley, Milt, *Hiking Trails of the Santa Monica Mountains,* Canyon Publishing Company, 1987.

Munz, Philip A., *Introduction to California Desert Wildflowers,* University of California Press, 2004.

———, *Introduction to California Mountain Wildflowers,* University of California Press, 2003.

———, *Introduction to California Spring Wildflowers of the Foothills, Valleys, and Coast,* University of California Press, 2004.

Peterson, P. Victor, *Native Trees of Southern California,* University of California Press, 1966.

Raven, Peter H., *Native Shrubs of Southern California,* University of California Press, 1974.

Robinson, John W., and David Money Harris, *San Bernardino Mountain Trails,* 7th edition, Wilderness Press, 2016.

Schad, Jerry, and David Harris, *Afoot & Afield in Los Angeles County,* 4th edition, Wilderness Press, 2019.

———. *Afoot & Afield in Orange County,* 4th edition, Wilderness Press, 2015.

Schad, Jerry, and Scott Turner. *Afoot & Afield in San Diego County,* 5th edition, Wilderness Press, 2017.

Randall, Laura, et al., *The Pacific Crest Trail: Southern California,* 7th edition, Wilderness Press, 2020.

Schoenherr, Allan A., *A Natural History of California,* University of California Press, 1995.

Sharp, Robert P., and Allen F. Glazner, *Geology Underfoot in Southern California,* Mountain Press Publishing Company, 1993.

Tway, Linda, *Tidepools of Southern California: An Guide to 92 Locations from Point Conception to Mexico,* 2nd edition, Wilderness Press, 2011.

Index

About the Authors

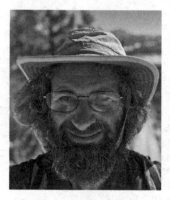

David Harris is a professor of engineering at Harvey Mudd College. He is the author or coauthor of seven hiking guidebooks and four engineering textbooks. David grew up rambling about the Desolation Wilderness as a toddler in his father's pack and later roamed the High Sierra as a Boy Scout. As a Sierra Club trip leader, he organized mountaineering trips throughout the Sierra Nevada. Since 1999, he has been exploring the mountains and deserts of Southern California. He lives with his three children in Upland, California, and delights in sharing his love of the outdoors with them.

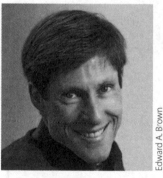

Edward A. Brown

Jerry Schad (1949–2011) was Southern California's leading outdoors writer. His 16 guidebooks, including the popular and comprehensive Afoot & Afield series, and his "Roam-O-Rama" column in the *San Diego Reader* have helped thousands of hikers discover the region's diverse wild places. Schad ran or hiked many thousands of miles of distinct trails throughout California, in the Southwest, and in Mexico. He was a sub-24-hour finisher of Northern California's 100-mile Western States Endurance Run and served in a leadership capacity for outdoor excursions around the world. He taught astronomy and physical science at San Diego Mesa College and chaired the Physical Sciences Department from 1999 until 2011. His sudden and untimely death from kidney cancer shocked and saddened the community.